Workbook

Textbook of

Radiographic Positioning and Related Anatomy

Seventh edition

Volume I
Chapters 1-13

Kenneth L. Bontrager, MA

John P. Lampignano, MEd, RT(R)(CT)

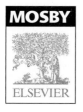

MOSBY

ELSEVIER

MOSBY
ELSEVIER

11830 Westline Industrial Drive
St. Louis, Missouri 63146

Workbook for Textbook of Radiographic Positioning and Related
Anatomy, Seventh Edition, Volume 1

ISBN: 978-0-323-05412-6

Notice

Knowledge and best practice in this field are constantly changing. As new research and experience broaden our knowledge, changes in practice, treatment and drug therapy may become necessary or appropriate. Readers are advised to check the most current information provided (i) on procedures featured or (ii) by the manufacturer of each product to be administered, to verify the recommended dose or formula, the method and duration of administration, and contraindications. It is the responsibility of practitioners, relying on their own experience and knowledge of the patient, to make diagnoses, to determine dosages and the best treatment for each individual patient, and to take all appropriate safety precautions. To the fullest extent of the law, neither the Publisher nor the Authors assumes any liability for any injury and/or damage to persons or property arising out of or related to any use of the material contained in this book.

The Publisher

ISBN 978-0-323-05412-6

Executive Editor: Jeanne R. Olson
Senior Developmental Editor: Becky Swisher
Publishing Services Manager: Catherine A. Jackson
Senior Project Manager: Karen M. Rehwinkel
Designer: Kimberly Denando

Working together to grow
libraries in developing countries

www.elsevier.com | www.bookaid.org | www.sabre.org

ELSEVIER   BOOK AID International   Sabre Foundation

Printed in the United States of America
Last digit is the print number: 9 8 7 6 5 4 3 2 1

Acknowledgments

I am pleased to acknowledge and recognize those persons who have made significant contributions to the seventh edition of this student workbook and laboratory manual.

I first want to thank John Lampignano, who as co-author expanded the objectives and content of each chapter by submitting additional questions for the new sections of the textbook. John is a very qualified and effective educator and has put a lot of effort and energy into this project. Thank you, John, for your excellent contributions.

I also thank Jeanne Olson, Karen Rehwinkel, and Rebecca Swisher of the Mosby/Elsevier staff for their help and support in the preparation of this manuscript.

Last and most important, I want to thank my family for their continued love, support, and encouragement and for bringing much joy and happiness into my life. I love each of you very much. Thanks Mary Lou, Neil, Troy, Kim, Robyn, Hallie, Alexis, Ashton, and Jonathan.

KLB

I would like to thank Ken Bontrager for his patience and mentorship in developing my skills as a writer. I've been honored to work with him over the past four editions. Ken has poured his heart and expertise into this text. Through his hard work and vision he has created a tremendous resource for students. Mary Lou Bontrager continues to provide the energy, technical support, and encouragement behind the scenes. Thank you, Mary Lou, for being there for both of us.

Ms. Rebecca Swisher, our developmental editor, deserves praise for her dedication and vision in coordinating this project. She kept us on task and focused but always with a smile and a gentle word. Special thanks also to Jeanne Olson for being a great editor and friend. Alissa Carden and Andrzej Lebiedzinski reviewed the exercises in the workbook. Special thanks to Karen Rehwinkel for her attention to detail and her professionalism during the editing phase of the text and workbooks.

I would like to thank the diagnostic medical imaging faculty and clinical instructors at Gateway Community College who provide a shining example of excellence each and every day for our students and community. To my students—past, present, and future—you have made teaching a rewarding experience! Without your energy, laughter, and enthusiasm, teaching and writing this text would have been a burden rather than a joy. To Debby Moore, my close friend and colleague, for her unshaken support over the years. Finally, to my close friend, Jerry Olson, who taught me everything about radiography and many things about life—you have made my life richer and more worthwhile.

My family—Deborah, Daniel, Molly, Chad, and Tatum—provide me with the greatest joy of all. I look at each of you and realize that I'm the luckiest person alive. Thank you for your love and support for the past 30 years. This book is dedicated to each of you.

JPL

Preface

The success of the first six editions of this workbook and laboratory manual and the accompanying textbook, along with the associated ancillary materials, is demonstrated by the many schools of radiologic technology throughout the United States, Canada, and other countries that have been using all or parts of these instructional media for more than 30 years.

NEW TO THIS EDITION

New illustrations and expanded questions have been added to reflect all the new content added to the seventh edition of *Textbook of Radiographic Positioning and Related Anatomy*. The use of visuals in these review exercises not only increases comprehension but also increases retention because most individuals retain information most effectively through visual images.

The detailed laboratory activities have been updated, and the positioning question and answer exercises have been expanded, with less emphasis on rote memory recall. More situational questions involving clinical applications have been added. These questions aid in the understanding of positioning principles and of which anatomical structures are best demonstrated on which projections. The clinical situational questions added to each chapter require students to think through and understand how application of this positioning information relates to specific clinical examples. New exercises and questions for new positions of the upper and lower limbs and shoulder girdle have been added.

Pathology questions have been expanded that will help students understand why they are performing specific exams and how exposure factors or positioning may be affected.

As in the textbook, updated information and concepts in digital radiography and surgical radiography have been added in this edition. The bone densitometry section has also been expanded and combined with mammography. Introductions to nuclear medicine, PET, radiation oncology, ultrasound imaging, and MRI have also been updated and expanded.

NEW BONTRAGER POCKET ATLAS HANDBOOK

The new seventh edition of the expanded *Bontrager's Handbook of Radiographic Positioning and Techniques* is now available from Elsevier as part of this comprehensive learning package on radiographic positioning and imaging. The new fifth edition of this handbook includes the unique added feature of a printed radiographic image of the position being described along with a basic critique checklist alongside each image. These primary critique checklist items are grouped in a consistent manner for all projections and are listed in more detail in the positioning pages of the textbook in the Radiographic Criteria section.

This unique handbook provides a guide for students to carry with them in the clinical setting as they learn what to look for when they evaluate each radiograph after it has been taken and processed. This critique checklist also provides a system for the clinical instructors to use in which they can check off each critique item for that radiograph and sign off that exam as a completed competency for that student.

INFORMATION FOR FACULTY

Instructor Resources

Electronic instructor resources are available on the Evolve website at http://evolve.elsevier.com/Bontrager and consist of the following four components:

- **Computerized Test Bank (CTB) in Exam View:** This test bank features more than 2000 questions divided into the 23 chapters. It has been updated, expanded, and revised into more registry-level questions that can be used as final evaluation exams for each chapter. The questions and related answers have been reviewed by the authors and a second-year imaging student. They can be used to produce paper-based exams, or they can be integrated into a Learning Management System (LMS) such as BlackBoard, Angel, or WebCT. Answer keys are provided for each examination.
- **Electronic Image Collection (EIC):** Also available is an updated and expanded electronic image collection of images from all 23 chapters of the seventh edition of the textbook. These nonannotated images can be used by instructors to create PowerPoint presentations or other web-based materials.
- **Electronic Instructional Presentation (EIP) in PowerPoint:** Now included is an updated and epanded electronic image PowerPoint program that is fully coordinated with all 23 chapters of the seventh edition textbook and workbooks.

These electronic images include text slides, some of which contain embedded anatomy and radiographic images, resulting in a visually led instructional narrative. This can then be used as a complete chapter-by-chapter preprogrammed PowerPoint lecture guide. Sections from the more advanced chapters can also be used for in-service training or with postgraduate presentations.

- **Instructor's Manual:** This resource links all parts of the educational package together by providing customizable lesson plans based on learning objectives. With these powerful resources at your fingertips, you'll save valuable preparation time and create a learning environment that fully engages students in classroom participation.

Student Instructions

The following information will show you how to correctly use this workbook and the accompanying textbook to help you master radiographic anatomy and positioning.

This course becomes the core of all your studies and your work as a radiologic technologist. This is one course that you must master. You cannot become a proficient technologist by marginally passing this course. Therefore please read these instructions carefully before beginning Chapter 1.

OBJECTIVES

Study the list of objectives carefully so that you will understand what you must know and be able to do after you complete each chapter.

TEXTBOOK AND WORKBOOK

Chapters 1 and *2* include a comprehensive introduction that prepares you for the remaining chapters of this positioning course. Your instructor may assign all or specific sections of these chapters at various times during your study of radiographic positioning and/or procedures.

Chapters 3-16 are specific positioning chapters that include the anatomy, positioning, and related procedures for all parts of the body.

Chapters 17-23 are more specialized procedures and modalities that are commonly studied later in a medical radiography program.

LEARNING EXERCISES

These exercises are the focal point of this workbook. Using them correctly will help you learn and remember the important information presented in each chapter of the textbook. To maximize the benefits from each exercise, follow the correct six-step order of activities as outlined below.

ANATOMY ACTIVITIES

Step 1 (Textbook)

Carefully read and learn the radiographic anatomy section of each of these chapters. Include the anatomic reviews on labeled radiographs provided in the textbook. Pay particular attention to those items in bold type and to the summary review boxes, where provided.

Step 2 (Workbook, Part I)

Complete Part I of the review exercises on radiographic anatomy. Do not look up the answers in the textbook or look at the answer sheet until you have answered as many of the questions as you can. Then refer to the textbook and/or the answer sheet and correct or complete those questions you missed. Reread those sections of the textbook in which you could not answer questions. Textbook page numbers are provided next to each review exercise in this workbook.

POSITIONING ACTIVITIES

Step 3 (Textbook)

Carefully read and study Part II on all of the parts on radiographic positioning. Note the general positioning considerations, alternate modalities, and pathologic indications for each chapter. Information from these sections will be seen on workbook review exercises, self-tests, and chapter evaluations. This is followed by the specific positioning pages, which include pathology demonstrated, technical factors, and the dose ranges of skin, midline, and specific organ doses, where provided. Pay particular attention to dose comparisons between different techniques, or anteroposterior (AP) versus posteroanterior (PA) projections. Learn the specific positioning steps, the central ray location and angle, and the four-part radiographic criteria for each projection or position.

Step 4 (Workbook, Part II)

Complete Part II of the review exercises, which include technical considerations and positioning. Also included is a section on problem solving for technical and positioning errors. As before, complete as many of the questions as you can before looking up the answers in the textbook or checking the answers on the answer sheet.

The last review exercise in each positioning chapter covers radiographic critique questions in the workbook. These questions may involve radiographic evaluation of images from the text. These important exercises will help you make the transition from factual knowledge to application and will help you prepare for clinical experience. Compare each critique radiograph that demonstrates errors with the correctly positioned radiographs in that chapter of the textbook and see if you can determine which radiographic criteria points could be improved and which are repeatable errors.

With digital images you will learn that in some cases postprocessing adjustments can be made to improve the exposures and the diagnostic value of the images rather than repeating the exam. Positioning errors, however, would still need to be repeated as they would with film-screen imaging and processing. Students who successfully complete these exercises will be ahead of those students who don't attempt them before coming to the classroom. The instructor will then explain and clarify the repeatable and nonrepeatable errors on each radiograph.

LABORATORY ACTIVITY

Step 5 (Workbook, Part III—Laboratory Activity)

These exercises must be performed in a radiographic laboratory using a phantom and/or a student (without making exposure), an energized radiographic unit, illuminators for viewing radiographs, and/or monitors for viewing digital images. Arrange for a time when you can use your radiographic laboratory or a diagnostic radiographic room in a clinic setting.

This is one of the most important aspects of this learning series and should not be neglected or underemphasized. Students frequently have difficulty transferring the information they have learned about positioning to effective use in a clinical setting. Therefore you must carry out the laboratory activities as described in each chapter. Your instructors and/or lab assistants will assist you as needed in these exercises.

Each radiograph taken of the phantom and/or other radiographs provided by your instructor should be evaluated as described in your lab manual. Critique and evaluate each radiograph for errors of less-than-optimal positioning or exposure factors based on radiographic criteria provided in the textbook. Also, with the help of your instructor, learn how to discriminate between less-than-optimal, but passable radiographs, and those that need to be repeated. This generally requires additional experience and practice before you can make these judgments without assistance from a supervising technologist or radiologist.

SELF-TEST

Step 6

You should take the self-test only after you have completed all of the preceding steps. Treat the self-test like an actual exam. After you have completed it, compare your answers with the answer sheet at the end of this workbook. If your score is less than 90% to 95%, you should go back and review the textbook again; pay special attention to the areas you missed before you take the final chapter evaluation exam provided by your instructor.

Warning: Statistics prove that students who diligently complete all the exercises described in this section will invariably get higher grades in their positioning courses and will perform better in the clinical setting than those who don't. Avoid the temptation of taking shortcuts. If you bypass some of these exercises or just fill in the answers from the answer sheets, your instructors will know by your grade and by your clinical performance that you have taken these shortcuts. Most importantly, you will know that you are not doing your best and you will have difficulty competing with better-prepared technologists in the job market when you graduate.

Go to it and enjoy the feeling of satisfaction and success that only comes when you know you're doing your best!

Contents

Contents

1 General Anatomy, Terminology, and Positioning Principles

CHAPTER OBJECTIVES

After you have successfully completed the activities in this chapter, you will be able to:

A. General, Systemic, and Skeletal Anatomy and Arthrology

_____ 1. List the four basic types of tissues.

_____ 2. List the 10 systems of the body.

_____ 3. Match specific bodily functions to their correct anatomic system.

_____ 4. List the four general classifications of bone.

_____ 5. Identify specific characteristics and aspects of bone.

_____ 6. Classify specific joints by their structure and function.

_____ 7. Classify specific synovial joints by their movement.

B. Positioning Terminology

_____ 1. Define general radiographic and anatomic relational terminology.

_____ 2. Define the imaginary planes, sections, and surfaces of the body used to describe central ray angles or relationships among body parts.

_____ 3. Distinguish among a radiographic projection, position, and view.

_____ 4. Given various hypothetical situations, identify the correct radiographic projection.

_____ 5. Given various hypothetical situations, identify the correct radiographic position.

_____ 6. List the antonyms (terms with opposite meanings) of specific terms related to movement.

C. Positioning Principles

_____ 1. Given a hypothetical clinical situation, identify the response as required in the professional code of ethics.

_____ 2. Identify the correct sequence of steps taken to perform a routine radiographic procedure.

_____ 3. Given a set of circumstances, apply the three general rules of radiography concerning the minimal number of projections required for specific regions of the body.

_____ 4. Identify the correct way to view a conventional radiograph, computed tomography (CT) image, and magnetic resonance (MR) image.

LEARNING ACTIVITY EXERCISES

The following review exercises should be completed only after careful study of the associated pages in the textbook as indicated by each exercise. Because certain topics may be too advanced for the entry-level student, the review exercises for Chapter 1 are divided into sections A through C. You can complete specific sections of review exercises, as directed by your instructor, to best meet your learning needs.

After completing each of these individual exercises, check your answers with the answers provided at the end of the review exercises.

REVIEW EXERCISE A: General, Systemic, and Skeletal Anatomy and Arthrology (see textbook pp. 2-13)

1. The lowest level of the structural organization of the human body is the _____.

2. List the four basic types of tissues in the body.

   A. _____   C. _____

   B. _____   D. _____

3. List the 10 systems of the human body.

   A. _____   F. _____

   B. _____   G. _____

   C. _____   H. _____

   D. _____   I. _____

   E. _____   J. _____

4. Match the following functions to the correct body system.

   _____ 1. Eliminates solid waste from the body   A. Skeletal system

   _____ 2. Regulates fluid and electrolyte balance and volume   B. Circulatory system

   _____ 3. Maintains posture   C. Digestive system

   _____ 4. Regulates body activities with electrical impulses   D. Respiratory system

   _____ 5. Regulates bodily activities through various hormones   E. Urinary system

   _____ 6. Eliminates carbon dioxide from blood   F. Reproductive system

   _____ 7. Receives stimuli, such as temperature, pressure, and pain   G. Nervous system

   _____ 8. Reproduces the organism   H. Muscular system

   _____ 9. Helps regulate body temperature   I. Endocrine system

   _____ 10. Supports and protects many soft tissues of the body   J. Integumentary system

5. True/False: One of the six functions of the circulatory system is to protect against disease.

6. Which of the following body systems regulate body temperature?
   A. Endocrine
   B. Integumentary
   C. Digestive
   D. Circulatory

7. What is the largest organ system in the body?
   A. Digestive
   B. Nervous
   C. Integumentary
   D. Respiratory

8. List the two divisions of the human skeletal system.

   A. _____   B. _____

9. True/False: The adult skeleton system contains 256 separate bones.

10. True/False: The scapula is part of the axial skeleton.

11. True/False: The skull is part of the axial skeleton.

12. True/False: The pelvis is part of the appendicular skeleton.

13. List the four classifications of bones.

   A. _____   C. _____

   B. _____   D. _____

14. The outer covering of a long bone, which is composed of a dense, fibrous membrane, is called what?
   A. Spongy or cancellous bone
   B. Compact bone
   C. Medullary aspect
   D. Periosteum

15. Which aspect of long bones is responsible for the production of red blood cells?
   A. Spongy or cancellous bone
   B. Compact bone
   C. Medullary aspect
   D. Periosteum

16. Which aspect of the long bone is essential for bone growth, repair, and nutrition?
   A. Medullary aspect
   B. Compact bone
   C. Periosteum
   D. Articular cartilage

17. Identify the primary and secondary growth centers for long bones.

   A. Primary growth center: _____

   B. Secondary growth center: _____

18. True/False: Epiphyseal fusion of the long bones is complete by the age of 16 years.

19. The study of joints or articulations is called _____.

20. List the three *functional* classifications of joints.

    A. _____

    B. _____

    C. _____

21. List the three *structural* classifications of joints.

    A. _____

    B. _____

    C. _____

22. Match the following joints to the correct structural classification.

    _____ 1. First carpometacarpal of thumb   A. Fibrous joint

    _____ 2. Roots around teeth   B. Cartilaginous joint

    _____ 3. Proximal radioulnar joint   C. Synovial joint

    _____ 4. Skull sutures

    _____ 5. Epiphyses

    _____ 6. Interphalangeal joints

    _____ 7. Distal tibiofibular joint

    _____ 8. Intervertebral disk space

    _____ 9. Symphysis pubis

    _____ 10. Hip joint

23. List the seven types of movement for synovial joints (give both the preferred terms).

    A. _____

    B. _____   E. _____

    C. _____   F. _____

    D. _____   G. _____

24. Match the following synovial joints to the correct type of movement.

_____ 1. First carpometacarpal joint   A. Plane

_____ 2. Elbow joint   B. Ginglymus

_____ 3. Shoulder joint   C. Trochoidal

_____ 4. Intercarpal joint   D. Ellipsoidal

_____ 5. Wrist joint   E. Sellar

_____ 6. Temporomandibular joint   F. Spheroidal

_____ 7. First and second cervical vertebra joint   G. Bicondylar

_____ 8. Second interphalangeal joint

_____ 9. Distal radioulnar joint

_____ 10. Ankle joint

_____ 11. Knee joint

_____ 12. Third metacarpophalangeal joint

REVIEW EXERCISE B: Positioning Terminology (see textbook pp. 14-28)

1. A(n) _____ is an image of a patient's anatomical part(s) as produced by the actions of x-rays on an image receptor (radiograph).

2. The _____ _____ is the aspect of an x-ray beam that has the least divergence (unless there is angulation).

3. An upright position with the arms abducted, palms forward, and head and feet directed straight ahead describes the

_____ position.

4. The vertical plane that divides the body into equal right and left parts is the _____ plane.

5. The vertical plane that divides the body into equal anterior and posterior parts is the _____ plane.

6. A plane taken at right angles along any point of the longitudinal axis of the body is the _____ plane.

7. True/False: The *base plane of the skull* is a plane located between the infraorbital margin of the orbit and the superior margin of the external auditory meatus.

8. True/False: The *Frankfort horizontal plane* is also referred to as *the mid-coronal plane.*

9. The direction or path of the central ray defines the following positioning term.
   A. Projection   C. Position
   B. View   D. Perspective

10. The positioning term that describes the general and specific body position is:
    A. Projection   C. Position
    B. View   D. Perspective

11. True/False: Oblique and lateral positions are described according to the side of the body closest to image receptor.

12. True/False: Decubitus positions always use a horizontal x-ray beam.

13. What is the name of the position in which the body is turned 90° from a true anteroposterior (AP) or posteroanterior

    (PA) projection? _____

14. **Situation:** A patient is erect with the back to the image receptor. The left side of the body is turned 45° toward the

    image receptor. What is this position?_____

15. **Situation:** A patient is recumbent facing the image receptor. The right side of the body is turned 15° toward the

    image receptor. What is this position? _____

16. **Situation:** The patient is lying on his or her back. The x-ray beam is directed horizontally and enters the right side
    of the body and exits the left side of the body. An image receptor is placed against the left side of the patient. Which
    specific position has been used?

17. **Situation:** The patient is erect with the right side of the body against the image receptor. The x-ray beam enters the left

    side and exits the right side of the body. Which specific position has been performed? _____

18. **Situation:** A patient is lying on the left side on a cart. The x-ray beam is directed horizontally and enters the posterior
    surface and exits the anterior aspect of the body. The image receptor is against the anterior surface. Which specific

    position has been performed? _____

19. Match the following definitions to the correct term (using each term only once).

    _____ 1. Palm of the hand   A. Posterior

    _____ 2. Lying on the back facing upward   B. Anterior

    _____ 3. An upright position   C. Plantar

    _____ 4. Lying down in any position   D. Dorsum pedis

    _____ 5. Front half of the patient   E. Trendelenburg

    _____ 6. Top or anterior surface of the foot   F. Erect

    _____ 7. Position in which head is higher than the feet   G. Supine

    _____ 8. Posterior aspect of foot   H. Palmar

    _____ 9. Position in which head is lower than feet   I. Recumbent

    _____ 10. Back half of the patient   J. Fowler's

20. What is the name of the projection in which the central ray enters the anterior surface and exits the posterior surface?

    _____

21. A projection using a CR angle of 10° or more directed parallel along the long axis of the body or body part is termed

    a/an _____ projection.

22. The specific position that demonstrates the apices of the lungs, without superimposition of the clavicles, is termed

    a/an _____ position.

23. True/False: Radiographic "view" is not a correct positioning term in the United States.

24. True/False: The term *varus* describes the bending of a part outward.

25. Match the following. (Indicate whether the following terms describe a **position** or **projection**.)

    _____ 1. Anteroposterior   A. Position

    _____ 2. Prone   B. Projection

    _____ 3. Trendelenburg

    _____ 4. Left posterior oblique

    _____ 5. Left lateral chest

    _____ 6. Mediolateral ankle

    _____ 7. Apical AP

    _____ 8. Lordotic

    _____ 9. Inferosuperior axial

    _____ 10. Left lateral decubitus

26. For each of the following terms, list the term that has the **opposite** meaning.

    A. Flexion: _____

    B. Ulnar deviation: _____

    C. Dorsiflexion: _____

    D. Eversion: _____

    E. Lateral (external) rotation: _____

    F. Abduction: _____

    G. Supination: _____

    H. Retraction: _____

    I. Depression: _____

27. Match the following relationship terms to the correct definition (using each term only once):

    _____ 1. Near the source or beginning   A. Caudad or inferior

    _____ 2. On the opposite side   B. Deep

    _____ 3. Toward the center   C. Distal

    _____ 4. Toward the head end of the body   D. Contralateral

    _____ 5. Away from the source or beginning   E. Cephalad or superior

    _____ 6. Outside or outward   F. Proximal

    _____ 7. On the same side   G. Medial

    _____ 8. Near the skin surface   H. Superficial

    _____ 9. Away from the head end   I. Ipsilateral

    _____ 10. Farther from the skin surface   J. Exterior

28. Moving or thrusting the jaw forward from the normal position is an example of _____.

29. To turn or bend the wrist toward the radius side is called _____.

30. Which two types of information should be imprinted on **every** radiographic image?

    A. _____

    B. _____

REVIEW EXERCISE C: Positioning Principles (see textbook pp. 29-34)

1. True/False: Technologists have the right to refuse to perform an examination on a patient whom they find offensive. (Refer to p. 31 in text.)

2. True/False: Technologists are responsible for the professional decisions they make during the care of the patient. (Refer to p. 31 in text.)

3. True/False: The technologist has the responsibility of communicating with the patient to obtain pertinent clinical information. (Refer to p. 31 in text.)

4. True/False: The technologist is expected to provide a preliminary interpretation of radiographic findings to the referring physician. (Refer to p. 31 in text.)

5. True/False: The technologist may reveal confidential information pertaining to a patient who is less than 18 years of age to the patient or guardian. (Refer to p. 31 in text.)

6. List the two rules or principles for determining positioning routines as they relate to the maximum number of projections required in a basic routine.

   A. _____   B. _____

7. Indicate the minimum number of projections required for each of the following anatomic regions.

   A. Foot _____   F. Fifth toe _____

   B. Chest _____   G. Postreduction of wrist (image of wrist in cast) _____

   C. Wrist _____   H. Left hip _____

   D. Tibia/fibula _____   I. Knee _____

   E. Humerus _____   J. Pelvis (nonhip injury) _____

8. **Situation**: A young child enters the emergency room with a fractured forearm. After one projection is completed, which confirms a fracture, the child refuses to move the forearm for any additional projections.

   A. What is the minimum number of projections that should be taken for this forearm study?
      (a) One   (c) Three
      (b) Four   (d) Two

   B. If additional projections are required for a routine forearm series, what should the technologist do with the young patient described in this situation?
      (a) Because only one projection is required for a fractured forearm, the technologist is not required to take additional projections.
      (b) With the help of a parent or guardian, gently but firmly move the forearm for each additional projection required.
      (c) Rather than move the forearm for a second projection, place the cassette and x-ray tube as needed for a second projection 90° from the first projection.
      (d) Ask the emergency room physician to move the forearm for a second projection. This eliminates any liability for the technologist in case the patient is injured further.

9. The physical localization of bony landmarks on a patient is called _____.

10. Which two landmarks may not palpated due to institutional policy?

    A. _____

    B. _____

11. True/False: Always place a radiograph for viewing as the image receptor "sees" the patient. (The patient's left is to the viewer's left on AP projections.)

12. True/False: Most CT images are viewed so that the patient's right is to the viewer's left.

This series of self-tests should be taken only after completing all of the readings, review exercises, and laboratory activities for a particular section. This self-test is divided into three sections. The purpose of this test is not only to provide a good learning exercise but also to serve as a strong indicator of what your final evaluation exam will cover. It is strongly suggested that if you do not get at least a 90% to 95% grade on each self-test, that you review those areas in which you missed questions before going to your instructor for the final evaluation exam.

SELF-TEST A: General, Systemic, and Skeletal Anatomy and Arthrology

1. Which of the following is (are) *not* one of the four basic types of tissue in the human body? (More than one answer is possible.)
   A. Integumentary
   B. Connective
   C. Nervous
   D. Osseous
   E. Muscular
   F. Epithelial

2. How many separate bones are found in the adult human body?
   A. 180
   B. 243
   C. 206
   D. 257

3. Which one of the following systems distributes oxygen and nutrients to the cells of the body?
   A. Digestive
   B. Circulatory
   C. Skeletal
   D. Urinary

4. Which one of the following systems maintains the acid-base balance in the body?
   A. Digestive
   B. Urinary
   C. Reproductive
   D. Circulatory

5. Which one of the following systems is considered to be the largest organ system in the human body?
   A. Muscular
   B. Endocrine
   C. Skeletal
   D. Integumentary

6. The two divisions of the human skeleton are:
   A. Bony and cartilaginous
   B. Axial and appendicular
   C. Vertebral and extremities
   D. Integumentary and appendicular

7. Which portion of the long bones is responsible for the production of red blood cells?
   A. Spongy or cancellous
   B. Periosteum
   C. Hyaline
   D. Compact aspect

8. What type of tissue covers the ends of the long bones?
   A. Spongy or cancellous
   B. Periosteum
   C. Hyaline or articular cartilage
   D. Compact aspect

9. The narrow space between the inner and outer table of the flat bones in the cranium is called the:
   A. Calvarium
   B. Periosteum
   C. Medullary portion
   D. Diploe

10. What is the primary center for endochondral ossification in long bones?
    A. Diaphysis (shaft)
    B. Epiphyseal plate
    C. Epiphyses
    D. Medulla

11. What is the name of secondary growth centers of endochondral ossification found in long bones?
    A. Diaphysis (shaft)
    B. Epiphyseal plate
    C. Epiphyses
    D. Medulla

12. A skull suture has the structural classification of a _____ joint.
    A. Fibrous
    B. Cartilaginous
    C. Synovial
    D. Diarthrosis

13. The symphysis pubis has the structural classification of a _____ joint.
    A. Fibrous
    B. Cartilaginous
    C. Synovial
    D. Synarthrosis

14. Which specific joint(s) is (are) the only true syndesmosis, amphiarthrodial, fibrous joint(s)?
    A. Joints between the roots of teeth and adjoining bone
    B. First carpometacarpal joint
    C. Distal tibiofibular joint
    D. Proximal and distal radioulnar joints

15. Match the following bones to their correct classification.

    _____ 1. Sternum   A. Long bone

    _____ 2. Femur   B. Short bone

    _____ 3. Tarsal bones   C. Flat bone

    _____ 4. Pelvic bones   D. Irregular bone

    _____ 5. Scapulae

    _____ 6. Humerus

    _____ 7. Vertebrae

    _____ 8. Calvarium

16. The three structural classifications of joints are synovial, cartilaginous, and:
    A. Amphiarthrodial
    B. Ellipsoidal
    C. Diarthrodial
    D. Fibrous

17. Classify the following synovial joints based on their type of movement.

_____ 1. First carpometacarpal joint   A. Plane (gliding)

_____ 2. Intercarpal joint   B. Ginglymus (hinge)

_____ 3. Hip joint   C. Trochoidal (pivot)

_____ 4. Proximal radioulnar joint   D. Ellipsoidal (condyloid)

_____ 5. Interphalangeal joint   E. Sellar (saddle)

_____ 6. Fourth metacarpophalangeal joint   F. Spheroidal (ball and socket)

_____ 7. Knee joint   G. Bicondylar

_____ 8. Wrist joint

_____ 9. Joint between C1 and C2

_____ 10. Ankle joint

SELF-TEST B: Positioning Terminology

1. Which plane divides the body into equal anterior and posterior parts?
   A. Midsagittal   B. Transverse   C. Midcoronal   D. Longitudinal

2. True/False: The terms *radiograph* and *image receptor* refer to the same thing.

3. A longitudinal plane that divides the body into right and left parts is the:
   A. Coronal plane   C. Sagittal plane
   B. Horizontal plane   D. Oblique plane

4. Match the following definitions to the correct term.

_____ 1. Near the source or beginning   A. Eversion

_____ 2. Away from head end of the body   B. Circumduction

_____ 3. Inside of something   C. Pronation

_____ 4. Increasing the angle of a joint   D. Contralateral

_____ 5. Outward stress of the foot   E. Proximal

_____ 6. Movement of an extremity away from the midline   F. Medial

_____ 7. Turning palm downward   G. Interior

_____ 8. A backward movement   H. Retraction

_____ 9. To move around in the form of a circle   I. Caudad

_____ 10. Toward the center   J. Extension

_____ 11. Away from the source or beginning   K. Abduction

_____ 12. On the opposite side of the body   L. Distal

5. Match the following definitions to the correct term.

_____ 1. Lying down in any position   A. Base plane of skull

_____ 2. Head lower than the feet position   B. Plantar

_____ 3. Upright position, palms forward   C. Palmar

_____ 4. Top of the foot   D. Fowler's position

_____ 5. Frankfort horizontal plane   E. Lithotomy position

_____ 6. A plane at right angles to the longitudinal plane   F. Anatomic position

_____ 7. Head higher than feet position   G. Trendelenburg position

_____ 8. Palm of hand   H. Horizontal plane

_____ 9. Sole of foot   I. Midcoronal plane

_____ 10. Front half of body   J. Dorsum pedis

_____ 11. A plane that divides body into anterior and posterior halves   K. Anterior

       L. Recumbent

_____ 12. A recumbent position with knees and hips flexed with support for legs

6. The direction or path of the central ray of the x-ray beam defines the positioning term:

  A. Position   C. Perspective

  B. View   D. Projection

7. **Situation:** A patient is placed in a recumbent position facing downward. The left side of the body is turned 30° toward the image receptor. Which specific position has been performed?

  A. LAO   C. LPO

  B. Left lateral decubitus   D. RAO

8. **Situation:** A patient is placed into a recumbent position facing downward. The x-ray tube is directed horizontally and enters the left side and exits the right side of the body. An image receptor is placed against the right side of the patient. Which position has been performed?

  A. Dorsal decubitus   C. Ventral decubitus

  B. Left lateral decubitus   D. Right lateral decubitus

9. **Situation:** A patient is erect with their back to the image receptor. The central ray enters the anterior aspect and exits the posterior aspect of the body. Which projection has been performed?

  A. Posteroanterior   C. Ventral decubitus

  B. Tangential   D. Anteroposterior

10. **Situation:** A patient is lying down facing upward with the posterior surface of the body against the image receptor. The right side of the body turned 45° toward the image receptor. The x-ray tube is directed vertically and enters the anterior surface of the body. Which position has been performed?
    - A. LPO
    - B. RAO
    - C. RPO
    - D. LAO

11. **Situation:** An elbow projection is taken with the posterior surface placed against the image receptor. The elbow is rotated 20° outwardly. Which specific projection has been performed?
    - A. PA oblique with medial rotation
    - B. PA oblique with lateral rotation
    - C. AP oblique with medial rotation
    - D. AP oblique with lateral rotation

12. **Situation:** A specific projection of the foot in which the central ray enters the anterior surface and exits the posterior surface is termed:
    - A. Dorsoplantar
    - B. Plantodorsal
    - C. Axioplantar
    - D. Posteroanterior

13. **Situation:** A patient is placed in a recumbent position with the body tilted so that the head is higher than the feet. The image receptor is under the patient and the x-ray tube is above the patient. Which is the general position of the patient?
    - A. Trendelenburg
    - B. Reid's
    - C. Sims'
    - D. Fowler's

14. **Situation:** The anterior surface of the right knee of the patient is facing the image receptor. The anterior aspect of the knee and lower leg is rotated 15° toward the midline. Which specific projection has been performed?
    - A. AP oblique with medial rotation
    - B. PA oblique with medial rotation
    - C. PA oblique with lateral rotation
    - D. AP oblique with lateral rotation

15. What is the name of the projection in which the central ray merely skims a body part?
    - A. Tangential
    - B. Decubitus
    - C. Axial
    - D. Trendelenburg

16. What is the name of the specific projection where the central ray enters the left side of the chest and exits the opposite side?
    - A. Parietoacanthial
    - B. Axial
    - C. Transthoracic
    - D. Lordotic

17. What is the specific projection that enters the posterior aspect of the skull and exits the acanthion?
    - A. Acanthioparietal
    - B. Tangential
    - C. Axial
    - D. Parietoacanthial

18. Which one of the following is an example of an axial projection?
    - A. Transthoracic lateral
    - B. Mediolateral ankle
    - C. AP Chest with 20° cephalic angle
    - D. AP abdomen with 30° rotation to left

19. Which one of the following positioning terms is no longer considered valid in the United States?
    - A. Radiographic view
    - B. Radiographic position
    - C. Radiographic projection
    - D. Semi-axial projection

20. Match each of the following positioning terms to the term that is its direct opposite.

_____ 1. Proximal   A. Kyphosis

_____ 2. Cephalad   B. Inferior

_____ 3. Ipsilateral   C. External

_____ 4. Medial   D. Distal

_____ 5. Superficial   E. Plantodorsal

_____ 6. Internal   F. Lateral

_____ 7. Lordosis   G. PA

_____ 8. AP   H. Caudad

_____ 9. Superior   I. Contralateral

_____ 10. Dorsoplantar   J. Deep

SELF-TEST C: Positioning Principles

1. True/False: If a patient is younger than 18 years of age, any confidential information obtained during the procedure must be shared with the parent or guardian.

2. True/False: The technologist must provide a preliminary interpretation of any radiographs if requested by the referring physician.

3. True/False: Personal patient information can be shared with another technologist even if they have no role in that patient's procedure.

4. True/False: The technologist can explain a radiographic procedure to the patient without permission from the referring physician or radiologist.

5. Indicate the minimum number of projections required for the following structures.

_____ 1. Knee   A. Two

_____ 2. Fourth finger   B. Three

_____ 3. Humerus

_____ 4. Sternum

_____ 5. Ankle

_____ 6. Tibia/fibula

_____ 7. Chest

_____ 8. Hand

_____ 9. Hip (proximal femur)

_____ 10. Forearm

6. Which of the following radiographic procedures requires a single AP projection be taken?
   A. Post-reduction forearm
   B. KUB
   C. Hand on a pediatric patient
   D. Ribs

7. **Situation:** A patient enters the emergency room with a fractured forearm. The fracture is set, or reduced. The orthopedic physician orders a postreduction series. How many projections are required?
   A. One
   B. Three
   C. Two
   D. Four

8. **Situation:** A patient enters the emergency room with a dislocated elbow. The patient is in extreme pain. What is the minimum number of projections that must be performed?
   A. One
   B. Three
   C. Two
   D. Four

9. **Situation:** A patient comes to radiology for a rib study. What is the minimum number of projections that must be performed?
   A. One
   B. Three
   C. Two
   D. Four

10. **Situation:** A patient enters the emergency room with possible fractured ankle. She can move it but is painful. What is the minimum number of projections that must be performed?
    A. One
    B. Three
    C. Two
    D. Four

11. **Situation:** A patient enters the emergency room with a small piece of wire embedded in the palm of the hand. What is the minimum number of projections required for this study?
    A. One
    B. Three
    C. Two
    D. Four

12. **Situation:** Patient has fallen on ice and has a possible fractured hip (proximal femur). What is the minumum number of projections that should be taken for this patient?
    A. One
    B. Three
    C. Two
    D. Five

13. **Situation:** A patient enters the emergency room with a possible fractured little (fifth) toe. What is the minimum number of projections that must be taken?
    A. One
    B. Three
    C. Two
    D. Five

14. Which of the following positioning routines should be performed for a wrist study?
    A. AP, PA, and lateral projections
    B. AP and lateral projections
    C. PA, oblique and lateral projections
    D. Oblique, axial and lateral projections

15. Which of the following positioning routines should be performed for a chest study?
    A. PA and lateral projections
    B. PA, oblique, and lateral projections
    C. AP, PA, and lateral projections
    D. PA, RAO, and LAO projections

16. The technique for localizing bony and soft tissue of radiographic landmarks is termed:
    A. Localization
    B. Tactile localization
    C. Physical assessment
    D. Palpation

2 Image Quality, Digital Technology, and Radiation Protection

CHAPTER OBJECTIVES

After you have successfully completed the activities in this chapter, you will be able to:

A. Image Quality in Film-Screen Imaging

_____ 1. Describe the major exposure factors that influence the diagnostic quality of the radiograph.

_____ 2. List the four image quality factors and their impact on a radiograph.

_____ 3. Define *radiographic density* and identify its controlling factors.

_____ 4. Given a hypothetical situation, select the correct factor to improve radiographic density.

_____ 5. Describe the correlation between radiographic density and the *anode heel effect*.

_____ 6. List three types of filters and which radiographic procedures are enhanced by their use.

_____ 7. Define *radiographic contrast* and identify its controlling factors.

_____ 8. Distinguish between long- and short-scale radiographic contrast.

_____ 9. Given a hypothetical situation, select the correct factor to improve radiographic contrast.

_____ 10. Given situations, identify the type of grid cut-off errors present and its impact on image quality.

_____ 11. Define resolution and identify its controlling factors.

_____ 12. List the three geometric factors that influence image sharpness.

_____ 13. Identify the best ways of controlling voluntary and involuntary motion.

_____ 14. Given a hypothetical situation, select the correct factor to improve radiographic detail.

_____ 15. Define radiographic distortion and identify its controlling factors.

_____ 16. Given a hypothetical situation, select the correct factor to minimize radiographic distortion.

B. Image Quality in Digital Radiography

_____ 1. List the six image quality factors specific to digital imaging.

_____ 2. Define *brightness* and identify its controlling factors in the digital image.

_____ 3. Define *contrast* and identify its controlling factors in the digital image.

_____ 4. List the two types of pixel sizes.

_____ 5. Define *resolution* and identify its controlling factors in the digital image.

_____ 6. Define *distortion* and identify its controlling factors in the digital image.

_____ 7. Define *exposure index* and describe its relationship to the amount of radiation striking the image receptor (IR).

_____ 8. Explain the concept of the signal-to-noise ratio (SNR).

_____ 9. Define specific terms related to the post-processing of the digital image.

C. Applications of Digital Technology

_____ 1. List the differences between computed tomography (CT) and conventional radiography.

_____ 2. List and briefly describe the two types of digital fluoroscopy systems.

_____ 3. Identify the major components of a digital fluoroscopy system.

_____ 4. List the major components of a computed radiography (CR) system.

_____ 5. Describe briefly how an image is recorded, processed, and viewed with a CR system.

_____ 6. Explain the importance of correct centering, collimation, use of lead masking, and use of grids to the overall quality of the CR image.

_____ 7. Identify specific differences and similarities between CR and digital radiography (DR).

_____ 8. Define the terms PACS, RIS, HIS, HL7, and DICOM.

_____ 9. Compare and contrast different size image receptors between metric and English units of measurement.

_____ 10. Define specific imaging terms and acronyms.

D. Radiation Protection

_____ 1. List and define the traditional units and International System of Units (SI units) of radiation measurement and the conversion factors used to convert between systems.

_____ 2. List the specific annual dose limiting recommendations of whole body effective dose for the general population and occupationally exposed workers.

_____ 3. Define ALARA.

_____ 4. Apply the principles of ALARA to any given hypothetical situation.

_____ 5. Define skin entrance exposure (SEE) and effective dose (ED).

_____ 6. Identify specific methods to reduce exposure to the technologist during fluoroscopic and radiographic procedures.

_____ 7. Describe the seven methods to reduce exposure to the patient during radiographic procedures.

_____ 8. Identify the major types of area and gonadal shields and the minimum lead equivalent thickness requirements of these shields.

_____ 9. Define the 10-day rule and describe its limitations.

_____ 10. Define patient dose terminology for specific regions of the body.

_____ 11. Identify methods to ensure a dose to the patient is minimized when using digital imaging systems.

LEARNING EXERCISES

The following review exercises should be completed only after careful study of the associated pages in the textbook as indicated by each exercise. The review exercises for Chapter 2 are divided into four sections. You can complete specific sections of review exercises, as directed by your instructor, to best meet your learning needs.

After completing each of these individual exercises, check your work with the answers provided at the end of the review exercises.

REVIEW EXERCISE A: Image Quality in Film-Screen Imaging (see textbook pp. 36-46)

1. The radiographic film image is composed of metallic _____ on a polyester base.

2. List the four image quality factors of a radiograph.

   A. _____   C. _____

   B. _____   D. _____

3. Which specific exposure factor controls the quality or penetrating ability of the x-ray beam?

   _____

4. Exposure time is usually expressed in units of _____.

5. The amount of blackness seen on a processed radiograph is called _____.

6. The primary controlling factor for the overall blackness on a radiograph is _____.

7. If the distance between the x-ray tube and image receptor is increased from 40 to 80 inches, what specific effect will it have on the radiographic density, if other factors are not changed?
   A. Increase density to 50%   C. No effect on density
   B. Decrease density to 25%   D. Decrease density to 50%

8. Which term is used to describe a radiograph that has too little density? _____

9. Doubling the mAs will result in _____ the density on the IR image.

10. True/False: kV must be altered to change radiographic density on the IR image.

11. When IR images, using manual technique settings, are underexposed or overexposed, a minimum change in mAs of

    _____ is required to make a visible difference in the radiographic density.
    A. 1% to 3%   C. 25% to 30%
    B. 10% to 15%   D. 50% to 100%

12. According to the anode heel effect, the x-ray beam is less intense at the _____ (cathode or anode) end of the x-ray tube.

13. To best use the anode heel effect, the thicker part of the anatomic structure should be placed under the

    _____ (cathode or anode) end of the x-ray tube.

14. What device or method (other than the anode heel effect) may be used to compensate for the anatomic part

    thickness difference and produce an acceptable density on the IR image? _____

15. List three common types of compensating filters.

    A. _____

    B. _____

    C. _____

16. Which type of compensating filter is used commonly for AP projections of the thoracic spine?

    _____ filter

17. Which type of compensating filter permits soft tissue and bony detail of the shoulder to be equally visualized?

    _____ filter

18. **Situation:** A radiograph of the foot is produced using conventional film-screen cassettes. The resulting radiograph demonstrates too little density and must be repeated. The original exposure was 5 mAs. What mAs is needed to correct the density on this radiograph? (Hint: Density needs to be doubled.)
    A. 5 mAs   C. 30 mAs
    B. 17.5 mAs   D. 10 mAs

19. The difference in density on adjacent areas of the radiograph defines _____.

20. What is the primary controlling factor for radiographic contrast? _____

21. List the two scales of radiographic contrast, and identify which is classified as high contrast and which is low contrast.

    A. _____   B. _____

22. Which scale of contrast is produced with a 110 kV technique? _____

23. True/False: A 50 kV technique will produce a high-contrast image.

24. True/False: A low-contrast image demonstrates more shades of gray on the radiograph.

25. Which one of the following sets of exposure factors will result in the least patient exposure and produce long-scale contrast on a PA chest radiographic image?
    A. 50 kV, 800 mAs   C. 80 kV, 100 mAs
    B. 70 kV, 200 mAs   D. 110 kV, 10 mAs

26. **Situation:** A radiograph of the hand is underexposed and must be repeated. The original technique used was 55 kV with 2.5 mAs. The technologist decides to keep the mAs at the same level but change the kV to increase radiographic density. How much of an increase is needed in kilovoltage (kV) to double the density?
    A. 3 to 5 kV increase   C. 10 to 15 kV increase
    B. 8 to 10 kV increase   D. 15 to 20 kV increase

27. If an anatomic part measures greater than _____ cm, a grid must be used.

28. Identify the type of grid cutoff that is created by the following situations:

    A. The central ray (CR) and face of grid are not perpendicular.
       1. Off-center grid cut-off
       2. Off-level grid cut-off
       3. Off-focus grid cut-off
       4. Upside down grid cut-off

    B. The SID is set beyond the focal range of the grid.
       1. Off-center grid cut-off
       2. Off-level grid cut-off
       3. Off-focus grid cut-off
       4. Upside down grid cut-off

    C. The back of the grid is facing the x-ray tube.
       1. Off-center grid cut-off
       2. Off-level grid cut-off
       3. Off-focus grid cut-off
       4. Upside down grid cut-off

29. The recorded sharpness of structures or objects on the radiograph defines _____.

30. The lack of visible sharpness is called _____.

31. List the three geometric factors that control or influence image resolution.

    A. _____

    B. _____

    C. _____

32. The term that describes the unsharp edges of the projected image is _____.

33. True/False: The use of a small focal spot will entirely eliminate the problem identified in the previous question.

34. The greatest contributor to image unsharpness as related to positioning is _____.

35. What is the best mechanism to control involuntary motion during an exposure?
    A. Use of a small focal spot
    B. Use of a grid
    C. Decrease object image receptor distance (OID)
    D. Shorten exposure time

36. Which one of the following changes will improve image resolution?
    A. Decrease OID
    B. Decrease source image receptor distance (SID)
    C. Use a large focal spot
    D. Use a higher kilovoltage

37. **Situation:** The technologist is performing an elbow series on a pediatric patient. Because of the nature of the injury, the technologist has been asked to produce radiographs that have the highest degree of recorded resolution possible. Which one of the following sets of factors will produce that level of detail?
    A. 0.3-mm focal spot and 30-inch SID
    B. 1.0-mm focal spot and 45-inch SID
    C. 0.5-mm focal spot and 40-inch SID
    D. 0.3-mm focal spot and 40-inch SID

38. The misrepresentation of an object size or shape projected onto a radiographic recording medium is called

    _____.

39. True/False: Through careful selection and control of exposure and geometric factors, it is possible to eliminate all image distortion.

40. List the four primary controlling factors for distortion.

    A. _____   C. _____

    B. _____   D. _____

41. True/False: A decrease in SID reduces distortion.

42. True/False: An increase in OID reduces distortion.

43. True/False: Distortion is reduced when the central ray (CR) is kept perpendicular to the plane of the image receptor.

44. The SID for general radiographic procedures resulting in maximum recorded resolution is:
    A. 40 inches (100 cm)
    B. 72 inches (180 cm)
    C. 44 inches (110 cm)
    D. 48 inches (120 cm)

45. **Situation:** A chest x-ray on a patient with an enlarged heart has been requested. Which SID is recommended for this study?
    A. 40 inches (100 cm)
    B. 72 inches (180 cm)
    C. 44 inches (110 cm)
    D. 48 inches (120 cm)

46. True/False: Every radiographic image reflects some degree of penumbra or unsharpness, even if the smallest focal spot is used.

47. True/False: As the distance between the object and the image receptor is increased, magnification is reduced.

48. True/False: Image distortion increases as the angle of divergence increases from the center of the x-ray beam to the outer edges.

49. True/False: The greater the angle of inclination of the object or the IR, the greater the amount of distortion.

50. True/False: Central ray alignment has little impact on image distortion.

1. True/False: Digital imaging requires that images be chemically processed.

2. True/False: Digital images are a numeric representation of the x-ray intensities that are transmitted through the patient.

3. True/False: Digital images viewed on a monitor are referred to as *hard-copies*.

4. Digital processing involves the systematic application of highly complex mathematical formulas called:
   A. Matrices   C. Analog-to-digital converters
   B. PACS   D. Algorithms

5. The range or level of image contrast in the digital image is primarily controlled by:
   A. kV   C. Digital processing
   B. mAs   D. Matrix size

6. Exposure latitude with digital imaging is more _____ (narrow or wide) when compared with film-screen imaging.

7. List the six image quality factors specific to digital images.

   A. _____   D. _____

   B. _____   E. _____

   C. _____   F. _____

8. In digital imaging, the term _____ replaces density as applied in IR-screen imaging.
   A. Brightness   C. Latitude
   B. Signal   D. Noise

9. True/False: Changes in mAs will not have a primary controlling effect on digital image brightness.

10. True/False: Brightness cannot be altered in the digital image once it has been processed.

11. A digital imaging system's ability to distinguish between similar tissues is termed:
    A. Brightness   C. Signal
    B. Image resolution   D. Contrast resolution

12. Radiographic contrast in the digital image is primarily affected by:
    A. kV   C. Application of processing algorithms
    B. Signal-to-noise ratio   D. Matrix size

13. The greater the bit depth of a digital imaging system, the greater the:
    A. Size of the matrix   C. Brightness
    B. Contrast resolution   D. Pixel size

14. List the terms describing the two pixel sizes used in digital imaging.

    A. _____

    B. _____

15. Which one of the two pixel sizes listed above is most critical in maintaining high-resolution digital images?

    _____

16. True/False: Focal spot size has no impact on the resolution of the digital image.

17. The current range of image resolution for digital general radiographic imaging is between:
    A. 1 to 5 microns
    B. 10 to 50 microns
    C. 50 to 75 microns
    D. 100 to 200 microns

18. Resolution in the digital image is primarily dependent on:
    A. kV
    B. Display capabilities of the monitor
    C. SID
    D. Use of a grid

19. True/False: The factors that affect image distortion for the digital image are different from those that affect film-screen systems.

20. A numeric value that is representative of the exposure the digital image receptor receives is termed the

    _____.

21. List the four factors that affect exposure index in the digital image.

    A. _____   C. _____

    B. _____   D. _____

22. The complete term for "S number," as used by several manufacturers of CR equipment, is _____.

23. An "S number" is _____ (directly or indirectly) proportional to the radiation exposing the

    patient; and an exposure index, as used by other manufacturers, is _____ (directly or indirectly) proportional.

24. If the recommended exposure index range for a well-exposed image is between 150 and 250, an "S number" of

    350 to 550 would indicate _____ (overexposure or underexposure) of the image.

25. If the recommended exposure index is between 2.0 to 2.4, an exposure index number of 1.2 would indicate

    _____ (overexposure or underexposure) of the image.

26. A random disturbance that obscures or reduces clarity is the definition for _____.

27. SNR is the acronym for the _____.

28. When insufficient mAs is applied in the production of a digital image, it will produce a _____ (high-SNR or low-SNR) image.

29. Another term for image noise is:
   A. Variance
   B. Static
   C. Mottle
   D. Digital spam

30. Changing or enhancing the electronic image to improve its diagnostic quality is called _____.

31. Identify the type of post-processing described by listing the correct term for the following definitions.

   A. Adding text to images: _____

   B. Increasing brightness along the edges of structures to increase the visibility of the edges:

   _____

   C. Reversing the dark and light pixel values of an image—the x-ray image reverses from a negative to a positive:

   _____

   D. Magnifying all or part of an image: _____

   E. Adjusting brightness values of adjacent pixels closer together: _____

   F. Removing background anatomy to allow visualization of contrast media–filled structures:

   _____

REVIEW EXERCISE C: Applications of Digital Technology (see textbook pp. 52-58)

1. List the three components of a CR system.

   A. _____

   B. _____

   C. _____

2. What material on the CR imaging plate captures the latent image? _____

3. With CR, the imaging plate (IP):
   A. Must be kept in a light-tight cassette and replaced with recharged plates daily
   B. Must be used in conjunction with light-sensitive IR
   C. Must be used in conjunction with intensifying screens
   D. None of the above

4. When using a CR image plate, patient data can be linked to the image by use of a(n):
   A. Bar code reader
   B. White light source
   C. Laser
   D. Ultraviolet light source

5. True/False: Once the CR image plate has had an image recorded on it, it must be discarded.

6. True/False: The latent image on a CR image plate is read line by line by a laser within the CR reader.

7. True/False: It takes approximately 20 seconds to process a CR image and reload the cassette with a clean imaging plate.

8. The latent image is erased on the CR image plate by applying:
   A. Bright light
   B. Heat
   C. Low-level radiation
   D. Microwaves

9. The process of transferring the CR image to a storage device is termed _____.

10. Which one of the following technical factors does *not* apply to CR (computed radiography)?
    A. Close collimation
    B. Accurate centering of part and IR
    C. Use of lead masks
    D. A minimum of 72 inches (183 cm) is required for all CR projections

11. When using CR, a minimum of _____ % of the IR must be exposed for an accurate exposure index.

12. True/False: The use of grids is optional with CR since the IP is not as sensitive to scatter radiation as film-screen radiography.

13. Which of the following imaging components is *not* required with direct digital radiography (DR)?
    A. IP
    B. Image reader
    C. Grid
    D. Both A and B

14. True/False: Patient dose may be lower with DR as compared with film-screen radiography and CR.

15. True/False: When using DR for most nongrid procedures, one reason the grid is generally not removed is its fragile construction.

16. True/False: The 30% collimation rule applies to direct digital radiography (DR).

17. Match the following metric measurements for image receptor sizes to the nearest equivalent traditional size.

Metric	**Traditional (English)**
_____ 1. 24 × 30 cm	A. 14 × 17 inches
_____ 2. 18 × 24 cm	B. 14 × 36 inches
_____ 3. 35 × 43 cm	C. 11 × 14 inches
_____ 4. 30 × 35 cm	D. 10 × 12 inches
_____ 5. 24 × 24 cm	E. 8 × 10 inches
_____ 6. 35 × 90 cm	F. 8 × 8 inches

18. True/False: The size of the image receptor used is dependent primarily on the size of the body part being examined.

19. Define the acronym PACS.

P : _____

A : _____

C : _____

S : _____

20. True/False: A PACS automatically transports conventional x-ray IRs to the chemical processor after they have been exposed.

21. What do the following acronyms represent? (Write the complete term.)

A. DICOM: _____

B. RIS: _____

C. HIS: _____

D. HL7: _____

22. The electronic transmission of diagnostic imaging studies is termed _____.

23. An elecronic, comprehensive database of all patient records and data is referred to as _____. (Include the acronym.)

24. Provide the correct term for the following definitions.

_____ A. Series of "boxes" that gives form to the image

_____ B. Range of exposure factors that will produce an acceptable image

_____ C. The user adjusting the window level and window width

_____ D. Unsharp edges of the projected image

_____ E. Numeric value that is representative of the exposure the image receptor received in digital radiography

_____ F. Representative of the number of shades of gray that can be demonstrated by each pixel

_____ G. Misrepresentation of object size or shape as projected onto radiographic recording media

_____ H. The energy of the x-ray photon

_____ I. Random disturbance that obscures or reduces clarity

_____ J. The delivery of health care services using telecommunications and computer technology

_____ K. Changing or enhancing the electronic image to view it from a different perspective or improve its diagnostic quality

25. List the complete term for the following acronyms.

   A. RIS: _____

   B. IR: _____

   C. OID: _____

   D. DR: _____

   E. AEC: _____

   F. HIS: _____

26. Match the following terms to the correct definition.

   _____ A. Windowing   1. Controls the brightness of a digital image (within a certain range).

   _____ B. Bit-depth   2. Range of exposure factors that will produce an acceptable image.

   _____ C. Noise   3. Random disturbance that obscures or reduces clarity.

   _____ D. Exposure latitude 4. A term used by some equipment manufacturers to indicate exposure index.

   _____ E. Level   5. The user adjusting the window level and window width.

   _____ F. Sensitivity number 6. Series of "boxes" that give form to the image.

   _____ G. Matrix   7. Representative of the number of shades of gray that can be demonstrated by each pixel.

REVIEW EXERCISE D: Radiation Protection (see textbook pp. 59-67)

1. Which traditional unit is used to measure radiation exposure in air? _____

2. Which traditional unit of measurement is used to describe patient dose? _____

3. What does the acronym ED stand for? _____

4. What is the whole body effective dose limit per year for a technologist (in traditional and SI units)?

   _____

5. What is the cumulative dose limit for a 35-year-old technologist (in traditional and SI units)?

   _____

6. For each of the following traditional units, list the equivalent SI unit of radiation measurement and its symbol.

   Traditional Unit   **SI Unit**

   A. Roentgen (R)   _____

   B. Radiation absorbed dose (rad)   _____

   C. Radiation equivalent man (rem)   _____

7. Convert the following doses, stated in traditional units, into the equivalent SI unit.

   A. 3 rad = _____ Gy   C. 38 rem = _____ Sv

   B. 448 mrad = _____ mGy   D. 15 rem = _____ mSv

8. What is the maximum dose limit for a pregnant technologist?

   A. Per month: _____

   B. For the entire gestational period: _____

9. The ED limit for minors under the age of 18 years is _____ per year.

10. Personnel monitoring devices must be worn if there is a possibility of acquiring _____ % of the annual annual, occupational effective dose limit.
    A. 1%   C. 15%
    B. 10%   D. 20%

11. Define the following dosimetry terms.

    A. TLD: _____

    B. OSL: _____

12. The acronym ALARA stands for _____.

13. **Situation:** A young child comes to the radiology department for a skull series. The child is combative and will not hold still for the procedure. Which one of the following individuals should be asked to restrain the patient?
    A. A family member (if not pregnant)   C. The oldest technologist
    B. A student technologist   D. A nuclear medicine technologist

14. True/False: With accurate and close collimation, area shields do not need to be used.

15. True/False: Skin entrance exposure (SEE) has the highest numeric value of all patient doses.

16. True/False: In radiography, SEE carries the least biologic significance.

17. True/False: ED describes gonadal dose levels only for each radiographic procedure.

18. What is the best method of reducing scatter to a worker's eyes and neck during fluoroscopy?

   _____

19. Which of the following is the best place for a technologist to stand during fluoroscopy to reduce occupational exposure?
    A. Head end of table
    B. Foot end of table
    C. Behind the radiologist
    D. Next to the radiologist

20. What is the federal set limit for exposure rates for intensified fluoroscopy units?
    A. 1 R/min
    B. 6 to 8 R/min
    C. 3 to 4 R/min
    D. 10 R/min

21. With most modern fluoroscopy equipment, the average exposure rate is:
    A. 0.5 R/min
    B. 3 to 4 R/min
    C. 1 R/min
    D. 10 R/min

22. What is one of the primary causes for repeat radiographs? (Select the *best* answer.)
    A. Excessive kilovoltage
    B. Wrong IR selection
    C. Poor communication between technologist and patient
    D. Distortion caused by incorrect SID

23. In addition to the primary cause identified in the previous question, what two other factors often lead to repeat exposures?

    A. _____   B. _____

24. Refer to the patient dose chart on p. 61 of the textbook to answer the following questions (A through G).

    A. The _____ (AP or PA) chest projection provides the greatest ED for females.

    B. _____ (Male or Female) patients receive a greater ED for an AP hip, with or without gonadal shielding.

    C. List the gonadal dose for male and female patients for an AP abdomen projection using 70 kV.

       Male, shielded: _____

       Male, unshielded: _____

       Female, unshielded: _____

    D. Which specific organ in each gender receives the greatest dose in AP, PA, and lateral upper GI projections:

       lungs, testes, ovaries, thyroid, marrow, or breast? _____

    E. List the gonadal doses for an AP hip projection for the following patients.

       Male, unshielded (testes): _____   Female, unshielded (ovaries): _____

       Male shielded: _____   Female shielded: _____

    F. Which radiographic procedure listed on the patient dose chart provides the least amount of SEE for males and

       females? _____ (Note the correlation among kilovoltage peak, milliampere seconds, and dose.)

G. Which procedure on the patient dose chart provides the greatest amount of

ED for a male patient? _____ For a female patient? _____

25. If a technologist receives 3.3 to 6.7 mR/min standing 1 foot from a fluoroscopy unit, what will the dose be if the technologist moves to a distance of 4 feet? (See Exposure Levels chart on p. 62 of the textbook.)
  A. Less than 0.25 mR/min
  B. 0.4 to 0.8 mR/min
  C. 0.8 to 1.7 mR/min
  D. 1.7 to 3 mR /min

26. List the two major forms of filtration found in x-ray tubes that affect the quality of the primary x-ray beam.

  A. _____

  B. _____

27. What is the most common metal used in filters for diagnostic radiology equipment? _____

28. List the two ways collimation will reduce patient exposure.

  A. _____

  B. _____

29. True/False: Safety standards require that collimators be accurate to within 10% of the selected SID.

30. True/False: Positive beam limitation (PBL) collimators restrict the size of the exposure field to the size of the cassette in a Bucky tray.

31. True/False: PBL collimators became optional on new equipment manufactured after May 1993 because of a change in Food and Drug Administration (FDA) regulations.

32. List the two general types of specific area shields.

  A. _____

  B. _____

33. The minimum thickness of a gonadal shield placed within the primary x-ray field should be:
  A. 0.1-mm lead equivalent
  B. 0.25-mm lead equivalent
  C. 1-mm lead equivalent
  D. 0.5-mm lead equivalent

34. If placed properly, gonadal shields absorb _____ of the primary beam in the 50 to 100 kV range.
  A. 95% to 99%
  B. 80% to 90%
  C. 70% to 80%
  D. 50% to 70%

35. An area shield should be used when radiation-sensitive tissues lie within _____ inches (or

_____ cm) of the primary beam.

36. Which type of area shield would be best suited for use during a sterile procedure? _____

37. True/False: The 10-day rule is considered by the International Commission on Radiological Protection (ICRP) and the American College of Radiology (ACR) to be obsolete.

38. **Situation:** A 20-year-old female enters the emergency room with a possible fracture of the pelvis. What should the technologist do in regard to gonadal shielding?
   A. Use it for all projections
   B. Use it for the AP projections only
   C. Ask the patient whether she is pregnant
   D. Do not use shielding for initial pelvis projection

39. What is the disadvantage of using faster-speed screens for all IR-screen radiographic procedures?

   _____

40. List the complete term for each of the following abbreviations used in patient dose icon boxes (found in the positioning pages of the textbook).

   A. Sk: _____

   B. ML: _____

   C. Gon: _____

   D. NDC: _____

41. True/False: Area shields must be used for all radiographic procedures with all patients.

42. What is the minimum lead equivalency recommended for a protective apron worn during fluoroscopy?

   _____

43. List the three cardinal principles for radiation protection.

   A. _____

   B. _____

   C. _____

44. True/False: The selection of kV and mAs factors are as critical for digital imaging as for film-based systems.

45. True/False: If the sensitivity number is outside of the established exposure index for that procedure, the exposure must be repeated.

This series of self-tests should be taken only after completing all of the readings, review exercises, and laboratory activities for a particular section. This self-test is divided into four sections. The purpose of this test is not only to provide a good learning exercise but also to serve as a strong indicator of what your final evaluation exam will cover. It is strongly suggested that if you do not get at least a 90% to 95% grade on each self-test that you review those areas in which you missed questions before going to your instructor for the final evaluation exam.

SELF-TEST A: Image Quality in Film-Screen Imaging

1. Which one of the following is not one of the four primary image quality factors?
   - A. Density
   - B. Contrast
   - C. Kilovoltage (kV)
   - D. Detail
   - E. Distortion

2. The amount of blackness on a processed radiograph is called:
   - A. Density
   - B. Milliampere seconds (mAs)
   - C. Contrast
   - D. Penumbra

3. Which of the following exposure factors primarily controls radiographic density?
   - A. kV
   - B. mAs
   - C. Focal spot size
   - D. Source image receptor distance (SID)

4. True/False: For an underexposed radiograph, the mAs must be increased by a factor of four to produce a visible change in radiographic density.

5. **Situation:** A radiograph of the knee reveals that it is overexposed and must be repeated. The original technique used 10 mAs. Which one of the following changes will improve the image during the repeat exposure?
   - A. Increase to 15 mAs
   - B. Decrease to 5 mAs
   - C. Increase to 20 mAs
   - D. Decrease to 2 mAs

6. The primary controlling factor for radiographic contrast is:
   - A. mAs
   - B. kV
   - C. Focal spot size
   - D. SID

7. **Situation:** Chest radiography requires long-scale contrast. Which set of exposure factors will produce this?
   - A. 50 kV, 20 mAs
   - B. 65 kV, 15 mAs
   - C. 110 kV, 2 mAs
   - D. 80 kV, 5 mAs

8. Which one of the following sets of exposure factors will produce the highest radiographic contrast?
   - A. 60 kV, 30 mAs
   - B. 80 kV, 20 mAs
   - C. 96 kV, 5 mAs
   - D. 120 kV, 2 mAs

9. True/False: Kilovoltage is a secondary controlling factor for radiographic density.

10. True/False: A low kilovoltage technique (50 kV) produces a long-scale contrast image.

11. **Situation:** A radiograph of the elbow reveals that it is overexposed. The technologist wants to adjust kV rather than mAs for the repeat exposure. This is contrary to common practice. The original exposure factors were 70 kV and 5 mAs. Which one of the following kV settings would reduce radiographic density by one-half?

   A. 80 kV and 5 mAs   C. 60 kV and 5 mAs

   B. 66 kV and 5 mAs   D. 56 kV and 5 mAs

12. Which one of the following techniques or devices will reduce the amount of scatter radiation striking the IR?

   A. Collimation   C. Grids

   B. Lower kV   D. All of the above

13. True/False: Recorded detail or image resolution is optimal with a long object image receptor distance (OID) and a short SID.

14. Which one of the following factors best controls involuntary cardiac motion artifact?

   A. Careful instructions given to the patient

   B. High kV technique

   C. Practicing with patient when to hold breath

   D. Shortening the exposure time

15. **Situation:** The technologist is asked to produce a high-quality image of the carpal (wrist) bones. The emergency room physician suspects that the patient has a very small fracture of one of the bones. Which one of following sets of technical factors will produce an image with the highest degree of radiographic resolution?

   A. 1.0-mm focal spot and 30-inch SID

   B. 2.0-mm focal spot and 36-inch SID

   C. 0.5-mm focal spot and 40-inch SID

   D. 0.3-mm focal spot and 40-inch SID

16. Rather than rely on the anode heel effect, what can be used to equalize density of specific anatomy?

   A. Inherent filtration   C. Added filtration

   B. Compensating filter   D. A diaphragm

17. Which type of compensating filter is recommended for an AP projection of the shoulder?

   A. Wedge   C. Trough

   B. Boomerang   D. Beveled

18. Which type of compensation filter is recommended for an axiolateral hip projection?

   A. Wedge   C. Trough

   B. Boomerang   D. Beveled

19. Which type of grid cut-off is created if the CR and the face of the grid are not perpendicular to each other?

   A. Off-level   C. Upside down grid

   B. Off-center   D. Off-focus

20. Which one of the following projections requires the use of a grid?

   A. PA hand   C. AP abdomen

   B. Axial calcaneus (heel)   D. AP elbow

21. The misrepresentation of an object's size or shape projected on a radiograph is called:

   A. Magnification   C. Unsharpness

   B. Blurring   D. Distortion

22. Which one of the following sets of factors minimizes radiographic distortion to the greatest degree?
    A. 40-inch SID and 8-inch OID
    B. 44-inch SID and 6-inch OID
    C. 72-inch SID and 3-inch OID
    D. 60-inch SID and 4-inch OID

23. True/False: To best use the anode heel effect, the thinner aspect of the anatomic part should be placed under the cathode aspect of the x-ray tube.

24. The best method to reduce distortion of the joints of the hand is to keep the fingers _____ to the IR.
    A. Perpendicular   C. at a 30° angle
    B. Parallel   D. Vertical

25. Which one of the following factors impacts image resolution to the greatest degree?
    A. Use of a grid   C. Focal spot size
    B. kV   D. mAs

SELF-TEST B: Image Quality in Digital Radiography

1. Each digital image is formed by two dimensional elements termed:
   A. Pixels   C. Voxels
   B. Matrix   D. Bytes

2. Highly complex mathematical formulas used in creating the digital image are termed:
   A. Digital reconstructions   C. Digital displays
   B. Bit processing matrices   D. Algorithms

3. True/False: Changes in kV have little impact on patient dose with digital imaging.

4. True/False: kV and mAs do not have the same direct effect on image quality with digital imaging as they do with IR-screen imaging.

5. True/False: A wide exposure latitude associated with digital imaging systems will lead to less repeat exposures.

6. The intensity of light that represents the individual pixels in the image on the monitor is termed:
   A. Latitude   C. Contrast
   B. Brightness   D. Resolution

7. The primary controlling factor of contrast in the digital image is:
   A. kV   C. Processing algorithms
   B. mAs   D. Use of a grid

8. The greater the bit depth of a digital system, the greater the:
   A. Contrast resolution   C. Resolution
   B. Brightness   D. Noise

9. Which one of the following terms describes the minimum pixel size that can be displayed by a monitor?
   A. Acquisition pixel size   C. Monitor latent pixel size
   B. Display pixel size   D. Reconstructed pixel size

10. True/False: OID and SID have little impact on resolution of the digital image.

11. True/False: The current range of resolution for digital general radiographic imaging is between approximately 100 to 200 microns (2.5 to 5 line pairs per mm).

12. A numeric value that is representative of the exposure the image receptor received is termed:
    A. Algorithm
    B. Noise
    C. Spatial resolution
    D. Exposure index

13. Random disturbance that obscures or reduces clarity is the definition for:
    A. Noise
    B. Signal
    C. Digital fluctuation
    D. Signal variation

14. True/False: If an acceptable exposure index range is between 2.0 and 2.4, an exposure index of 4.0 would indicate overexposure of the image.

15. True/False: A high SNR results when insufficient mAs is used in creating a digital image.

16. Which one of the following factors will result in an increase in noise?
    A. Excessive mAs
    B. Scatter radiation
    C. Excessive kV
    D. Decrease in pixel size

17. Changing or enhancing the electronic image to improve its diagnostic quality describes:
    A. Noise reduction
    B. Smoothing
    C. Post-processing
    D. Edge enhancement

18. _____ adjusts brightness values of adjacent pixels closer together.
    A. Smoothing
    B. Edge enhancement
    C. Brightness gain
    D. Magnification

19. Window width controls the _____ of the digital image.
    A. Edge enhancement
    B. Contrast
    C. Smoothing
    D. Brightness

20. True/False: Post-processing can correct for a low-SNR image.

SELF-TEST C: Applications of Digital Technology

1. Which one of the following statements is true in regard to computed radiography?
   A. CR provides a wide exposure latitude
   B. AEC can not be used with CR
   C. Collimation should not be used
   D. A longer SID must be used with CR over film-screen systems

2. Which one of the following processes is used to erase the CR imaging plate following exposure?
   A. Ultraviolet light
   B. Low-level x-rays
   C. Bright light
   D. Laser

3. Patient information may be linked to the image on the CR imaging plate by:
   A. Light source
   B. Laser
   C. X-ray source
   D. Bar code reader

4. The CR imaging plate is composed of:
   A. Calcium tungstate phosphor
   B. Zinc cadmium sulfate phosphor
   C. Silicon phosphor
   D. Photostimulable phosphor

5. The latent image recorded on the CR image plate is read by a(n):
   A. Laser
   B. Bright light source
   C. Microwave source
   D. Ultraviolet light source

6. True/False: Close collimation must be avoided when acquiring an image on a CR IP.

7. A minimum of _____ % of the CR imaging plate must be exposed to produce an accurate exposure index.
   A. 10
   B. 20
   C. 30
   D. 50

8. True /False: Grids must not be used with a CR system.

9. True/False: Grids are often used for extremity exams when using DR.

10. True/False: DR requires less exposure as compared with CR and film-screen systems.

11. True/False: Close collimation should be avoided when using DR.

12. True/False: DR produces less dose for most procedures as compared with CR.

13. True/False: PACS is a digital network that permits viewing and storage of both digital and film-screen produced images.

14. The acronym RIS stands for:
    A. Rapid imaging system
    B. Radiology imaging system
    C. Radiology information system
    D. Reusable imaging system

15. The acronym DICOM refers to:
    A. A set of standards to ensure communication among digital imaging systems
    B. A new direct digital "flat plate" receptor system
    C. A digital image transmission system
    D. A new-generation CR system

16. A digital transmission system for transferring radiographic images to remote locations by telephone, by satellite, or by the Web is:
    A. PACS
    B. Direct DR
    C. HIS
    D. Teleradiology

17. _____ is the unsharp edges of the projected image.
    A. Noise
    B. Penumbra
    C. Mottle
    D. Electronic noise

18. A series of "boxes" that give form to the image is the definition for:
    A. Pixels
    B. Voxels
    C. Display matrices
    D. Acquisition matrices

19. A 30 × 35 cm IR is equivalent to a:
    A. 14 × 17 in IR
    B. 11 × 14 in IR
    C. 8 × 10 in IR
    D. 10 × 12 in IR

20. A post-processing technique that adjusts brightness values of adjacent pixels closer together is the definition for:
    A. Windowing
    B. Edge enhancement
    C. Window width
    D. Smoothing

SELF-TEST D: RADIATION PROTECTION

1. What is the SI unit of radiation measurement for absorbed dose?
   A. Seivert
   B. Gray
   C. Coulombs per kilogram of air
   D. Roentgen

2. What traditional unit measures radiation exposure in air?
   A. Seivert
   B. Gray
   C. Coulombs per kilogram of air
   D. Roentgen

3. What is the annual whole body effective dose (ED) for a technologist?
   A. 10 rem, or 100 mSv
   B. 0.1 rem, or 1 mSv
   C. 1 rem, or 10 mSv
   D. 5 rem, or 50 mSv

4. What is the cumulative lifetime ED for a 25-year-old technologist?
   A. 250 mSv
   B. 25 mSv
   C. 500 mSv
   D. 2500 mSv

5. What is the annual ED limit for an individual younger than 18 years of age?
   A. 5 rem, or 50 mSv
   B. 0.1 rem, or 1 mSv
   C. 1 rem, or 1 mSv
   D. 10 rem, or 100 mSv

6. The federal set maximum limit on exposure rates for intensified fluoroscopy units is:
   A. 3 to 4 R/min
   B. 0.5 R/min
   C. 1 R/min
   D. 10 R/min

7. For most modern equipment, the average fluoroscopy rate is:
   A. 10 R/min
   B. 5 to 8 R/min
   C. 3 to 4 R/min
   D. 15 to 20 R/min

8. What is the primary purpose of x-ray tube filtration?
   A. Absorb lower energy x-rays
   B. Harden the x-ray beam
   C. Increase penetrability of the x-ray beam
   D. All of the above

9. Which of the following results in the highest ED for females (assuming no specific area shields are used)?
   A. Anteroposterior (AP) thoracic spine (7- × 17-inch collimation)
   B. AP thoracic spine (14- × 17-inch collimation)
   C. AP hip (10- × 12-inch collimation)
   D. AP chest (14- × 17-inch collimation)

10. The use of a gonadal shield reduces the gonadal dose by _____ if the gonads are within the primary x-ray field.
   A. 20% to 30%   C. 50% to 90%
   B. 40% to 50%   D. 100%

11. Which type of shield is ideal when the affected tissue is part of a sterile field?
   A. Contact shield   C. Shadow shield
   B. Lead masking   D. Gonadal shaped shield

12. True/False: Low kV and high mAs techniques greatly reduce patient dose compared with high kV and low mAs techniques.

13. True/False: The total ED for females on an AP chest projection is more than double that for a PA chest.

14. True/False: The use of a positive beam limiting (PBL) collimator is no longer required by the FDA for new x-ray equipment manufactured after 1994.

15. True/False: Collimators must be accurate within 5% of the selected SID.

16. Which one of the following is not one of the cardinal principles of radiation protection?
   A. Distance   C. Time
   B. Shielding   D. Collimation

17. Which one of the following changes will best reduce patient dose?
   A. Decrease kV and increase mAs   C. Increase kV and lower mAs
   B. Using a grid   D. Increase mAs and lower kV

18. Where is the safest place for the technologist to stand during a fluoroscopic procedure?
   A. Head end of table
   B. Foot end of table
   C. On floor behind the fluoroscopic tower
   D. Behind radiologist

19. Which one of the following protection devices must be employed during a fluoroscopic procedure?
   A. Bucky slot shield   C. Compensating filter
   B. Lead gloves   D. Restraining devices

20. The ED for a pregnant technologist per month is:
   A. 0.1 rem (1 mSv)   C. 500 mrem (5 mSv)
   B. 0.05 rem (0.5 mSv)   D. 5 rem (50 mSv)

21. True/False: A second personnel dosimeter is required and must be worn by a pregnant technologist.

22. True/False: All radiology staff must wear a personnel dosimeter even if not involved with patient care directly.

23. True/False: The ICRP and ACR has determined that the "10-day rule" is obsolete for procedures of the abdomen and pelvis.

24. Which one of the following statement is false in regard to digital imaging?

   A. The use of higher kV and lower mAs is recommended

   B. A longer SID is encouraged with CR and DR procedures

   C. All radiographs must be within the exposure index

   D. ALARA does not apply to digital imaging

25. True/False: Using a different algorithm to process an overexposed CR image is an acceptable practice.

3 Chest

CHAPTER OBJECTIVES

After you have successfully completed the activities in this chapter, you will be able to:

_____ 1. List the parts of the bony thorax.

_____ 2. List specific topographic positioning landmarks of the chest.

_____ 3. Identify the parts and function of specific structures of the respiratory system.

_____ 4. List the four organs of the mediastinum.

_____ 5. Identify specific structures of the chest on line drawings.

_____ 6. Identify specific structures of the chest on posteroanterior (PA) and lateral radiographs.

_____ 7. Identify specific structures of the chest on a computed tomography (CT), transverse image.

_____ 8. Describe the methods to ensure proper degree of inspiration during chest radiography.

_____ 9. Describe the importance of using close collimation, gonadal shielding, and anatomic side markers during chest radiography.

_____ 10. Identify the correct exposure factors to be used during chest radiography.

_____ 11. Identify alterations in positioning routine and exposure factors specific to pediatric and geriatric patients.

_____ 12. List three reasons for taking chest radiographs with the patient in the erect position whenever possible.

_____ 13. Describe the three important positioning criteria that must be present on chest radiographs using erect PA and lateral positions.

_____ 14. Describe the advantages of the central ray placement method compared with the traditional method of centering for the PA and lateral chest positions.

_____ 15. Identify advantages and disadvantages in using CT, sonography, nuclear medicine, and magnetic resonance imaging (MRI) to demonstrate specific types of pathologic conditions in the chest.

_____ 16. Match various types of pathologic chest conditions to their correct definition.

_____ 17. For specific forms of pathologic chest conditions, indicate whether manual exposure factors need to be increased, decreased, or remain the same.

_____ 18. List the correct central ray placement, part position, and criteria for specific chest positions.

_____ 19. List the patient dose ranges for skin, midline, thyroid, and breast for specific projections of the chest and upper airway.

_____ 20. Given a hypothetical situation, identify the correct modifications of position, exposure factors, or both to improve the radiographic image.

_____ 21. Given a hypothetical situation, identify the correct position for a radiograph of specific pathologic conditions.

POSITIONING AND RADIOGRAPHIC CRITIQUE

_____ 1. Using a peer, position the patient for posteroanterior (PA), anteroposterior (AP), and lateral chest projections.

_____ 2. Using a chest phantom, use routine PA and lateral chest positions to produce satisfactory radiographs (if equipment is available).

_____ 3. Determine whether rotation is present on PA and lateral chest radiographs.

_____ 4. Critique and evaluate chest radiographs based on the four divisions of radiographic criteria: (1) structures shown, (2) position, (3) collimation and central ray, and (4) exposure criteria.

_____ 5. Distinguish between acceptable and unacceptable chest radiographs based on exposure factors, motion, collimation, positioning, or other errors.

LEARNING EXERCISES

Complete the following review exercises after reading the associated pages in Chapter 3 of the textbook as indicated by each exercise. Answers to each review exercise are given at the end of the review exercises and laboratory activities.

PART I: RADIOGRAPHIC ANATOMY
Review Exercise A: Radiographic Anatomy of the Chest (see textbook pp. 70-77)

1. The bony thorax consists of (A) the single _____ anteriorly, (B) two _____,

   (C) two _____, (D) twelve pairs of _____, and (E) twelve _____

   posteriorly.

2. The two important bony landmarks of the thorax that are used for locating the central ray on a posteroanterior

   (PA) and anteroposterior (AP) chest projection are the (A) _____ and

   (B) _____, respectively.

3. The four divisions of the respiratory system are:

   A. _____   C. _____

   B. _____   D. _____

4. Identify correct anatomic terms for the following structures.

   A. Adam's apple _____   D. Shoulder blade _____

   B. Voice box _____   E. Collar bone _____

   C. Breastbone _____

5. List the three divisions of the structure located proximally to the larynx that serve as a common passageway for both food and air.

   A. _____   C. _____

   B. _____

6. What is the name of the structure that acts as a lid over the larynx to prevent foreign objects such as food particles

   from entering the respiratory system? _____

7. The trachea is located _____ (anteriorly or posteriorly) to the esophagus.

8. The _____ bone is seen in the anterior portion of the neck and is found just below the tongue or floor of the mouth.

9. If a person accidentally inhales a food particle, which bronchus is it most likely to enter, and why?

   A. The _____ bronchus

   B. Why? _____

10. A. What is the name of the prominence, or ridge, seen when looking down into the bronchus where it divides

   into the right and left bronchi? _____

   B. This prominence, or ridge, is approximately at the level of the _____ vertebra.

11. What is the term for the small air sacs located at the distal ends of the bronchioles, in which oxygen and carbon

   dioxide are exchanged in the blood? _____

12. A. The delicate, double-walled sac or membrane containing the the lungs is called the _____.

   B. The outer layer of this membrane adhering to the inner surface of the chest wall and diaphragm is the

   _____.

   C. The inner layer adhering to the surface of the lungs is the _____ or

   _____.

   D. The potential space between these two layers (identified in B and C) is called the _____.

   E. Air or gas that enters the space identified in D results in a condition called _____.

13. Fill in the correct terms for the following portions of the lungs.

   A. Lower, concave portion: _____

   B. Central area in which bronchi and blood vessels enter the lungs: _____

   C. Upper, rounded portion above the level of the clavicles: _____

   D. Extreme, outermost lower corner of the lungs: _____

14. Explain why the right lung is smaller than the left lung and the right hemidiaphragm is positioned higher than the

   left hemidiaphragm. _____

15. List the four important structures located in the mediastinum.

   A. _____   C. _____

   B. _____   D. _____

16. Identify the following structures in Fig. 3-1.

   A. _____
      gland

   B. _____

   C. _____

   D. _____

   E. _____

   F. _____
      gland

   G. _____

   H. _____

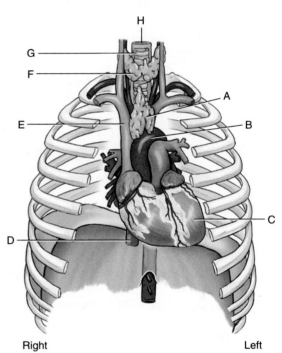

Right   Left

Fig. 3-1. Structures within the mediastinum.

17. The heart is enclosed in a double-walled membrane called the _____.

18. The three parts of the aorta are the _____, _____, and _____.

19. Identify the following labeled structures as seen on PA and lateral chest radiographs in Figs. 3-2 and 3-3.

A. _____

B. _____

C. _____

D. _____

E. _____

F. _____

G. _____

H. _____

I. _____

J. _____

K. _____

L. _____

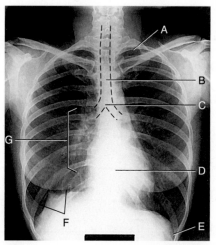

Fig. 3-2. Posteroanterior (PA) chest radiograph.

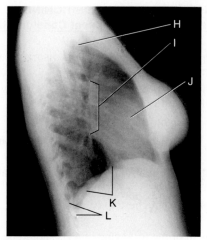

Fig. 3-3. Lateral chest radiograph.

20. Identify the labeled parts on this computed tomography (CT) image (Fig. 3-4) of a transverse section of the thorax at the level of T5, the fifth thoracic vertebra, which is also the level of the carina. (HINT: B, G, and H are major blood vessels.)

A. _____

B. _____

C. _____

D. _____

E. _____

F. _____

G. _____

H. _____

I. _____

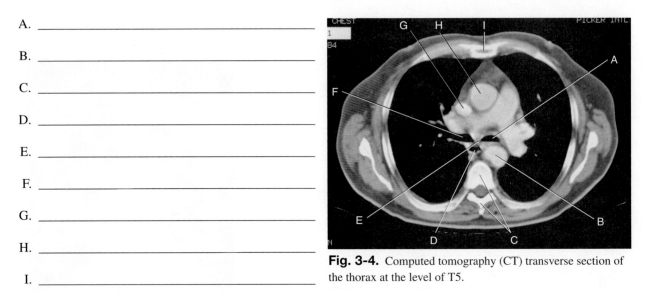

Fig. 3-4. Computed tomography (CT) transverse section of the thorax at the level of T5.

PART II: RADIOGRAPHIC POSITIONING
Review Exercise B: Technical Considerations (see textbook pp. 78-85)

1. Which type of body habitus is associated with a broad and deep thorax? _____

2. Which one of the following types of body habitus may cause the costophrenic angles to be cut off if careful vertical collimation is not used?
   A. Hypersthenic   C. Sthenic
   B. Hyposthenic   D. Hyposthenic and asthenic

3. What is the minimum number of ribs that should be demonstrated above the diaphragm on a PA radiograph of an

   average adult chest with full inspiration? _____

4. Which of the following objects should be removed (or moved) before chest radiography? (Choose all that apply.)
   A. Necklace   D. Dentures   F. Hair fasteners
   B. Bra   E. Pants   G. Oxygen lines
   C. Religious medallion around neck

5. True/False: Chest radiography is the most commonly repeated radiographic procedure because of poor positioning or exposure factor selection errors.

6. True/False: Generally, you do not need to use radiographic grids for adult patients for PA or lateral chest radiographs.

7. Chest radiography for the adult patient usually employs a kilovoltage peak of _____ to

   _____ kV.

8. Optimal technical factor selection ensures proper penetration of the:
    A. Heart
    B. Great vessels
    C. Lung regions
    D. Hilar region
    E. All of the above

9. Describe the way optimum density of the lungs and mediastinal structures can be determined on a PA chest

   radiograph _____.

10. True/False: Because the heart is always located in the left thorax, the use of anatomic side markers on a PA chest projection may not be necessary.

11. Which one of the following devices should be used for the erect PA and lateral chest projections for an infant?
    A. Upright chest device
    B. Supine table Bucky
    C. Pigg-O-Stat
    D. Plexiglas restraint board

12. Which one of the following sets of exposure factors is recommended for a chest examination of a young pediatric patient?
    A. 60 to 70 kV, short exposure time
    B. 90 to 100 kV, medium exposure time
    C. 100 to 120 kV, short exposure time
    D. 120 to 150 kV, long exposure time

13. True/False: Because they have shallower (superior-inferior dimension) lung fields, the central ray is often centered higher for geriatric patients.

14. To ensure better lung inspiration during chest radiography, exposure should be made during the

   _____ inspiration.

15. List four possible pathologic conditions that would suggest the need for both inspiration and expiration PA chest radiographs (five were given in the textbook).

    A. _____   C. _____

    B. _____   D. _____

16. List and explain briefly the three reasons that chest radiographs should be taken with the patient in the erect position (when the patient's condition permits).

    A. _____   C. _____

    B. _____

17. Explain the primary purpose and benefit of performing chest radiography using a 72-inch source image-receptor

   distance (SID). _____

18. Why do the lungs tend to expand more with the patient in an erect position than in a supine position?

   _____

19. What is a common radiographic sign seen on a chest radiograph for a patient with respiratory distress syndrome (RDS)?
    A. Enlargement of heart   C. Elevated diaphragms
    B. Fluid in apices   D. Air bronchogram

20. Which one of the following anatomic structures is examined to determine rotation on a PA chest radiograph?
    A. Appearance of ribs   C. Symmetric appearance of sternoclavicular joints
    B. Shape of heart   D. Symmetric appearance of costophrenic angles

21. Which positioning tip will help you prevent the patient's chin from being superimposed over the upper airway and apices of the lungs for a PA chest radiograph?

    _____

    _____

22. For patients with the following clinical histories, which lateral position would you perform—right or left?

    A. Patient with severe pains in left side of chest _____

    B. Patient with no chest pain but recent history of pneumonia in right lung _____

    C. Patient with no chest pain or history of heart trouble _____

23. Why is it important to raise the patient's arms above the head for lateral chest projections?

    _____

    _____

24. The traditional central ray centering technique for the chest is to place the top of the image receptor (cassette)

    _____ inches (_____ cm) above the shoulders.

25. A recommended central ray centering technique for a PA chest projection requires the technologist to palpate

    the _____ and measure down from that bony landmark _____ inches (_____ cm) for a male

    and _____ inches (_____ cm) for a female patient.

26. A. Should the 14- × 17-inch (35- × 43-cm) image receptor be aligned lengthwise or crosswise for a PA chest

    projection of a hypersthenic patient? _____

    B. For a hyposthenic patient? _____

27. True/False: With most digital chest units, the question of IR placement into either vertical or crosswise positions is eliminated because of the larger IR.

28. Which one of the following bony landmarks is palpated for centering of the AP chest position?
    A. Vertebra prominens   C. Thyroid cartilage
    B. Jugular notch   D. Sternal angle

29. True/False: In general, for an average patient more collimation should be visible on the lower margin of the chest image than on the top for a PA or lateral chest projection.

30. True/False: For most patients, the central ray level for a PA chest projection is near the inferior angle of the scapula.

31. True/False: The height, or vertical dimension, of the average-to-large person's chest is greater than the width, or horizontal dimension.

32. True/False: Single-photon emission computed tomography (SPECT) is frequently used to diagnose myocardial infarction.

33. True/False: Ultrasound is not an effective modality to detect pleural effusion.

34. True/False: Echocardiography and electrocardiography are basically the same procedure.

35. Match each of the following descriptions of pathologic indicators to its correct term.

_____ 1. One of the most common inherited diseases	A. Atelectasis
_____ 2. Condition most frequently associated with congestive heart failure	B. Bronchiectasis
	C. Bronchitis
_____ 3. Coughing up blood	
	D. Chronic obstructive pulmonary disease (COPD)
_____ 4. Accumulation of air in pleural cavity	
	E. Hemoptysis
_____ 5. Accumulation of pus in pleural cavity	
	F. Cystic fibrosis
_____ 6. A form of occupational lung disease	
	G. Empyema
_____ 7. A contagious disease caused by an airborne bacterium	
	H. Pleurisy
_____ 8. Irreversible dilation of bronchioles	I. Pneumothorax
_____ 9. Most common form is emphysema	J. Pulmonary edema
_____ 10. Acute or chronic irritation of bronchi	K. Tuberculosis
_____ 11. Collapse of all or portion of lung	L. Silicosis
_____ 12. Inflammation of pleura	

36. For the following types of pathologic conditions, indicate whether manual exposure factors would be increased (+), decreased (−), or generally remain the same (0) as compared with standard chest exposure factors.

_____ Left lung atelectasis

_____ Lung neoplasm

_____ Severe pulmonary edema

_____ Respiratory distress syndrome (RDS) or adult respiratory distress syndrome (ARDS), known as hyaline membrane disease (HMD) in infants

_____ Secondary tuberculosis

_____ Advanced emphysema

_____ Large pneumothorax

_____ Pulmonary emboli

_____ Primary tuberculosis

_____ Advanced asbestosis

37. Which one of the following is not a form of occupational lung disease?
   A. Anthracosis
   B. Myocosis
   C. Silicosis
   D. Asbestosis

38. Which one of the following chest projections is recommended to detect calcifications or cavitations within the upper lung region near the clavicles?
   A. Left lateral decubitus
   B. PA
   C. RPO and LPO
   D. AP lordotic

Review Exercise C: Positioning of the Chest (see textbook pp. 90-100)

1. Why is a PA chest preferred to an AP projection? _____

2. The CR is placed at the level of the _____ vertebra for a PA chest projection.

3. The shoulders need to be rolled forward for the PA projection to allow the _____ to move laterally and to be clear of the lung fields.

4. When the automatic exposure control system (AEC) is being used for the PA projection, which ionization chambers should be activated?
   A. Left chamber
   B. Center chamber
   C. Right chamber
   D. Left and right chambers

5. What is the midline dose range for a PA projection of the chest for an average-size female?
   A. 10 to 100 mrad
   B. Greater than 100 mrad
   C. Less than 10 mrad
   D. 0.5 to 1 rad

6. True/False: The average breast dose and thyroid dose for a PA chest projection are approximately the same.

7. The average female breast dose on an AP chest projection is approximately _____ times that for a PA chest dose.

   A. 1.5   B. 4   C. 10   D. 30

8. How much separation of the posterior ribs on a lateral chest projection indicates excessive rotation from a true lateral position? _____ (NOTE: Less separation than this is caused by the divergent x-rays.)

9. To prevent the clavicles from obscuring the apices on an AP projection of the chest, the central ray should be angled (A) _____ (caudad or cephalad) so that it is perpendicular to the (B) _____ .

10. What is the name of the condition characterized by fluid entering the pleural cavity? _____

11. Which specific position would be used if a patient were unable to stand but the physician suspected the patient had fluid in the left lung? _____

12. What is the name of the condition characterized by free air entering the pleural cavity?

   _____

13. Which specific position would be used if the patient were unable to stand but the physician suspected the patient had free air in the left pleural cavity? _____

14. What circumstances or clinical indications suggest that an AP lordotic projection should be ordered?

   _____

15. What position/projection would be used for a patient who is too ill or weak to stand for an AP lordotic projection?

   _____

16. A. Which anterior oblique position would best demonstrate the left lung—right anterior oblique (RAO) or left anterior oblique (LAO)? _____

   B. Which posterior oblique position would best demonstrate the left lung—RPO or LPO?

   _____

17. For certain studies of the heart, the _____ (right or left) anterior oblique requires a rotation of _____ °.

18. Which AEC ionization chamber(s) should be activated for an LAO chest projection? _____

19. Where is the central ray placed for a lateral projection of the upper airway? _____

20. Which one of the following tissues receives the greatest dose during an AP projection of the upper airway?

A. Thyroid   C. Midline structures

B. Breast   D. Gonads

Review Exercise D: Problem Solving for Technical and Positioning Errors

The following radiographic problems involve technical and positioning errors that lead to substandard images. Other questions involve situations pertaining to various conditions and pathologic findings. As you analyze these problems and situations, use your textbook to help you find solutions to these questions.

1. A radiograph of a PA view of the chest reveals that the sternoclavicular (SC) joints are not the same distance from the spine. The right SC joint is closer to the midline than is the left SC joint. What is the positioning error?

   _____

2. A radiograph of a PA projection of the chest shows only seven posterior ribs above the diaphragm. What caused this

   problem, and how could it be prevented on the repeat exposures? _____

   _____

3. A radiograph of a PA and left lateral projection of the chest reveals that the mediastinum of the chest is underpenetrated. The technologist used the following factors for the radiograph: a 72-inch SID, an upright Bucky, a full-inspiration exposure, 75 kV and 600 mA, and a $\frac{1}{60}$-second exposure time.

   A. Which one of these factors is the most likely cause of the problem? Briefly explain.

   _____

   B. How can the technologist improve the image when making the repeat exposure? _____

4. A radiograph of a PA projection of the chest reveals that the top of the apices are cut off and a wide collimation border can be seen below the diaphragm. In what way can this be corrected during the repeat radiograph?

   _____

5. **Situation:** A patient with a clinical history of advanced emphysema comes to the radiology department for a chest x-ray. AEC will not be used. How should the technologist alter the manual exposure settings for this patient?

   A. Do not alter them. Use the standard exposure factors.

   B. Decrease the kV moderately (– –).

   C. Increase the kV slightly (+).

   D. Increase the kV moderately (++).

6. **Situation:** A patient with severe pleural effusion comes to the radiology department for a chest x-ray. AEC will not be used. How should the technologist alter the manual exposure settings for this patient?

   A. Do not alter them. Use the standard exposure factors.

   B. Decrease the kV moderately (– –).

   C. Increase the kV slightly (+).

   D. Increase the kV moderately (++).

7. **Situation:** A patient comes to the radiology department for a presurgical chest examination. The clinical history indicates a possible situs inversus of the thorax (transposition of structures within the thorax). Which positioning step or action must be taken to perform a successful chest examination?

_____

8. A radiograph of a lateral projection of the chest reveals that the posterior ribs and costophrenic angles are separated more than ½ inch, or 1 cm, indicating excessive rotation. Describe a possible method of determining the direction of

   rotation. _____

9. **Situation:** A patient enters the emergency room with a possible hemothorax in the right lung caused by a motor vehicle accident (MVA). The patient is unable to stand or sit erect. Which specific position would best diagnose this

   condition, and why? _____

   _____

10. **Situation:** A young child enters the emergency room with a possible foreign body in one of the bronchi of the lung. The foreign body, a peanut, cannot be seen on the PA and lateral projections of the chest projection. Which additional projection(s) could the technologist perform to locate the foreign body?

   _____

11. **Situation:** A routine chest study indicates a possible mass beneath a patient's right clavicle. The PA and lateral projections are inconclusive. What additional projection(s) could be taken to rule out this condition?

   _____

12. **Situation:** A patient has a possible small pneumothorax. Routine chest projections (PA and lateral) fail to reveal the pneumothorax conclusively. Which additional projections could be taken to rule out this condition?

   _____

13. **Situation:** A patient with a history of pleurisy comes to the radiology department. Which one of the following positioning routines should be used?
   A. Soft tissue lateral of the upper airway   C. Erect PA and lateral
   B. Right and left lateral decubitus   D. CT scan of the chest

14. **Situation:** A patient with a possible neoplasm in the right lung apex comes to the radiology department for a chest examination. The PA and lateral projections do not clearly demonstrate the neoplasm because of superimposition of the clavicle over the apex. The patient is unable to stand or sit erect. Which additional projection can be taken to clearly demonstrate the neoplasm and eliminate the superimposition of the clavicle and the left lung apex?

   _____

15. **Situation:** PA and left lateral projections demonstrate a suspicious region in the left lung. The radiologist orders an oblique that will best demonstrate or "elongate" the left lung. Which specific oblique projections will best elongate the left lung? (More than one oblique projection will accomplish this goal.)

   _____

PART III: LABORATORY ACTIVITIES

You must gain experience in chest positioning before performing the following exams on actual patients. You can get experience in positioning and radiographic evaluation of these projections by performing exercises using radiographic phantoms and practicing on other students (although not taking actual exposures).

The following suggested activities assume that your teaching institution has an energized lab and radiographic phantoms. If not, perform only Laboratory Exercise B, the physical positioning activities. (Check off each step and projection as you complete it.)

Laboratory Exercise A: Energized Laboratory

1. Using the chest radiographic phantom, produce radiographs using:

   _____ PA and AP projections _____ Lateral projection

2. Evaluate the radiographs you produced above, additional radiographs provided by your instructor, or both for the following criteria.

   _____ Rotation   _____ Anatomic side markers

   _____ Collimation   _____ Proper exposure factors

   _____ Part and central ray centering   _____ Motion

Laboratory Exercise B: Physical Positioning

1. On another person, simulate taking all of the following basic and special projections of the chest. Follow the suggested positioning steps and sequence as listed below and as described in Chapter 1 of your textbook:

   _____ PA chest   _____ AP supine or semisupine

   _____ Anterior and posterior obliques   _____ Lateral decubitus

   _____ Lateral chest   _____ AP lordotic

   _____ AP and lateral upper airway

Step 1. General Patient Positioning

_____ Select the size and number of cassettes needed.

_____ Prepare the radiographic room. Check that tube is centered to the center of the IR holder (or the centerline of the table for Bucky exams).

_____ Correctly identify the patient and bring the patient into the room.

_____ Explain to the patient what you will be doing.

_____ Assist the patient to the proper place and position for the first radiograph.

Step 2. Measuring Part Thickness

_____ Measure the body part being radiographed and set correct exposure factors (manual technique). (If using an AEC system, select the correct chamber cells on the control panel.)

Step 3. Part Positioning

_____ Align and center the body part to the central ray or vice versa for chest positioning with the chest board. (For Bucky exams on a table, move the patient and table top together as needed [with floating-type table top]). (NOTE: In cases in which the correct central ray position is of primary importance, the central ray icon is included in the textbook on the appropriate positioning page.)

Step 4. Image Receptor (IR) Centering

_____ After the part has been centered to the central ray, the IR (cassette) is also centered to the central ray. (NOTE: This step can be omitted on most chest units where the x-ray tube and IR unit are attached and move together.)

Additional Steps or Actions

_____ 1. Collimate accurately to include only the area of interest.

_____ 2. Place the correct side marker within the exposure field (so that you do not superimpose pertinent anatomic structures).

_____ 3. Restrain or provide support for the body part to prevent motion.

_____ 4. Use contact lead shielding as needed (e.g., gonadal, breast, thyroid).

_____ 5. Give clear breathing instructions and make the exposure while watching patient through window.

This self-test should be taken only after completing all of the readings, review exercises, and laboratory activities for a particular section. The purpose of this test is not only to provide a good learning exercise but also to serve as a strong indicator of what your final unit evaluation exam will cover. It is strongly suggested that if you do not get at least a 90% to 95% grade on each self-test that you review those areas in which you missed questions before going to your instructor for the final unit evaluation exam.

1. Match each of the following structures with its correct anatomic term.

   _____ 1. Breastbone   A. Clavicle

   _____ 2. Adam's apple   B. Larynx

   _____ 3. Shoulder blade   C. Thyroid cartilage

   _____ 4. Voice box   D. Scapula

   _____ 5. Collar bone   E. Sternum

2. The correct term for the seventh cervical vertebrae is:
   A. Xiphoid process   C. Axis
   B. Jugular notch   D. Vertebra prominens

3. A notch, or depression, located on the superior portion of the sternum is called the:
   A. Sternal notch   C. Jugular notch
   B. Xiphoid notch   D. Sternal angle

4. The trachea bifurcates and forms the:
   A. Right and left bronchi   C. Costophrenic angles
   B. Right and left hilum   D. Pulmonary arteries

5. A specific prominence, or ridge, found at the point where the internal distal trachea divides into the right and left bronchi is called the:
   A. Hilum   C. Epiglottis
   B. Carina   D. Alveoli

6. The area of each lung where the bronchi and blood vessels enter and leave is called the:
   A. Carina   C. Base
   B. Apex   D. Hilum

7. The structures within the lung where oxygen and carbon dioxide gas exchange occurs are called:
   A. Carina   C. Hilum
   B. Alveoli   D. Bronchi

8. Which of the following is *not* an aspect of the pleura?
   A. Parietal pleura   C. Pleural cavity
   B. Hilar pleura   D. Pulmonary pleura

9. The condition in which blood fills the potential space between the layers of pleura is called:
   A. Pneumothorax   C. Atelectasis
   B. Hemothorax   D. Empyema

10. The extreme, outermost lower corner of each lung is called the:
    A. Costophrenic angle   C. Base
    B. Apex   D. Hilar region

11. Which one of the following structures is *not* found in the mediastinum?
    A. Thymus gland   C. Epiglottis
    B. Heart and great vessels   D. Trachea

12. A narrow thorax that is shallow from the front to back but very long in the vertical dimension is characteristic of

    a(n) _____ body habitus.
    A. Hypersthenic   C. Hyposthenic
    B. Sthenic   D. Asthenic

13. Identify the best technique for chest radiography from the following choices.
    A. 85 kV, 300 mA, ⅟₃₀ second, 40-inch SID
    B. 110 kV, 100 mA, ⅟₁₀ second, 40-inch SID
    C. 120 kV, 600 mA, ⅟₆₀ second, 60-inch SID
    D. 125 kV, 600 mA, ⅟₆₀ second, 72-inch SID

14. Match the correct answers for the structures labeled on this midsagittal section of the pharynx and upper airway (Fig. 3-5).

    _____ A.   1. Laryngopharynx

    _____ B.   2. Uvula

    _____ C.   3. Epiglottis

    _____ D.   4. Esophagus

    _____ E.   5. Spinal cord

    _____ F.   6. Oral cavity

    _____ G.   7. Hyoid bone

    _____ H.   8. Nasopharynx

    _____ I.   9. Thyroid gland

    _____ J.   10. Oropharynx

    _____ K.   11. Larynx

    _____ L.   12. Hard palate

    _____ M.   13. Thyroid cartilage

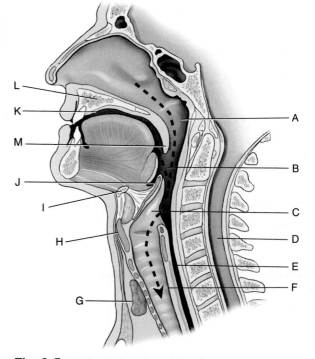

Fig. 3-5. Midsagittal section of the pharynx and upper airway.

15. Identify the structures labeled on this computed tomography (CT) axial section of the thorax at the level of T3 (the third thoracic vertebra) (Fig. 3-6).

A. _____

B. _____

C. _____

D. _____

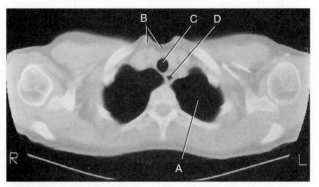

Fig. 3-6. Computed tomography (CT) axial section of the thorax at the level of T3.

16. Identify the structures on this CT axial section of the thorax at the approximate level of T4-T5, 1 cm proximal to carina (HINT: B, E, and F are major blood vessels) (Fig 3-7).

A. _____

B. _____

C. _____

D. _____

E. _____

F. _____

G. _____

H. _____

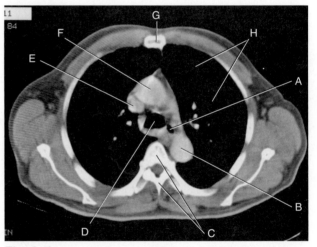

Fig. 3-7. Computed tomography (CT) axial section of the thorax at the approximate level of T4-T5.

17. What is the name of the special immobilization device used for pediatric chest studies?
   A. Pigg-O-Stat
   B. Restraining chair
   C. Chest immobilizer
   D. Franklin unit

18. Which one of the following exposure factors is recommended for a chest study of a young pediatric patient?
   A. 110 kV, short exposure time
   B. 90 kV, medium exposure time
   C. 65 kV, short exposure time
   D. 60 kV, long exposure time

19. Which of the following is *not* a valid reason to perform chest projections with the patient in the erect position?
    A. To reduce patient dose
    B. To demonstrate air and fluid levels
    C. To allow the diaphragm to move down farther
    D. To prevent hyperemia of pulmonary vessels

20. Why are the shoulders pressed downward and toward the IR for a posteroanterior (PA) projection of the chest?
    A. To remove scapulae from lung fields
    B. To prevent hyperemia of pulmonary vessels
    C. To allow the diaphragm to move down farther
    D. To reduce chest rotation

21. Why are the shoulders rolled forward for a PA projection of the chest?
    A. To remove scapulae from lung fields
    B. To prevent hyperemia of pulmonary vessels
    C. To allow the diaphragm to move down farther
    D. To reduce chest rotation

22. Where is the central ray placed for an anteroposterior (AP) supine projection of the chest?
    A. 7 to 8 inches (18 to 20 cm) below vertebra prominens
    B. 1 to 2 inches (2.5 to 5 cm) below jugular notch
    C. 3 to 4 inches (8 to 10 cm) below jugular notch
    D. 3 to 4 inches (8 to 10 cm) below thyroid cartilage

23. Which one of the following terms is defined as a "shortness of breath"?
    A. Dyspnea   C. Pleurisy
    B. Bronchiectasis   D. Atelectasis

24. A condition in which all or a portion of the lung is collapsed is:
    A. Atelectasis   C. Pneumothorax
    B. Pleural effusion D. Pneumoconiosis

25. A condition in which excess fluid builds in the lungs as a result of obstruction of the pulmonary circulation is termed:
    A. Pulmonary emboli C. Pulmonary edema
    B. Pneumothorax   D. Bronchopneumonia

26. A sudden blockage of an artery in the lung is called:
    A. Pleurisy   C. Adult respiratory distress syndrome (ARDS)
    B. Pulmonary emboli D. Chronic obstructive pulmonary disease (COPD)

27. Which one of the following is *not* a form of occupational lung disease?
    A. Asbestosis   C. Anthracosis
    B. Silicosis   D. Tuberculosis

28. Manual exposure factors for a patient with a large pneumothorax should:
    A. Be reduced   C. Be increased
    B. Remain the same   D. Change from automatic exposure control (AEC) to manual technique

29. A PA chest radiograph reveals that the left sternoclavicular joint is superimposed over the spine (in comparison with the right joint). What specific positioning error is involved?

 A. Poor inspiration

 B. Rotation into a right anterior oblique (RAO) position

 C. Rotation into a left anterior oblique (LAO) position

 D. Tilting of the chest toward the left

30. A PA chest radiograph shows 10 posterior ribs above the diaphragm.

 Is this an acceptable degree of inspiration ? _____ Yes _____ No

31. A PA and lateral chest radiographic study has been completed. The PA projection reveals that the right costophrenic angle was collimated off, but both angles are included on the lateral projection.

 Would you repeat the PA projection? _____ Yes _____ No

32. A lateral chest radiograph demonstrates that the soft tissue of the upper limbs is superimposed over the apices of the lungs. How can this situation be prevented?

 A. Deeper inspiration   C. Slight rotation to the patient's left

 B. Extend chin   D. Raise upper limbs higher

33. A lateral chest radiograph reveals that the posterior ribs and costophrenic angles are separated by approximately

 ½ inch (slightly less than 1 cm). Should the technologist repeat this projection? _____ Yes _____ No

34. **Situation:** A radiograph of an AP lordotic projection reveals that the clavicles are projected within the apices. The clinical instructor informs the student technologist that the study is unacceptable, but during the repeat exposure, the patient complains of being too unsteady to lean backward for another projection. What other options are available if the student wants to complete the study?

 A. Perform the PA lordotic projection   C. Perform both lateral decubitus projections

 B. Perform an AP semiaxial projection   D. Perform inspiration and expiration PA projections

35. **Situation:** An ambulatory patient with a clinical history of advanced emphysema enters the emergency room. The patient is having difficulty breathing and is receiving oxygen. The physician has ordered a PA and lateral chest study. Should the technologist alter the typical exposure factors for this patient?

 A. No. Use the standard exposure factors.

 B. Yes. Increase the exposure factors.

 C. Yes. Decrease the exposure factors.

 D. No. Increase the SID instead of changing the exposure factors.

36. **Situation:** A patient enters the ER with an injury to the chest. The ER physician suspects a pneumothorax may be present in the right lung. The patient is unable to stand or sit erect. Which specific position or projection can be performed to confirm the presence of the pneumothorax?

 A. Left lateral decubitus   C. Right lateral decubitus

 B. Inspiration and expiration PA   D. AP lordotic

37. **Situation:** A PA and lateral chest study reveals a suspicious mass located near the heart in the right lung. The radiologist would like a radiograph of the patient in an anterior oblique position to delineate the mass from the heart. Which position or projection should the technologist use to accomplish this objective?

 A. 45° LAO   C. 60° LAO

 B. 45° RAO   D. AP lordotic

38. **Situation:** A patient with a history of pulmonary edema comes to the radiology department and is unable to stand. The physician suspects fluid in the left lung. Which specific position should be used to confirm this diagnosis?

A. Right lateral decubitus   C. AP lordotic

B. AP semiaxial   D. Left lateral decubitus

39. For the following critique questions, refer to textbook p. 101 (Fig. C3-90) (PA chest).

A. Which positioning error(s) is(are) visible on this radiograph? (More than one answer may be selected.)

(a) All essential anatomic structures are not demonstrated.

(b) Central ray is incorrectly centered.

(c) Collimation is not evident.

(d) Exposure factors are incorrect.

(e) No anatomic side marker is visible.

(f) Rotation into the RAO position is evident. (The spine is shifted to the right.)

(g) Rotation into the LAO position is evident. (The spine is shifted to the left.)

(h) The chin is not elevated.

B. Which error(s) on this radiograph is(are) considered "repeatable"?

C. Which of the following modifications must be made during the repeat exposure? (More than one answer may be selected.)

(a) Increase closer collimation.

(b) Center CR correctly to T7.

(c) Decrease exposure factors.

(d) Increase exposure factors.

(e) Place anatomic side marker on IR before exposure.

(f) Correct for rotation of shoulders and hips.

(g) Place image receptor crosswise.

(h) Elevate chin higher.

40. For the following critique questions, refer to Fig. C3-92 in textbook. (Lateral chest)

A. What positioning error(s) is(are) seen on this radiograph? (More than one answer may be selected.)

(a) All essential anatomy is not demonstrated on the radiograph.

(b) CR centering is incorrect.

(c) Collimation is not evident.

(d) Exposure factors are incorrect.

(e) No anatomic side marker is seen on radiograph.

(f) Excessive rotation of the chest is demonstrated.

B. Which error(s) on this radiograph is(are) considered "repeatable"?

C. Which of the following modifications must be made during the repeat exposure? (More than one answer may be selected.)

(a) Center the central ray correctly—to T7.

(b) Decrease the exposure factors.

(c) Increase the exposure factors.

(d) Place an anatomic marker correctly on the IR before exposure.

(e) Ensure that the shoulders and hips are superimposed to eliminate rotation.

(f) Raise the upper limbs higher.

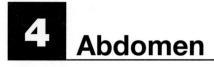

Abdomen

After you have successfully completed the activities in this chapter, you will be able to:

_____ 1. List the location of the three muscles of the abdomen that are important in abdominal radiography.

_____ 2. List the major organs and structures of the digestive and urinary systems.

_____ 3. Using drawings and radiographs, identify the principle structures of the digestive system, biliary system, urinary system, and accessory organs involved in digestion.

_____ 4. Identify whether select organs of the abdomen are intraperitoneal, retroperitoneal, or infraperitoneal.

_____ 5. Identify the correct quadrant or region of the abdomen where specific organs are located.

_____ 6. Identify specific bony topographic landmarks used for positioning of the abdomen.

_____ 7. Using drawings, radiographs, and computed tomography (CT) images, identify the major bony and soft tissue structures of the abdomen.

_____ 8. List specific types of pathologic findings that are clinical indications for an acute abdominal series.

_____ 9. List specific methods for controlling involuntary and voluntary motion during abdominal radiography.

_____ 10. Describe the factors that affect collimation and the use of gonadal shielding during abdominal radiography.

_____ 11. Identify the correct exposure factors to be used during abdominal radiography.

_____ 12. Identify alterations in positioning routine and exposure factors for pediatric and geriatric patients.

_____ 13. Identify the pathologic conditions and diseases of the abdomen that are best demonstrated with CT, sonography, nuclear medicine, and magnetic resonance imaging (MRI).

_____ 14. Match various types of abdominal pathologic findings to their correct definition.

_____ 15. Match specific types of abdominal pathologic findings to their correct radiographic appearance.

_____ 16. Describe variations in cassette and central ray placement that can be used to accommodate differences in body habitus.

_____ 17. List the dose ranges for skin, midline, and gonadal doses for the various projections of the abdomen on an average-size patient.

_____ 18. Identify the reason for the difference in female ovarian doses on an anteroposterior (AP) versus a posteroanterior (PA) abdomen projection with the same exposure factors.

_____ 19. List the correct central ray placement, part position, and radiographic criteria for specific abdomen positions.

_____ 20. List the pathologic indications for the acute abdominal series.

_____ 21. List the projections taken for the acute abdominal series and variations that can be used to accommodate specific patient conditions.

_____ 22. Given various hypothetical situations, identify the correct modification of position, exposure factors, or both to improve the radiographic image.

_____ 23. Given various hypothetical situations, identify the correct position for a specific pathologic feature or condition.

POSITIONING AND RADIOGRAPHIC CRITIQUE

_____ 1. Use another student as a model to practice putting a patient in supine, erect, and lateral decubitus abdominal positions.

_____ 2. Using an abdomen phantom, produce an AP projection of the abdomen that results in a satisfactory radiograph (if equipment is available).

_____ 3. Determine whether rotation, tilt, or both are present on a radiograph of an AP projection of the abdomen.

_____ 4. Critique and evaluate abdominal radiographs based on the four divisions of radiographic criteria: (1) structures shown, (2) position, (3) collimation and central ray, and (4) exposure criteria.

_____ 5. Distinguish between acceptable and unacceptable abdominal radiographs based on exposure factors, motion, collimation, positioning, or other errors.

_____ 6. Identify specific bony and soft tissue structures seen radiographically.

_____ 7. Discriminate among radiographs taken in supine, erect, or lateral decubitus positions.

LEARNING EXERCISES

Complete the following review exercises after reading the associated pages in Chapter 4 of the textbook as indicated by each exercise. Answers to each review exercise are given at the end of the review exercises.

PART I: RADIOGRAPHIC ANATOMY
Review Exercise A: Abdominopelvic Anatomy (see textbook pp. 104-111)

1. The two large muscles that are found in the posterior abdomen adjacent to the lumbar vertebra and are usually visible

   on an anteroposterior (AP) radiograph are called the _____.

2. The medical prefix for stomach is _____.

3. List the three parts of the small intestine.

   A. _____   B. _____   C. _____

4. Which portion of the small intestine is considered to be the longest? _____

5. The large intestine begins in the _____ quadrant with a saclike area called the

   _____.

6. The sigmoid colon is located between the _____ and _____ of the large intestine.

7. List the three accessory digestive organs.

   A. _____   B. _____   C. _____

8. Circle the correct term. The pancreas is located **anteriorly** or **posteriorly** to the stomach.

9. Which one of the following organs is *not* directly associated with the digestive system?
   A. Gallbladder   C. Jejunum
   B. Spleen   D. Pancreas

10. Which one of the following organs is considered to be part of the lymphatic system?
    A. Liver   C. Pancreas
    B. Spleen   D. Gallbladder

11. Why is the right kidney found in a more inferior position than the left kidney?

    _____

12. Which endocrine glands are superomedial to each kidney?

    _____

13. True/False: The correct term for the radiographic study of the urinary system is intravenous pyelogram (IVP).

14. The double-walled membrane lining the abdominopelvic cavity is called the _____.

15. The organs located posteriorly to, or behind, the serous membrane lining of the abdominopelvic cavity are referred

    to as _____.

16. Which one of the following structures helps stabilize and support the small intestine?
    A. Omentum   C. Viscera
    B. Peritoneum   D. Mesentery

17. Which one of the following structures is a double fold of peritoneum that connects the transverse colon to the greater curvature of the stomach?
    A. Mesocolon   C. Greater omentum
    B. Lesser omentum   D. Mesentery

18. Match the following structures to the correct location of the peritoneum.

_____ 1. Liver   A. Intraperitoneum

_____ 2. Urinary bladder   B. Retroperitoneum

_____ 3. Kidneys   C. Infraperitoneum

_____ 4. Spleen

_____ 5. Ovaries

_____ 6. Duodenum

_____ 7. Transverse colon

_____ 8. Testes

_____ 9. Adrenal glands

_____ 10. Stomach

_____ 11. Pancreas

_____ 12. Ascending and descending colon

19. For each of the following organs, identify the correct abdominal quadrant in which the organ is found—left upper quadrant (LUQ), left lower quadrant (LLQ), right lower quadrant (RLQ), or right upper quadrant (RUQ).

A. Liver _____

B. Spleen _____

C. Sigmoid colon _____

D. Left colic flexure _____

E. Stomach _____

F. Appendix _____

G. Two-thirds of jejunum _____

20. What is the correct name for the abdominal region found directly in the middle of the abdomen?
    A. Epigastric   C. Umbilical
    B. Inguinal   D. Pubic

21. Which one of the following abdominal regions contains the rectum?
    A. Pubic   D. Epigastric
    B. Inguinal   E. Hypochondriac
    C. Umbilical   F. Lumbar

22. Identify the bony landmarks in Fig. 4-1.

   A. _____

   B. _____

   C. _____

   D. _____

   E. _____

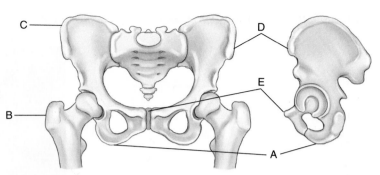

Fig. 4-1. Osteology of the pelvis.

23. The superior margin of the greater trochanter is about _____ inches (_____ cm) _____ (superior or inferior) to the

    level of the symphysis pubis, and the ischial tuberosity is about _____ inches (_____ cm) _____ (superior or inferior) to the superior aspect of the symphysis pubis.

24. Which topographic landmark corresponds to the inferior margin of the abdomen and is formed by the anterior

    junction of the two pelvic bones? _____

25. Which topographic landmark is found at the level of L2-L3? _____

26. The iliac crest is at the level of the _____ vertebra.

27. Identify the labeled parts of the digestive system (Fig. 4-2).

   A. _____

   B. _____

   C. _____

   D. _____ valve

   E. _____

   F. _____

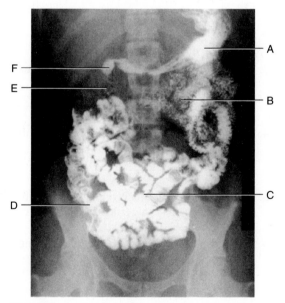

Fig. 4-2. Radiograph of the digestive tract.

28. Identify the labeled structures present on the computed tomography (CT) image (Fig. 4-3).

A. _____

B. _____

C. _____

D. _____

E. _____

F. _____

G. _____

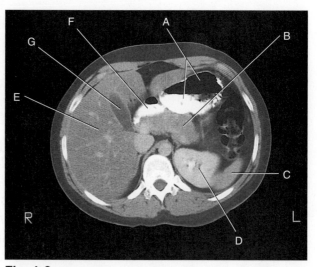

Fig. 4-3. Computed tomography (CT) cross-sectional image of abdomen at the level of L1 or L2.

PART II: RADIOGRAPHIC POSITIONING AND OTHER PATIENT CONSIDERATIONS
Review Exercise B: Shielding, Patient Dose, Pathology, Exposure Factors, and Positioning (see textbook pp. 112-114)

1. What are the two causes of voluntary motion?

   A. _____   B. _____

2. Voluntary motion can best be prevented by _____ to the patient.

3. What is the primary cause for involuntary motion in the abdomen?

   _____

4. What is the best mechanism to control involuntary motion?

   _____

5. True/False: Because the liver margin is visible in the right upper quadrant of the abdomen, it is not necessary to place a right or left anatomic side marker on the cassette before exposure.

6. Gonadal shielding should *not* be used during abdomen radiography if:
   A. It obscures essential anatomy
   B. The patient requests that it not be used
   C. The technologist does not elect to use it
   D. The patient is 40 years or older

7. True/False: For an adult abdomen, a collimation margin must be visible on all four sides of the radiograph.

8. Gonadal shielding for _____ may be impossible for studies of the lower abdominopelvic region.
   A. Males
   B. Females
   C. Both males and females
   D. Small children

9. Gonadal shielding for females involves placing the top of the shield at or slightly above the level of the

_____, with the bottom at the _____.

10. Which one of the following exposure factors would be most ideal for an AP abdomen of a small- to average-size adult?
   A. 110 kV, 200 mA, ¼ second, grid, 40-inch SID
   B. 85 kV, 300 mA, ⅕ second, grid, 40-inch SID
   C. 75 kV, 600 mA, ¹⁄₃₀ second, grid, 40-inch SID
   D. 60 kV, 400 mA, ¹⁄₁₅ second, grid, 40-inch SID

11. Which of the following technical factors is essential when performing abdomen studies on a young pediatric patient?
   A. Short exposure times   C. High milliamperage
   B. High-speed image receptor   D. All of the above

12. True/False: A radiolucent pad should be placed underneath geriatric patients for added comfort.

13. With the use of iodinated contrast media, _____ is able to distinguish between a simple cyst or tumor of the liver.
   A. Ultrasound   C. CT
   B. Nuclear medicine   D. MRI

14. _____ is being used to evaluate patients with acute appendicitis.
   A. Ultrasound   C. CT
   B. Nuclear medicine   D. MRI

15. The preferred imaging modality for examining the gallbladder quickly is:
   A. Ultrasound   C. Barium enema study
   B. Nuclear medicine   D. MRI

16. Match the following definitions to the correct pathologic indicator.

   _____ 1. Free air or gas in the peritoneal cavity   A. Volvulus

   _____ 2. Inflammatory condition of the colon   B. Adynamic ileus

   _____ 3. Telescoping of a section of bowel into another loop of bowel   C. Ascites

   _____ 4. Abnormal accumulation of fluid in the peritoneal cavity   D. Ulcerative colitis

   _____ 5. Bowel obstruction caused by a lack of intestinal peristalsis   E. Pneumoperitoneum

   _____ 6. A twisting of a loop of bowel creating an obstruction   F. Intussusception

   _____ 7. Chronic inflammation of the intestinal wall that may result in   G. Crohn's disease
            bowel obstruction

17. Match each of the following radiographic appearances of the abdomen to its corresponding type of pathologic condition.

_____ 1. Distended loops of air-filled small intestine   A. Ascites

_____ 2. Air-filled "coiled spring" appearance   B. Volvulus

_____ 3. General abdominal haziness   C. Pneumoperitoneum

_____ 4. Thin crest-shaped radiolucency underneath diaphragm   D. Ulcerative colitis

_____ 5. Deep air-filled mucosal protrusions of colon wall   E. Intussusception

_____ 6. Large amount of air trapped in sigmoid colon   F. Crohn's disease
         with a tapered narrowing at the site of obstruction

18. The central ray is centered to the level of the _____ for a supine AP projection of the abdomen.

19. Exposure for an AP projection of the abdomen should be taken on _____ (inspiration or expiration).

20. Rotation can be determined on a KUB radiograph by the loss of symmetric appearance of:

A. _____   C. _____

B. _____   D. _____

21. Which type of body habitus may require two crosswise images to be taken if the entire abdomen is to be included?

_____

22. True/False: A tall asthenic patient may require two 14- × 17-inch (35- × 43-cm) image receptors placed lengthwise if the entire abdomen is to be included.

23. Which of the following generates the largest gonadal dose?
A. Female AP abdomen   C. Female posteroanterior (PA) abdomen
B. Male lateral decubitus abdomen   D. Male erect AP abdomen

24. What is the gonadal dose range for an average-size female patient with an AP projection of the abdomen?
A. 1 to 5 mrad   C. 35 to 75 mrad
B. 5 to 10 mrad   D. 200 to 300 mrad

25. Which one of the following abdominal structures is not visible on a properly exposed KUB?
A. Kidneys   C. Pancreas
B. Margin of liver processes   D. Lumbar transverse processes

26. Why may the PA projection of a KUB generally be less desirable than the AP projection?

_____

27. Which decubitus position of the abdomen best demonstrates intraperitoneal air in the abdomen?

_____

28. Why should a patient be placed in the decubitus position for a minimum of 5 minutes before exposure?

_____

29. Which decubitus position best demonstrates possible aneurysms, calcifications of the aorta, or umbilical hernias?

_____

30. Which position best demonstrates a possible aortic aneurysm in the prevertebral region of the abdomen?

_____

31. List the projections commonly performed for an acute abdominal series or three-way abdomen series.

A. _____   B. _____   C. _____

32. Which position of the three-way acute abdominal series best demonstrates free air under the diaphragm?

_____

33. Which positioning routine should be used for an acute abdominal series if the patient is too ill to stand?

_____

34. To ensure that the diaphragm is included on an erect abdomen projection, the central ray should be at the level of

_____, which places the top of the 14- × 17-inch (35- × 43-cm) cassette at the level of the

_____.

35. Which one of the following projections involves a kV setting of 110 to 125 ?
    A. Erect abdomen for ascites
    B. Supine abdomen for intraabdominal mass
    C. PA, erect chest for free air under diaphragm
    D. Dorsal decubitus abdomen for calcified aorta

36. When using automatic exposure control (AEC) systems, which ionization chamber(s) should be activated for an average- to large-size patient when performing an AP projection of the abdomen?

_____

37. True/False: A larger patient receives a greater amount of skin dose and midline dose as compared with a smaller patient during an AP projection of the abdomen.

Review Exercise C: Problem Solving for Technical and Positioning Errors
The following radiographic problems involve technical and positioning errors that may lead to substandard images. As you analyze these problems, review your textbook to find solutions to these questions.

Other questions involve situations pertaining to various patient conditions and pathologic findings. If you need more information about a particular pathologic condition, review your textbook or a medical dictionary to learn more about it.

1. A KUB radiograph reveals that the symphysis pubis was cut off along the bottom of the image. Is this an acceptable radiograph? If it is not, how can this problem be prevented during the repeat exposure?

_____

_____

2. A radiograph of an AP projection of an average-size adult abdomen was produced using the following exposure factors: 90 kV, 400 mA, $\frac{1}{10}$ second, grid, and 40-inch SID. The overall density of the radiograph was acceptable, but the soft tissue structures, such as the psoas muscles and kidneys, were not visible. Which adjustment to the technical factors will enhance the visibility of these structures on the repeat exposure?

_____

_____

3. A radiograph image of an AP projection of the abdomen demonstrates motion. The following exposure factors were selected: 78 kV, 200 mA, $\frac{2}{10}$ second, grid, and 40-inch SID. The technologist is sure that the patient didn't breathe or move during the exposure. What may have caused this blurriness? What can be done to correct this problem on the repeat exposure?

_____

_____

4. A radiograph of an AP abdomen reveals that the left iliac wing is more narrowed than the right. What specific positioning error caused this?

_____

_____

5. **Situation:** A patient with a possible dynamic ileus enters the emergency room. The patient is able to stand. The physician has ordered an acute abdominal series. What specific positioning routine should be used?

_____

_____

6. **Situation:** A patient with a possible perforated duodenal ulcer enters the emergency room. The ER physician is concerned about the presence of free air in the abdomen. The patient is in severe pain and *cannot* stand. What positioning routine should be used to diagnose this condition?

_____

_____

7. **Situation:** The ER physician suspects a patient has a kidney stone. The patient is sent to the radiology department to confirm the diagnosis. What specific positioning routine would be used to rule out the presence of a kidney stone?

_____

_____

8. **Situation:** A patient in intensive care may have developed intraabdominal bleeding. The patient is in critical condition and cannot go to the radiology department. The physician has ordered a portable study of the abdomen. Which specific position or projection can be used to determine the extent of the bleeding?

_____

_____

9. **Situation:** A patient with a history of ascites comes to the radiology department. Which one of the following positions best demonstrates this condition?

   A. Erect AP abdomen   B. Erect PA chest   C. Supine KUB   D. Prone KUB

10. **Situation:** A KUB radiograph reveals that the gonadal shielding is superior to the upper margin of the symphysis pubis. The female patient has a history of kidney stones. What is the next step the technologist should take?

    A. Accept the radiograph because the kidneys were not obscured by the shielding.

    B. Repeat the exposure without using gonadal shielding.

    C. Repeat the exposure only if the patient complains of pain in the lower abdomen.

    D. Repeat the exposure with gonadal shielding, but position it below the symphysis pubis.

11. **Situation:** A hypersthenic patient comes to the radiology department for a KUB. The radiograph reveals that the symphysis pubis is included on the image, but the upper abdomen, including the kidneys, is cut off. What is the next step the technologist should take?

    A. Accept the radiograph.

    B. Repeat the exposure, but expose it during inspiration to force the kidneys lower into the abdomen.

    C. Ask the radiologist whether the upper abdomen really needs to be seen. Repeat only if requested.

    D. Repeat the exposure. Use two 14- × 17-inch (35- × 43-cm) cassettes crosswise to include the entire abdomen.

12. **Situation:** A patient comes from the ER with a large distended abdomen caused by an ileus. The physician suspects that the distention is caused by a large amount of bowel gas that is trapped in the small intestine. The standard technique for a KUB on an adult is 76 kV, 30 mAs. Should the technologist change any of these exposure factors for this patient? (AEC is not being used.)

    A. No. Use the standard exposure settings.

    B. Yes. Decrease the milliamperage seconds (mAs).

    C. Yes. Increase the milliamperage seconds (mAs).

    D. Yes. Increase the kilovoltage (kV).

13. **Situation:** A child goes to radiology for an abdomen study. It is possible that he swallowed a coin. The ER physician believes it may be in the upper GI tract. Which of the the following routines would best identify the location of the coin?

    A. KUB and left lateral decubitus

    B. Acute abdominal series

    C. KUB and lateral abdomen

    D. Supine and erect KUB

PART III: LABORATORY EXERCISES

You must gain experience in chest positioning before performing the following exams on actual patients. You can get experience in positioning and radiographic evaluation of these projections by performing exercises using radiographic phantoms and practicing on other students (although you will not be taking actual exposures).

The following suggested activities assume that your teaching institution has an energized lab and radiographic phantoms. If not, perform only Laboratory Exercise B, the physical positioning activities. (Check off each step and projection as you complete it.)

Laboratory Exercise A: Energized Laboratory

1. Using the abdominal radiographic phantom, produce a radiograph of:

   _____ KUB

2. Evaluate the KUB radiograph, additional radiographs provided by your instructor, or both for the following criteria:

   _____ Rotation   _____ Part and central ray centering

   _____ Proper exposure factors   _____ Motion

   _____ Collimation   _____ Anatomic side markers

Laboratory Exercise B: Physical Positioning

1. On another person, simulate taking all of the following basic and special projections of the chest. Follow the suggested positioning steps and sequence as listed below and as described in Chapter 1 of your textbook.

   _____ KUB of the abdomen   _____ Dorsal decubitus

   _____ Left lateral decubitus   _____ Acute abdominal series to include: AP supine, AP erect, PA chest

Step 1. General Patient Positioning

_____ Select the size and number of cassettes needed.

_____ Prepare the radiographic room. Check that x-ray tube is centered to the center of the IR holder (or the centerline of the table for Bucky exams).

_____ Correctly identify the patient and bring the patient into the room.

_____ Explain to the patient what you will be doing.

_____ Assist the patient to the proper place and position for the first radiograph.

Step 2. Measuring Part Thickness

_____ Measure the body part being radiographed and set correct exposure factors (technique). (If using an AEC system, select the correct chamber cells on the control panel.)

Step 3. Part Positioning

_____ Align and center the body part to the central ray or vice versa. For Bucky exams on a table, move the patient and table top together as needed (with floating type of table top). (NOTE: In cases in which the correct central ray position is of primary importance, the central ray icon is included in the textbook on the appropriate positioning page.)

Step 4. IR Centering

_____ After the part has been centered to the central ray, the IR (cassette) is also centered to the central ray.

Additional Steps or Actions

_____ 1. Collimate accurately to include only the area of interest.

_____ 2. Place the correct marker within the exposure field (so that you do not superimpose pertinent anatomic structures).

_____ 3. Restrain or provide support for the body part to prevent motion.

_____ 4. Use contact lead shielding as needed.

_____ 5. Give clear breathing instructions and make the exposure while watching the patient through the window.

MY SCORE = _____ %

This self-test should be taken only after completing all of the readings, review exercises, and laboratory activities for a particular section. The self-test is divided into six sections. The purpose of this test is not only to provide a good learning exercise but also to serve as a strong indicator of what your final unit evaluation exam will cover. It is strongly suggested that if you do not get at least a 90% to 95% grade on each self-test that you review those areas in which you missed questions before going to your instructor for the final unit evaluation exam.

1. The double-walled membrane lining the abdominal cavity is called the:
   A. Greater omentum   C. Lesser omentum
   B. Mesentery   D. Peritoneum

2. Which of the following soft tissue structures are seen on a properly exposed KUB?
   A. Spleen   C. Psoas muscles
   B. Pancreas   D. Stomach

3. The first portion of the small intestine is called the:
   A. Duodenum   C. Jejunum
   B. Ileum   D. Pylorus

4. At the junction of the small and large intestine is the:
   A. Sigmoid colon   C. Ileocecal valve
   B. Rectum   D. Ascending colon

5. Match the correct answers to the structures labeled on Fig. 4-4.

   _____ 1.   A. Sigmoid colon

   _____ 2.   B. Liver

   _____ 3.   C. Jejunum

   _____ 4.   D. Oral cavity

   _____ 5.   E. Spleen

   _____ 6.   F. Stomach

   _____ 7.   G. Esophagus

   _____ 8.   H. Oropharynx

   _____ 9.   I. Pancreas

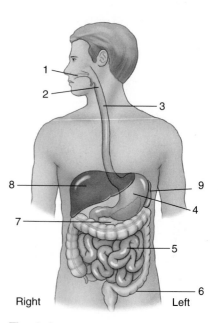

Fig. 4-4. Digestive tract and surrounding structures.

6. Which one of the following is not an accessory organ of digestion?
    A. Liver   C. Pancreas
    B. Gallbladder   D. Kidney

7. The kidneys are connected to the bladder by way of the:

    A. Urethra   B. Renal artery   C. Ureter   D. Renal vein

8. Which structure stores and releases bile?

    A. Liver   B. Spleen   C. Pancreas   D. Gallbladder

9. Which one of the following structures connects the small intestine to the posterior abdominal wall?
    A. Greater omentum   C. Lesser omentum
    B. Peritoneum   D. Mesentery

10. For each of the following organs, identify the correct abdominal quadrant(s) in which the organ would be found on an average sthenic patient—left upper quadrant (LUQ), left lower quadrant (LLQ), right lower quadrant (RLQ), or right upper quadrant (RUQ) (NOTE: Some organs may be found in more than one quadrant).

    A. Cecum _____

    B. Liver _____

    C. Spleen _____

    D. Stomach _____

    E. Right colic flexure _____

    F. Sigmoid colon _____

    G. Appendix _____

    H. Pancreas _____

    I. Gallbladder _____

11. Which region of the abdomen would contain the spleen?
    A. Epigastric   C. Left hypochondriac
    B. Umbilical   D. Left inguinal

12. Match the following structures to the correct compartment of the peritoneum.

　　_____ 1. Cecum 　　　　　　A. Intraperitoneum

　　_____ 2. Jejunum 　　　　　B. Retroperitoneum

　　_____ 3. Ascending colon 　C. Infraperitoneum

　　_____ 4. Liver

　　_____ 5. Adrenal glands

　　_____ 6. Gallbladder

　　_____ 7. Ovaries

　　_____ 8. Duodenum

　　_____ 9. Urinary bladder

　　_____ 10. Pancreas

13. The xiphoid process corresponds with which vertebral level?
   A. T9-10 　　　　　　C. L2-3
   B. L4-5 　　　　　　 D. T4-5

14. Identify the topographic positioning landmarks as labeled on Figs. 4-5 and 4-6.

　　_____ 1. Iliac crest

　　_____ 2. Ischial tuberosity

　　_____ 3. Xiphoid process

　　_____ 4. Pubic symphysis

　　_____ 5. Greater trochanter

　　_____ 6. Lower costal margin

　　_____ 7. Anterior superior iliac spine
　　　　　　 (ASIS)

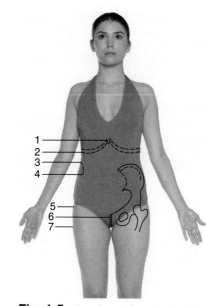

Fig. 4-5. Anterior surface landmarks.

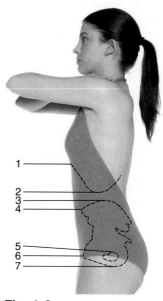

Fig. 4-6. Lateral surface landmarks.

15. To identify the inferior margin of the abdomen, the technologist can palpate the symphysis pubis or:
    A. Iliac crest   C. ASIS
    B. Greater trochanter   D. Ischial tuberosity

16. An important anatomic landmark that is commonly used to locate the center of the abdomen is the:
    A. Iliac crest   C. ASIS
    B. Greater trochanter   D. Ischial tuberosity

17. Which one of the following factors best controls the involuntary motion of a young, pediatric patient during abdominal radiography?
    A. Short exposure time
    B. High kV (100 to 125)
    C. Clear, concise breathing instructions
    D. Use of compression band across the abdomen

18. An abnormal accumulation of fluid in the abdominal cavity is called:
    A. Ileus   C. Volvulus
    B. Ulcerative colitis   D. Ascites

19. Another term describing a nonmechanical bowel obstruction is:
    A. Pneumoperitoneum   C. Ascites
    B. Paralytic Ileus   D. Intussusception

20. The telescoping of a section of bowel into another loop is called:
    A. Intussusception   C. Volvulus
    B. Ascites   D. Ulcerative colitis

21. A chronic disease involving inflammation of the large intestine is:
    A. Ascites   C. Crohn's disease
    B. Volvulus   D. Ulcerative colitis

22. Free air or gas in the peritoneal cavity is:
    A. Pneumothorax   C. Pneumoperitoneum
    B. Ileus   D. Volvulus

23. Free air in the intraabdominal cavity rises to the level of the _____ in a patient who is in the erect position.
    A. Greater omentum   C. Intraperitoneal cavity
    B. Diaphragm   D. Liver

24. Which one of the following conditions is demonstrated radiographically as general abdominal haziness?
    A. Pneumoperitoneum   C. Ileus
    B. Ascites   D. Volvulus

25. Which one of the following conditions is demonstrated radiographically as distended, air-filled loops of the small bowel?
    A. Ascites   C. Pneumoperitoneum
    B. Ulcerative colitis   D. Ileus

26. Identify the structures labeled on this AP KUB radiograph (Fig. 4-7).

A. _____

B. _____

C. _____

D. _____

E. _____

F. _____

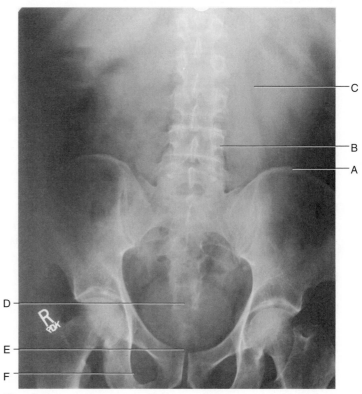

Fig. 4-7. Anteroposterior (AP) KUB radiograph.

27. Identify the organs or structures labeled on this computed tomography (CT) scan (Fig. 4-8) at the level of L1 or L2.

A. _____

B. _____

C. _____

D. _____

E. _____

F. _____

G. _____

H. _____

Major blood vessels.

I. _____

J. _____

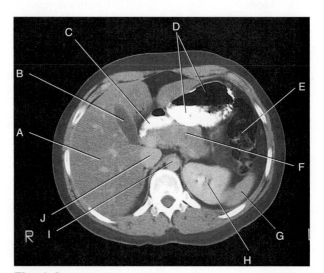

Fig. 4-8. Computed tomography (CT) cross-sectional image at the level of L1 or L2.

28. Which one of the following sets of exposure factors would be the best for abdominal radiography (for an average-size adult)?

    A. 110 kV, 400 mA, 1/20 second, grid, 40-inch SID

    B. 78 kV, 600 mA, 1/30 second, grid, 40-inch SID

    C. 78 kV, 200 mA, 1/10 second, grid, 40-inch SID

    D. 65 kV, 600 mA, 1/15 second, grid, 40-inch SID

29. A radiograph of an AP projection of the abdomen reveals that the right iliac wing is wider than the left. What type of positioning error was involved?

    A. Rotation toward the left   C. Rotation toward the right

    B. Tilt to the left   D. Tilt to the right

30. Most abdominal projections are taken:

    A. Upon expiration   C. Upon inspiration

    B. During shallow breathing   D. During deep breathing

31. A KUB radiograph on a large hypersthenic patient reveals that the entire abdomen is not included on the 35 × 43-cm (14 × 17-inch) IR. What can be done to correct this on the repeat radiograph?

    A. Use two cassettes placed lengthwise.   C. Expose during deep inspiration.

    B. Use two cassettes placed crosswise.   D. Perform KUB with patient in the erect position.

32. What is the minimum amount of time a patient should be upright before taking a projection to demonstrate intraabdominal free air?

    A. 20 minutes   C. 2 minutes

    B. 30 minutes   D. 5 minutes

33. If the posteroanterior (PA) chest projection is *not* performed for the acute abdomen series, centering for the erect abdomen projection *must* include the:

    A. Inferior liver margin   C. Entire kidneys

    B. Diaphragm   D. Bladder

34. Which specific decubitus position of the abdomen should be used in an acute abdomen series if the patient cannot stand?

    A. Left lateral decubitus   C. Right lateral decubitus

    B. Dorsal decubitus   D. Ventral decubitus

35. **Situation:** A patient with a possible ileus enters the emergency room. The physician orders an acute abdominal series. The patient can stand. Which specific position best demonstrates air/fluid levels in the abdomen?

    A. AP supine abdomen   C. Dorsal decubitus

    B. Right lateral decubitus   D. AP erect abdomen

36. **Situation:** A patient with a possible perforated bowel caused by trauma enters the ER. The patient is unable to stand. Which projection would best demonstrate any possible free air within the abdomen?

    A. Dorsal decubitus   C. AP supine abdomen

    B. Left lateral decubitus   D. Right lateral decubitus

37. **Situation:** A patient with a clinical history of a possible umbilical hernia comes to the radiology department. The KUB is inconclusive. Which additional projection can be taken to help confirm the diagnosis?

    A. AP erect abdomen   C. Dorsal decubitus

    B. Left lateral decubitus   D. Ventral decubitus

38. **Situation:** A patient comes to the radiology department with a clinical history of pneumoperitoneum. The patient is able to stand. Which one of the following projections will best demonstrate this condition?

    A. AP supine abdomen
    B. AP erect abdomen
    C. Dorsal decubitus
    D. Left lateral decubitus

39. **Situation:** A patient comes to the radiology department with a clinical history of ascites. The patient is unable to stand or sit erect. Which one of the following projections will best demonstrate this condition?

    A. AP supine abdomen
    B. Left lateral decubitus
    C. Dorsal decubitus
    D. AP supine chest

40. **Situation:** A patient comes in the ER with possible gallstones. The patient is in severe pain. Which of the following imaging modalities or projections would provide the quickest method for confirming the presence of gallstones?

    A. Sonography
    B. Acute abdomen series
    C. MRI
    D. KUB

41. Which one of the following alternative imaging modalities is most effectively used to evaluate GI motility and reflux?

    A. CT
    B. MRI
    C. Sonography
    D. Nuclear medicine

42. Which one of the following technical factors is essential when using computed radiography (CR) to ensure a high-quality image is produced?

    A. Low kV
    B. 72-in (180-cm) SID
    C. Large focal spot
    D. Close collimation

43. True/False: Identify whether each of the following statements concerning average-size patient doses for abdominal radiographs is true or false.

    _____ A. The female ovarian dose on a PA abdomen is close to the midline dose (±10%).

    _____ B. The skin dose for an average-size AP or PA abdomen is in the 50 to 75 mrad range.

    _____ C. The female ovarian dose for an AP abdomen is about double that for a PA projection.

    _____ D. The male testes dose is less than one-tenth that of the female ovarian dose with proper collimation.

44. For the following critique questions, refer to the textbook, p. ••• (Fig. C4-49) (AP supine KUB).

    A. Which positioning error(s) is (are) visible on this radiograph? (More than one answer may be selected.)

    (a) All essential anatomic structures are not demonstrated.
    (b) CR-to-IR centering is incorrect.
    (c) CR-to-anatomy centering is incorrect.
    (d) Collimation is not evident.
    (e) Exposure factors are incorrect.
    (f) No marker is seen on the radiograph.
    (g) Rotation is toward the right.
    (h) Rotation is toward the left.

    B. Which error(s) on this radiograph is(are) considered "repeatable"?

C. Which of the following modifications must be made during the repeat exposure? (More than one answer may be selected.)

(a) Open up collimation.

(b) Center CR-to-IR correctly.

(c) Center CR-to-anatomy correctly.

(d) Decrease exposure factors.

(e) Increase exposure factors.

(f) Place marker on IR before exposure.

(g) Ensure that ASISs are equal distance from table top to eliminate rotation.

45. For the following critique questions, refer to Fig. C4-51 (AP erect abdomen) on p. 122 in your textbook.

A. Which positioning error(s) is(are) visible on this radiograph? (More than one answer may be selected.)

(a) All essential anatomic structures are not demonstrated.

(b) CR-to-IR centering is incorrect.

(c) Collimation is not evident.

(d) Exposure factors are incorrect.

(e) No marker is seen on the radiograph.

(f) Rotation is toward the right.

(g) Rotation is toward the left.

B. Which error(s) on this radiograph is(are) considered "repeatable"?

_____

C. Which of the following modifications must be made during the repeat exposure? More than one answer may be selected.

(a) Open up collimation.

(b) Center CR-to-IR correctly.

(c) Decrease exposure factors.

(d) Increase exposure factors.

(e) Place marker on IR before exposure.

(f) Ensure that ASISs are equal distance from table top to eliminate rotation.

5 Upper Limb

CHAPTER OBJECTIVES

After you have successfully completed the activities in this chapter, you will be able to:

_____ 1. List the total number of bones of the hand and wrist.

_____ 2. Identify specific aspects of the phalanges, metacarpals, and carpal bones.

_____ 3. On drawings and radiographs, identify specific anatomic structures of the hand and wrist.

_____ 4. List and describe the location, size, and shape of each carpal bone of the wrist.

_____ 5. Match specific joints of the hand and wrist according to classification and movement type.

_____ 6. List four specific ligaments of the wrist.

_____ 7. On drawings and radiographs, identify specific fat pads and stripes of the upper limb.

_____ 8. Distinguish between ulnar and radial deviation wrist movements.

_____ 9. Identify specific parts of the forearm, elbow, and distal humerus.

_____ 10. On drawings and radiographs, identify specific anatomic structures of the forearm, elbow, and distal humerus.

_____ 11. List the technical factors commonly used for upper limb radiography.

_____ 12. Match specific pathologic features of the upper limb to their correct definition.

_____ 13. Match specific pathologic features of the upper limb to their correct radiographic appearance.

_____ 14. For select pathologic conditions of the upper limb, indicate whether manual exposure factors should be increased or decreased or remain the same.

_____ 15. Identify the correct central ray placement, part position, and radiographic criteria for specific positions of the fingers, thumb, hand, wrist, forearm, and elbow.

_____ 16. Identify which structures are best seen with each basic and special projection of the upper limb.

_____ 17. Based on clinical situations, describe the preferred positioning routine to assist the physician with the diagnosis of a specific condition or disease process.

_____ 18. Identify and apply the exposure conversion chart for various sizes of plaster and fiberglass casts.

_____ 19. List the three radiographic criteria for a true lateral elbow position.

_____ 20. List the skin and midline dose ranges and the relative differences among these doses for each body part of the upper limb.

_____ 21. Given various hypothetical situations, identify the correct modification of a position, exposure factors, or both to improve the radiographic image.

_____ 22. Given various hypothetical situations, identify the correct position for a specific condition or pathologic feature.

_____ 23. Given radiographs of specific upper limb positions, identify specific positioning and exposure factor errors.

POSITIONING AND RADIOGRAPHIC CRITIQUE

_____ 1. Using another student as a model, practice basic and special projections of the upper limb.

_____ 2. Using a hand and elbow radiographic phantom, produce satisfactory radiographs of the hand, thumb, wrist, and elbow (if equipment is available).

_____ 3. Critique and evaluate upper limb radiographs based on the four divisions of radiographic criteria: (1) structures shown, (2) position, (3) collimation and central ray, and (4) exposure criteria.

_____ 4. Distinguish between acceptable and unacceptable upper limb radiographs based on exposure factors, motion, collimation, positioning, or other errors.

LEARNING EXERCISES

Complete the following review exercises after reading the associated pages in the textbook as indicated by each exercise. Answers to each review exercise are given at the end of the review exercises.

PART I: RADIOGRAPHIC ANATOMY
Review Exercise A: Anatomy of the Hand and Wrist (see textbook pp. 124-127)

1. Identify the number of bones for each of the following.

   A. Phalanges (fingers and thumb) _____   C. Carpals (wrist) _____

   B. Metacarpals (palm) _____   D. Total _____

2. The two portions of the thumb (first digit) are the:

   A. _____

   B. _____

3. The three portions of each finger (second through fifth digits) are the:

   A. _____

   B. _____

   C. _____

4. The three parts of each phalanx, starting distally, are the:

A. _____ B. _____ C. _____

5. List the three parts of each metacarpal, starting proximally:

A. _____ B. _____ C. _____

6. The name of the joint between the proximal and distal phalanges of the first digit is the _____.

7. The joints between metacarpals and phalanges are the: _____.

8. Fill in the names and parts of the following bones and joints of the right hand as labeled on Fig. 5-1. Include abbreviations for joints if applicable.

A. _____

B. _____

C. _____

D. _____

E. _____

F. _____

G. _____

H. _____

I. _____

J. _____

K. _____

L. _____

M. _____

N. _____

O. _____

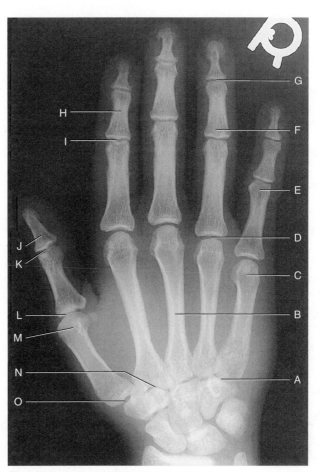

Fig. 5-1. Posteroanterior (PA) right hand.

9. Match each of the carpal bones labeled in Figs. 5-2 and 5-3 with its correct name.

_____ A.   1. Lunate

_____ B.   2. Hamate

_____ C.   3. Trapezium

_____ D.   4. Pisiform

_____ E.   5. Triquetrum

_____ F.   6. Trapezoid

_____ G.   7. Capitate

_____ H.   8. Scaphoid

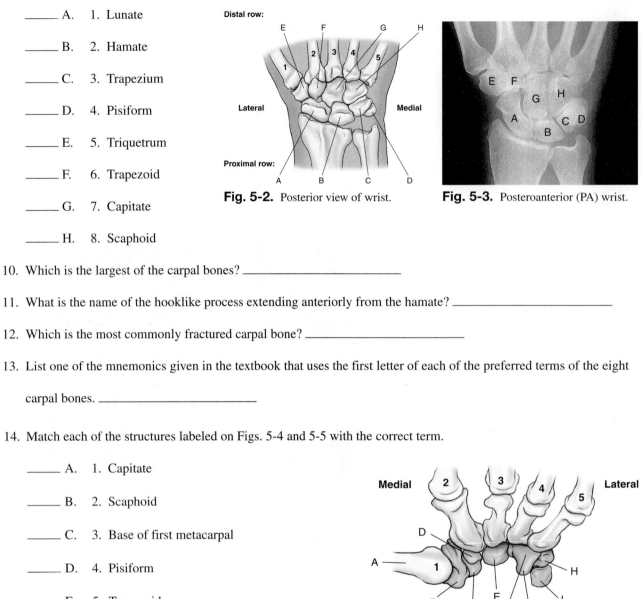

Fig. 5-2. Posterior view of wrist.   **Fig. 5-3.** Posteroanterior (PA) wrist.

10. Which is the largest of the carpal bones? _____

11. What is the name of the hooklike process extending anteriorly from the hamate? _____

12. Which is the most commonly fractured carpal bone? _____

13. List one of the mnemonics given in the textbook that uses the first letter of each of the preferred terms of the eight

carpal bones. _____

14. Match each of the structures labeled on Figs. 5-4 and 5-5 with the correct term.

_____ A.   1. Capitate

_____ B.   2. Scaphoid

_____ C.   3. Base of first metacarpal

_____ D.   4. Pisiform

_____ E.   5. Trapezoid

_____ F.   6. Hamulus (hamular process)

_____ G.   7. Triquetrum

_____ H.   8. Hamate

_____ I.   9. Trapezium

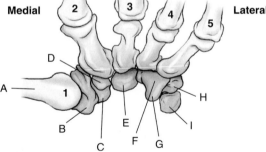

Fig. 5-4. Carpal tunnel view.

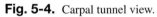

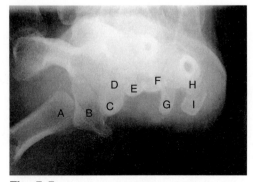

Fig. 5-5. carpal canal, inferosuperior projection.

15. Identify the carpals and other structures labeled on Fig. 5-6.

A. _____

B. _____

C. _____

D. _____

E. _____

F. _____

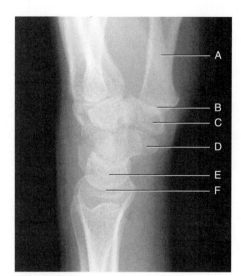

Fig. 5-6. Lateral wrist.

REVIEW EXERCISE B: Anatomy of the Forearm, Elbow, and Distal Humerus (see textbook pp. 128-130)

1. A. In the anatomic position, which of the bones of the forearm is located on the lateral (thumb) side? _____

   B. Which is on the medial side? _____

2. Indicate whether the following structures are part of the radius (R), ulna (U), or distal humerus (H) by listing the appropriate letter next to the structure.

   _____ A. Trochlear notch   _____ E. Coronoid tubercle

   _____ B. Radial notch   _____ F. Coronoid process

   _____ C. Olecranon fossa   _____ G. Olecranon process

   _____ D. Trochlea   _____ H. Coronoid fossa

3. Which two joints of the forearm allow it to rotate during pronation? _____

4. A. The articular portion of the medial aspect of the distal humerus is called the _____.

   B. The similar structure found on the lateral aspect of the distal humerus is called the _____.

5. The deep depression located on the posterior aspect of the distal humerus is the _____.

6. The criteria for evaluating a true lateral position of the elbow are the appearance of three concentric arcs (Fig. 5-7). These arcs include:

A. The first and smallest of the arcs: _____

B. The intermediate double arc, consisting of the outer ridges of:

   (a) The smaller arc: _____

   (b) The larger arc: _____

C. The third arc, which is part of the ulna:

   _____

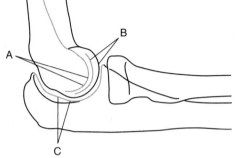

Fig. 5-7. True lateral elbow. Three concentric circles.

7. Match the following articulations with the correct joint movement types.

_____ A. Interphalangeal   1. Ginglymus

_____ B. Carpometacarpal of first digit   2. Ellipsoidal

_____ C. Elbow joint (humeroulnar and humeroradial) 3. Trochoidal

_____ D. Metacarpophalangeal of second to fifth digits 4. Plane

_____ E. Radiocarpal   5. Sellar

_____ F. Intercarpal

_____ G. Elbow joint

_____ H. Proximal and distal radioulnar joint

8. Ellipsoidal joints are classified as freely movable, or _____, and allow movement in

   _____ directions.

9. True/False: In addition to the ulnar and radial collateral ligaments, the following five additional ligaments are also important in stability of the wrist joint.

A. Dorsal radiocarpal   D. Scapulolunate
B. Palmar radiocarpal   E. Lunotriquetral
C. Triangular fibrocartilage complex (TFCC)

10. Which ligament of the wrist extends from the styloid process of the radius to the lateral aspect of the scaphoid and

    trapezium bones? _____

11. What is the name of the two special turning or bending positions of the hand and wrist that demonstrate medial and
    lateral aspects of the carpal region?

    A. _____   B. _____

12. Of the two positions listed in the previous question, which one is most commonly performed to detect a fracture of

    the scaphoid bone? _____

13. How does the forearm appear radiographically if pronated for a posteroanterior (PA) projection?

    _____

14. The two important fat stripes or bands around the wrist joint are the:

    A. _____   B. _____

15. The fat pads around the elbow joint are valuable diagnostic indicators if the following three technical/positioning
    requirements are met with the lateral position.

    A. _____

    B. _____

    C. _____

16. True/False: If the posterior fat pad of the elbow is not visible radiographically, it suggests that a nonobvious radial
    head or neck fracture is present.

17. True/False: If the elbow is flexed correctly at 90°, the posterior fat pad is visible if pathologic elbow trauma is present.

18. True/False: Trauma or infection makes the anterior fat pad more difficult to see on a lateral elbow radiograph.

19. Which projections best demonstrate the scaphoid fat pad? _____

20. Which projection best demonstrates the pronator fat stripe? _____

21. Identify the parts labeled on Figs. 5-8 and 5-9.

A. _____

B. _____

C. _____

D. _____

E. _____

F. _____

G. _____

H. _____

I. _____

J. _____

K. _____

L. _____

M. _____

N.* _____

O.* _____

P.* _____

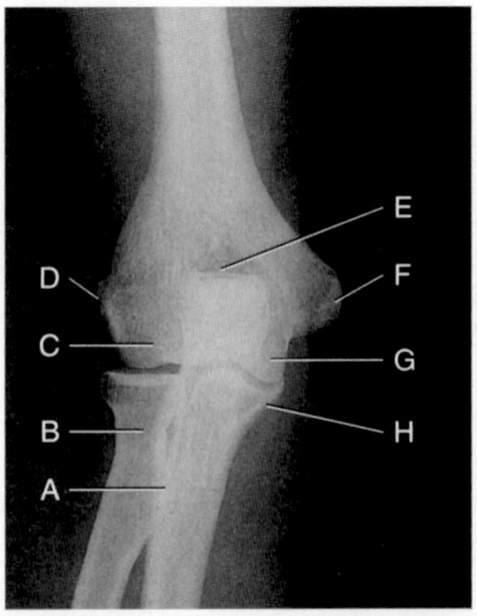

_____

*Hint: These are concentric arcs as evidence of a true lateral position.

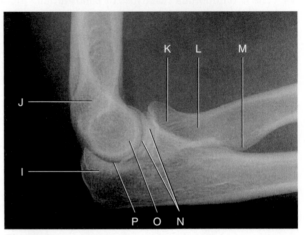

Fig. 5-8. Anteroposterior (AP) elbow.

Fig. 5-9. Lateral elbow.

22. Identify the parts labeled on Figs. 5-10 and 5-11.

A. _____

B. _____

C. _____

D. _____

E. _____

F. _____

G. _____

H. _____

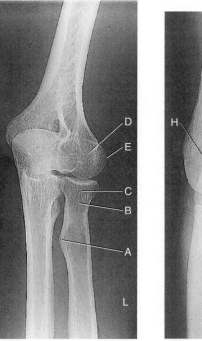 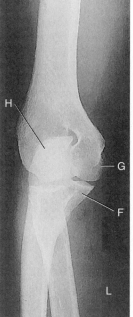

Fig. 5-10. Lateral (external) rotation of the elbow.

Fig. 5-11. Medial (internal) rotation of the elbow.

PART II: RADIOGRAPHIC POSITIONING
Review Exercise C: Positioning of the Fingers, Thumb, Hand, and Wrist (see textbook pp. 139-159)

1. Identify the following technical factors most commonly used for upper limb radiography.

A. Kilovoltage (kV) range: _____

B. Long or short exposure time? _____

C. Large or small focal spot? _____

D. Most common minimum source image receptor distance (SID): _____

E. Grids are used if the body part measures more than _____ cm.

F. Type of intensification screens most commonly used: _____

G. Small to medium dry plaster casts: Increase _____ kV.

H. Large plaster casts: Increase _____ kV or _____ % milliamperage seconds.

I. Fiberglass casts: Increase _____ kV or _____ %
milliamperage seconds.

J. Correctly exposed radiographs: Visualize _____ margins and

_____ markings of all bones.

2. The general rule for collimation for upper limb radiography states: _____

3. Circle all pertinent factors that help control distortion during upper limb radiography.
   A. Kilovoltage (kV)
   B. 40 to 44 inches (100 to 110 cm) SID
   C. Milliamperage seconds (mAs)
   D. Minimal object image receptor distance (OID)
   E. Correct central ray placement
   F. Use of small focal spot

4. Gonadal shielding is especially important for upper limbs on all persons who are _____.

5. True/False: Guardians of young pediatric patients who are having upper limb studies can be asked to hold their child during the radiographic study.

6. _____ is a radiographic procedure that uses contrast media injected into the joint capsule to visualize soft tissue pathology of the wrist, elbow, and shoulder joints.

7. What is the basic positioning routine for the second through fifth digits of the hand?

   _____

   _____

8. How much of the metacarpals should be included for PA projection of the digits?

   _____

   _____

9. List the two radiographic criteria used to determine whether rotation is present on the PA projection of the digits.

   A. _____

   B. _____

10. Identify which positioning modification(s) may be used for a study of the second digit to improve definition for each of the following:

    A. PA oblique projection: _____

    B. Lateral position: _____

11. Where is the central ray centered for a PA oblique projection of the second digit? _____

12. Why is it important to keep the affected digit parallel to the image receptor (IR) for the PA oblique and lateral projections?

    A. To prevent distortion of the phalanx   C. To demonstrate small, nondisplaced fractures near the joint

    B. To prevent distortion of the joints   D. All of the above

13. Why is the anteroposterior (AP) position of the thumb recommended instead of the PA?

    _____

14. Which projection of the thumb is achieved naturally by placing the palmar surface of the hand in contact with the

    cassette? _____

15. Which IR size should be used for a thumb routine? _____

16. A sesamoid bone is frequently found adjacent to the _____ joint of the thumb.

17. True/False: The entire metacarpal and trapezium must be demonstrated on all projections of the thumb.

18. Where is the central ray centered for an AP projection of the thumb?

    A. First interphalangeal (IP) joint   C. First metacarpophalangeal (MCP) joint

    B. Midaspect of proximal phalanx   D. First proximal interphalangeal (PIP) joint

19. A Bennett's fracture involves:

    A. Base of first metacarpal   C. Scaphoid bone

    B. Trapezium bone   D. Fracture extending through first IP joint

20. A. Which special positioning method can be performed to demonstrate a Bennett's fracture?

    _____

    B. Which central ray angulation is required for this projection? _____

21. Where is the central ray centered for a PA projection of the hand?

    A. Third MCP joint   C. Second MCP joint

    B. Midaspect of third metacarpal   D. Third PIP joint

22. A minimum of _____ inch(es) (_____ cm) of the forearm should be included radiographically for a PA projection of the hand.

23. True/False: Some superimposition of the distal third, fourth, and fifth metacarpals is expected with a well-positioned PA oblique projection of the hand.

24. Which preferred lateral position of the hand best demonstrates the phalanges without excessive superimposition?

    _____

25. Which lateral projection of the hand best demonstrates a possible foreign body in the palm of the hand?

    _____

26. What is the proper name for the position referred to as the "ball-catcher's position?" _____

27. The "ball-catcher's position" is commonly used to evaluate for early signs of:
   A. Osteoporosis   C. Osteopetrosis
   B. Osteomyelitis   D. Rheumatoid arthritis

28. The elbow generally should be flexed _____° for the basic positions of the wrist.

29. How much rotation is required for an oblique projection of the wrist? _____

30. Which alternative projection to the routine PA wrist best demonstrates the intercarpal joint spaces and wrist joint?

   _____

31. Which positioning error is involved if significant aspects of the third, fourth, and fifth metacarpals are superimposed in an oblique wrist projection? _____

32. Which one of the following fractures is not demonstrated in a wrist routine?
   A. Barton   C. Smith
   B. Pott   D. Colles'

33. During the PA axial scaphoid projection with central ray angle and ulnar flexion, the central ray must be angled

   _____° _____ (**distally** or **proximally**).

34. How much are the hand and wrist elevated from the IR for the modified Stecher method?
   A. None   C. 20°
   B. 10°   D. 15°

35. How much central ray angulation to the long axis of the hand is required for the carpal canal (tunnel) projection?

   _____

36. Which special projection of the wrist best demonstrates the interspaces on the ulnar side of the wrist between the

   lunate, triquetrum, pisiform, and hamate bones? _____

37. Which special projection of the wrist helps rule out abnormal calcifications in the carpal sulcus?

   _____

38. How much central ray angulation from the long axis of the forearm is required for the carpal bridge (tangential)

   projection? _____

39. What is the approximate difference in mrad between skin and midline doses for the hand and wrist?

   _____

Review Exercise D: Pathologic Features of the Fingers, Thumb, Hand, and Wrist (see textbook p. 136)

1. List the correct pathology term for each of the following definitions.

   A. _____ Fracture and dislocation of the posterior lip of the distal radius

   B. _____ Most common type of primary malignant tumor occurring in bone

   C. _____ Reduction in the quantity of bone or atrophy of skeletal tissue

   D. _____ Sprain or tear of the ulnar collateral ligament

   E. _____ An abnormality of the cartilage affecting long bones

   F. _____ Transverse fracture extending through the distal aspect of the metacarpal neck

   G. _____ Hereditary condition marked by abnormally dense bone

   H. _____ Transverse fracture of the distal radius with posterior displacement of the distal fragment

2. Match the pathologic condition or disease to its radiographic appearance.

   _____ A. Narrowing of joint space with periosteal growths on the joint margins   1. Osteomyelitis

   _____ B. Fluid-filled joint space with possible calcification   2. Bursitis

   _____ C. Possible calcification in the carpal sulcus   3. Carpal tunnel syndrome

   _____ D. Soft tissue swelling and loss of fat-pad detail visibility   4. Osteoarthritis

   _____ E. Mixed areas of sclerotic and cortical thickening along with   5. Osteopetrosis
            radiolucent lesions

3. For the following types of pathologic conditions, indicate whether the manual exposure factors should be increased (+), decreased (−), or remain the same (0) as compared with the standard exposure factors.

   _____ Advanced Paget's disease   _____ Osteoporosis

   _____ Joint effusion   _____ Osteopetrosis

   _____ Advanced rheumatoid arthritis   _____ Bursitis

Review Exercise E: Positioning of the Forearm, Elbow, and Humerus (see textbook pp. 160-169)

1. Which basic projections are required for a study of the forearm? _____

2. True/False: For a forearm study, the technologist needs to include only the joint closest to the site of the injury.

3. To properly position the patient for an AP projection of the elbow, the epicondyles must be _____ to the IR.

4. If the patient cannot fully extend the elbow for the AP projection, what alternative projection(s) should be performed? _____

5. Which basic projection of the elbow best demonstrates the radial head, neck, and tuberosity without any superimposition of the ulna? _____

6. True/False: Gonadal shielding is not required for upper limb radiographs if the patient can sit upright for these exams.

7. Which projection of the elbow best demonstrates the coronoid process in profile? _____

8. The best position to evaluate the posterior fat pads of the elbow joint is _____ .

9. Which special projection(s) of the elbow should be performed instead of the basic AP if the patient's elbow is tightly flexed and cannot be extended at all? _____

10. How much is the upper limb rotated for a lateral (rotation) oblique projection of the elbow? _____

11. What is a proper name for the acute flexion projection of the elbow? _____

12. How much and in which direction should the central ray be angled for the Coyle method involving the radial head?

_____

13. How much and in which direction should the central ray be angled for the Coyle method involving the coronoid process? _____

14. What is the only difference among the four radial head lateral projections of the elbow?

_____

15. Match the nearest skin dose for each of the following.

_____ A. PA finger   1. 5 mrad

_____ B. AP forearm   2. 10 mrad

_____ C. Lateral humerus   3. 15 mrad

_____ D. Lateral hand   4. 20 mrad

_____ E. Carpal canal wrist   5. 25 mrad

_____ F. PA hand   6. 30 mrad

Review Exercise F: Problem Solving for Technical and Positioning Errors

The following radiographic problems involve technical and positioning errors that may lead to substandard images. As you analyze these problems, review your textbook to find solutions to these questions.

Other questions involve situations pertaining to various patient conditions and pathologic findings. If you need more information about a particular pathologic condition, review your textbook or a medical dictionary to learn more about it.

1. A three-projection study of the hand was taken using the following exposure factors: 64 kV, 1000 mA, $\frac{1}{100}$ second, large focal spot, 36-inch (91-cm) SID, and high-speed screens. Which of these factors should be changed on future hand studies to produce more optimal images?

   _____

2. A radiograph of a PA projection of the second digit reveals that the phalanges are not symmetric on both sides of the bony shafts. Which specific positioning error is involved?

   _____

3. A radiograph of a PA oblique projection of the hand reveals that the midshafts of the fourth and fifth metacarpals are superimposed. Which specific positioning error is involved?

   _____

4. In a radiographic study of the forearm, the proximal radius crossed over the ulna in the frontal projection. Which specific positioning error led to this radiographic outcome?

   _____

5. A PA axial scaphoid projection of the wrist using a 15° distal central ray angle and ulnar flexion was performed. The resulting radiograph reveals that the scaphoid bone is foreshortened. How must this projection be modified to produce a more diagnostic image of the scaphoid?

   _____

6. A radiograph of an AP elbow projection reveals considerable superimposition between the proximal radius and ulna. Which specific positioning error is involved?

   _____

7. A routine radiograph of an AP oblique elbow with lateral rotation reveals that the radial tuberosity is partially superimposed on the ulna. In what way must this position be modified during the repeat exposure?

   _____

8. A radiograph of a lateral projection of the elbow reveals that the humeral epicondyles are not superimposed and the trochlear notch is not clearly demonstrated. Which specific type of positioning error is involved?

   _____

9. **Situation:** A patient with a possible fracture of the radial head enters the emergency room. When the technologist attempts to place the arm in the AP oblique-lateral rotation position, the patient is unable to extend or rotate the elbow laterally. Which other positions can be used to demonstrate the radial head and neck without superimposition on the proximal ulna?

   _____

10. **Situation:** A patient with a metallic foreign body in the palm of the hand enters the emergency room. Which specific positions should be used to locate the foreign body?

_____

11. **Situation:** A patient with a trauma injury enters the ER with an evident Colles' fracture. Which positioning routine should be used to determine the extent of the injury?

_____

12. **Situation:** A patient with a dislocated elbow enters the ER. The patient has the elbow tightly flexed and is careful not to move it. Which specific positioning routine can be used to determine the extent of the injury?

_____

13. **Situation:** A patient with a possible fracture of the trapezium enters the ER. The routine projections do not clearly demonstrate a possible fracture. Which other special projection can be taken?

_____

14. **Situation:** A patient with a history of carpal tunnel syndrome comes to the radiology department. The orthopedic physician suspects that bony changes in the carpal sulcus may be causing compression of the median nerve. Which special projection best demonstrates this region of the wrist?

_____

15. **Situation:** A patient comes to the radiology department for a hand series to evaluate early evidence of rheumatoid arthritis. Which special position can be used in addition to the basic hand projections to evaluate this patient?

_____

16. **Situation:** A patient is referred to radiology with a possible injury to the ulnar collateral ligament. The patient complains of pain near the first MCP joint. Initial radiographs of the hand do not indicate any fracture or dislocation. Which special projection can be performed to rule out an injury to the ulnar collateral ligament?

_____

17. **Situation:** A patient enters the ER with a possible foreign body in the dorsal aspect of the wrist. Initial wrist radiographs are inconclusive in demonstrating the location of the foreign body. What additional projection can be performed to demonstrate this region of the wrist?

_____

18. **Situation:** A patient has a basic elbow series performed. The AP projection indicates a possible deformity or fracture of the coronoid process. However, the patient is unable to pronate the upper limb for the AP oblique-medial rotation projection because of an arthritic condition. What other projection could be performed to demonstrate the coronoid process?

_____

Review Exercise G: Critique Radiographs of the Upper Limb (see textbook p. 170)

The following questions relate to the radiographs found at the end of Chapter 5 in the textbook. Evaluate these radiographs for the radiographic criteria categories (A through F) that follow. Describe the corrections needed to improve the overall image. The major, or "repeatable," errors are specific errors that indicate the need for a repeat exposure, regardless of the nature of the other errors.

A. PA hand (Fig. C5-159)

Description of possible error:

1. Structures shown: _____

2. Part positioning: _____

3. Collimation and central ray: _____

4. Exposure criteria: _____

5. Anatomic side markers: _____

Repeatable error(s): _____

B. Lateral wrist (Fig. C5-160)

Description of possible error:

1. Structures shown: _____

2. Part positioning: _____

3. Collimation and central ray: _____

4. Exposure criteria: _____

5. Anatomic side markers: _____

Repeatable error(s): _____

C. AP elbow (Fig. C5-161)

Description of possible error:

1. Structures shown: _____

2. Part positioning: _____

3. Collimation and central ray: _____

4. Exposure criteria: _____

5. Anatomic side markers: _____

Repeatable error(s): _____

D. PA wrist (Fig. C5-162)

Which special wrist projection is demonstrated on this radiograph?

Description of possible error:

   1. Structures shown: _____

   2. Part positioning: _____

   3. Collimation and central ray: _____

   4. Exposure criteria: _____

   5. Anatomic side markers: _____

Repeatable error(s): _____

E. PA forearm (Fig. C5-163)

Description of possible error:

   1. Structures shown: _____

   2. Part positioning: _____

   3. Collimation and central ray: _____

   4. Exposure criteria: _____

   5. Anatomic side markers: _____

Repeatable error(s): _____

F. Lateral elbow (Fig. C5-164)

Description of possible error:

   1. Structures shown: _____

   2. Part positioning: _____

   3. Collimation and central ray: _____

   4. Exposure criteria: _____

   5. Anatomic side markers: _____

Repeatable error(s): _____

PART III: LABORATORY EXERCISES

You must gain experience in upper limb positioning before performing the following exams on actual patients. You can get experience in positioning and radiographic evaluation of these projections by performing exercises using radiographic phantoms and practicing on other students (although you will not be taking actual exposures).

The following suggested activities assume that your teaching institution has an energized lab and radiographic phantoms. If not, perform Laboratory Exercises B and C, the radiographic evaluation and the physical positioning exercises. (Check off each step and projection as you complete it.)

Laboratory Exercise A: Energized Laboratory

1. Using the hand radiographic phantom, produce radiographs of the following basic routines:

    _____ Hand (PA, oblique, lateral)   _____ Thumb (AP, oblique, lateral)

    _____ Wrist (PA, oblique, lateral)

2. Using the elbow radiographic phantom, produce radiographs of the following basic routines:

    _____ AP   _____ AP oblique, medial rotation

    _____ Lateral elbow   _____ AP oblique, lateral rotation

Laboratory Exercise B: Radiographic Evaluation

1. Evaluate and critique the radiographs produced above, additional radiographs provided by your instructor, or both. Evaluate each radiograph for the following points:

    _____ Evaluate the completeness of the study. (Are all of the pertinent anatomic structures included on the radiograph?)

    _____ Evaluate for positioning or centering errors (e.g., rotation, off centering).

    _____ Evaluate for correct exposure factors and possible motion. (Are the density and contrast of the images acceptable?)

    _____ Determine whether anatomic side markers and an acceptable degree of collimation and/or area shielding are seen on the images.

Laboratory Exercise C: Physical Positioning

1. On another person, simulate performing all of the following basic and special projections of the upper limb. Include the six steps listed below and described in the textbook. (Check off each step when completed satisfactorily.)

   Step 1. Appropriate size and type of IR with correct side markers

   Step 2. Correct central ray placement and centering of part to central ray and/or IR

   Step 3. Accurate collimation

   Step 4. Area shielding of patient where advisable

   Step 5. Use of proper immobilizing devices when needed

   Step 6. Approximate correct exposure factors, breathing instructions where applicable, and initiating exposure

Projections	*Step 1*	*Step 2*	*Step 3*	*Step 4*	*Step 5*	*Step 6*
● Second to fifth digit routines (PA, oblique, lateral)	___	___	___	___	___	___
● Thumb routine (AP, oblique, lateral)	___	___	___	___	___	___
● Hand (PA, oblique, lateral)	___	___	___	___	___	___
● Wrist basic routine (PA, oblique, lateral)	___	___	___	___	___	___
● Scaphoid, carpal canal, and carpal bridge projections	___	___	___	___	___	___
● Elbow routine (AP, oblique, lateral)	___	___	___	___	___	___
● Partial flexion APs	___	___	___	___	___	___
● Acute flexion (Jones)	___	___	___	___	___	___
● Trauma axial laterals (Coyle)	___	___	___	___	___	___
● Radial head projections	___	___	___	___	___	___
● Forearm routine (AP, lateral)	___	___	___	___	___	___

This self-test should be taken only after completing all of the readings, review exercises, and laboratory activities for a particular section. The purpose of this test is not only to provide a good learning exercise but also to serve as a strong indicator of what your final unit evaluation exam will cover. It is strongly suggested that if you do not get at least a 90% to 95% grade on each self-test that you review those areas in which you missed questions before going to your instructor for the final unit evaluation exam.

1. A. How many bones make up the phalanges of the hand?
   A. 14   C. 5
   B. 8   D. 16

   B. How many bones make up the carpal region?
   A. 14   C. 5
   B. 8   D. 7

   C. What is the total number of bones that make up the hand and wrist?
   A. 21   C. 26
   B. 27   D. 32

2. Match the following joint locations with the correct term.

_____ A. Between the two phalanges of the first digit (thumb)   1. Radiocarpal

_____ B. Between the first metacarpal and the proximal phalanx of the thumb   2. Fourth DIP

_____ C. Between the middle and distal phalanges of the fourth digit   3. Fourth PIP

_____ D. Between the carpals and the first metacarpal   4. First MCP

_____ E. Between the forearm and the carpals   5. First CMC

_____ F. Between the distal radius and ulna   6. Distal radioulnar

                                              7. IP

3. Match each of the structures labeled on Fig. 5-12 to its correct term.

    _____ A.   1. Distal phalanx of fourth digit

    _____ B.   2. Head of fifth metacarpal

    _____ C.   3. Base of fourth metacarpal

    _____ D.   4. Scaphoid

    _____ E.   5. Base of first metacarpal

    _____ F.   6. Pisiform

    _____ G.   7. Trapezoid

    _____ H.   8. Body of proximal phalanx of fifth digit

    _____ I.   9. Fifth carpometacarpal joint

    _____ J.   10. Triquetrum

    _____ K.   11. Radius

    _____ L.   12. Proximal phalanx of first digit

    _____ M.   13. Radiocarpal joint

    _____ N.   14. Hamate

    _____ O.   15. Capitate

    _____ P.   16. Distal interphalangeal joint of fifth digit

    _____ Q.   17. Trapezium

    _____ R.   18. First metacarpophalangeal joint

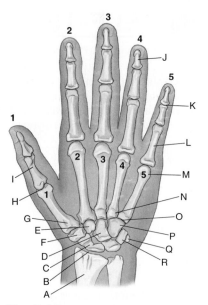

Fig. 5-12. Osteology of the hand and wrist.

4. Which carpal contains a "hooklike" process?
   A. Scaphoid   C. Hamate
   B. Trapezium   D. Pisiform

5. Which carpal articulates with the thumb?
   A. Scaphoid   C. Trapezoid
   B. Lunate   D. Trapezium

6. Which carpal is most commonly fractured?
   A. Scaphoid   C. Trapezium
   B. Capitate   D. Triquetrum

7. Which two carpal bones are located most anteriorly as seen on a lateral wrist radiograph? (HINT: They are on the radial side of the wrist.)
   A. Hamate and pisiform   C. Capitate and lunate
   B. Trapezium and trapezoid   D. Scaphoid and trapezium

8. Match each of the structures of the wrist labeled on Figs. 5-13, 5-14, and 5-15 to its correct term.

_____ A.   1. Pisiform

_____ B.   2. Trapezoid

_____ C.   3. Scaphoid

_____ D.   4. Triquetrum

_____ E.   5. Base of first metacarpal

_____ F.   6. Radius

_____ G.   7. Lunate

_____ H.   8. Trapezium

_____ I.   9. Hamate

_____ J.   10. Ulna

_____ K.   11. Capitate

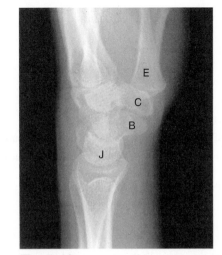

Fig. 5-13. Lateral wrist.

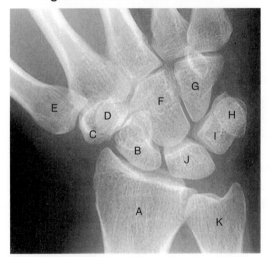

Fig. 5-14. Wrist.

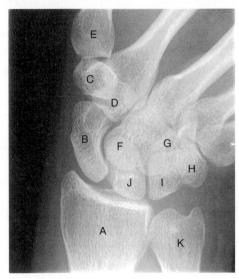

Fig. 5-15. Wrist.

9. Which wrist projection does Fig. 5-14 represent?
   A. PA wrist
   B. PA—ulnar deviation
   C. PA—radial deviation
   D. Carpal canal

10. Which one of the following carpals is *not* well seen in the projection in Fig. 5-14?
    A. Pisiform
    B. Lunate
    C. Scaphoid
    D. Triquetrum

11. Which projection does Fig. 5-15 represent?
    A. PA—ulnar deviation
    B. Carpal canal
    C. PA—radial deviation
    D. Modified Stecher method

12. Which one of the following carpal bones is best demonstrated in the projection in Fig. 5-15?
    A. Trapezium
    B. Scaphoid
    C. Trapezoid
    D. Hamate

13. Which bone of the upper limb contains the coronoid process?
    A. Humerus
    B. First metacarpal
    C. Radius
    D. Ulna

14. Where are the coronoid and radial fossae located?
    A. Anterior aspect of distal humerus
    B. Posterior aspect of distal humerus
    C. Proximal radius and ulna
    D. Distal end of radius

15. Which two bony landmarks are palpated to assist with positioning of the upper limb?
    A. Coronoid and olecranon processes
    B. Pisiform and hamate
    C. Lateral and medial epicondyle
    D. Radial and ulnar styloid processes

16. Where is the coronoid tubercle located?
    A. Medial aspect of coronoid process
    B. Anterior aspect of distal humerus
    C. Lateral aspect of proximal radius
    D. Posterior aspect of distal humerus

17. In an erect anatomic position, which one of the following structures is considered to be most inferior or distal?
    A. Head of ulna
    B. Olecranon process
    C. Radial tuberosity
    D. Head of radius

18. Match the following articulations to the correct joint movement type (each joint movement type may be used more than once).

    _____ A. Intercarpal joints   1. Sellar

    _____ B. Radiocarpal joint   2. Ginglymus

    _____ C. Elbow joint   3. Ellipsoidal

    _____ D. First carpometacarpal joint   4. Plane

    _____ E. Third carpometacarpal joint

110

19. The following four radiographs represent the most common routine or basic projections for the elbow. Match each of these projections to the correct figure number.

_____ A. Fig. 5-16   1. AP projection

_____ B. Fig. 5-17   2. Lateral position

_____ C. Fig. 5-18   3. AP oblique—lateral rotation

_____ D. Fig. 5-19   4. AP oblique—medial rotation

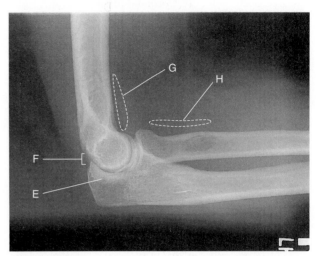

Fig. 5-16.

Identify the soft tissue and bony structures labeled on Figs. 5-16, 5-17, 5-18, and 5-19 (terms may be used more than once).

_____ E.   1. Trochlea

_____ F.   2. Olecranon process

_____ G.   3. Coronoid process

_____ H.   4. Medial epicondyle

_____ I.   5. Supinator fat pad

_____ J.   6. Capitulum

_____ K.   7. Anterior fat pad

_____ L.   8. Radial head and neck

_____ M.   9. Region of posterior fat pad

_____ N.   10. Coronoid tubercle

_____ O.

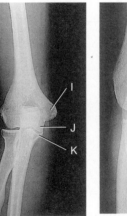

Fig. 5-17.   **Fig. 5-18.**   **Fig. 5-19.**

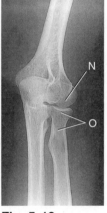

20. Identify each of the structures labeled on Figs. 5-20 and 5-21 with its correct term.

_____ A.   1. Coronoid fossa

_____ B.   2. Medial epicondyle

_____ C.   3. Head of radius

_____ D.   4. Trochlea

_____ E.*   5. Radial tuberosity

_____ F.*   6. Coronoid process

_____ G.   7. Lateral epicondyle

_____ H.   8. Capitulum

_____ I.   9. Trochlear sulcus

_____ J.   10. Coronoid tubercle

_____ K.   11. Radial fossa

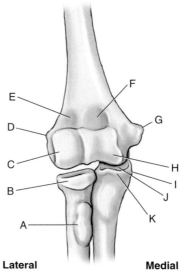

Lateral   **Medial**

Fig. 5-20. Anterior view of the elbow.

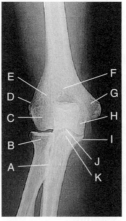

Fig. 5-21. Elbow. Anteroposterior (AP) extended.

21. True/False: To visualize fat pads surrounding the elbow, exposure factors must be adjusted to see both bony and soft tissue structures.

22. True/False: Fat pads of the elbow are normally seen on correctly positioned and correctly exposed anteroposterior (AP) elbow projections.

23. Why should a forearm never be taken as a PA projection?
    A. Too painful for the patient
    B. Causes the proximal radius to cross over the ulna
    C. Causes the distal radius to cross over the ulna
    D. Increases the object image receptor distance (OID) of the distal radius

---

*Not visible on radiograph

24. In what position should the hand be for an AP elbow projection?
    A. Supinated   C. Rotated 20° from supinated position
    B. Pronated   D. True lateral position

25. In what position should the hand be for an AP medial rotation oblique elbow position?
    A. Supinated   C. Rotated 20° from supinated position
    B. Pronated   D. True lateral position

26. Match the projection of the elbow that best demonstrates each of the following structures:

    _____ A. Coronoid process in profile   1. Lateral elbow

    _____ B. Radial head and tuberosity without superimposition   2. AP elbow

    _____ C. Olecranon process in profile   3. AP, medial rotation oblique

    _____ D. Coronoid tubercle   4. AP, lateral rotation oblique

    _____ E. Trochlear notch in profile

    _____ F. Capitulum and lateral epicondyle in profile

    _____ G. Olecranon process seated in olecranon fossa

27. True/False: Lead masking is not required when placing multiple images on the same digital image receptor (IR) plate.

28. The long axis of the anatomic part being imaged should be placed:
    A. Perpendicular to the long axis of the IR
    B. Parallel to the long axis of the IR
    C. 30° angle to the long axis of the IR
    D. Any way that will accommodate multiple images being placed on a single IR

29. *Arthrography* is a radiographic study of:
    A. Fat pads and stripes
    B. Epiphyses of long bones
    C. Medullary aspect of long bones
    D. Soft tissues structures within certain synovial joints

30. Match each of the following pathologic terms to its correct definition.

_____ 1. Accumulated fluid within the joint cavity   A. Skier's thumb

_____ 2. A reduction in the quantity of bone or atrophy of skeletal tissue   B. Bursitis

_____ 3. Local or generalized infection of bone or bone marrow   C. Carpal tunnel syndrome

_____ 4. Reverse of a Colles' fracture   D. Bennett's fracture

_____ 5. Inflammation of the fluid-filled sacs enclosing the joints   E. Smith fracture

_____ 6. Fracture of the base of the first metacarpal   F. Joint effusion

_____ 7. Sprain or tear of the ulnar collateral ligament   G. Osteomyelitis

_____ 8. Painful disorder of hand and wrist from compression of the median resulting nerve   H. Osteoporosis

31. Which one of the following pathologic indications requires a decrease in manual exposure factors?
    A. Paget's disease
    B. Advanced osteopetrosis
    C. Advanced osteoporosis
    D. Joint effusion

32. Where is the central ray centered for a PA projection of the second digit?
    A. Affected PIP joint
    B. Affected middle phalanx
    C. Affected MCP joint
    D. Affected CMC joint

33. Why is it important to keep the long axis of the digit parallel to the IR?
    A. To reduce distortion of the phalanges
    B. To properly visualize joints
    C. To demonstrate small fractures
    D. All of the above

34. Where is the central ray placed for a PA projection of the hand?
    A. Second MCP joint
    B. Third MCP joint
    C. Middle phalanx of third digit
    D. Third PIP joint

35. What is the major disadvantage of performing a PA projection of the thumb rather than an AP?
    A. Increased OID
    B. Increase in patient dose
    C. More painful for patient
    D. Awkward position for patient

36. What type of fracture is best demonstrated with a modified Robert's method?
    A. Barton fracture
    B. Colles' fracture
    C. Bennett's fracture
    D. Smith fracture

37. True/False: Both hands are examined with one single exposure when using the Norgaard method.

38. True/False: The hand(s) is (are) placed in a true PA position when using the Norgaard method.

39. Choose the *best* set of exposure factors for upper limb radiography.
    A. 75 kV, 200 mA, ½₀ second, small focal spot, 40-inch (102-cm) SID, high-speed screens
    B. 75 kV, 600 mA, ½₀ second, large focal spot, 40-inch (102-cm) SID, detail-speed screens
    C. 64 kV, 100 mA, ⅒ second, small focal spot, 40-inch (102-cm) SID, high-speed screens
    D. 64 kV, 200 mA, ½₀ second, small focal spot, 40-inch (102-cm) SID, detail-speed screens

40. True/False: The midline dose for a lateral forearm is greater than the skin dose for a PA finger.

41. A radiograph of a PA oblique of the hand reveals that the midaspect of the third, fourth, and fifth metacarpals is slightly superimposed. What must be done to correct this positioning problem on the repeat exposure?
    A. Increase obliquity of the hand   C. Decrease obliquity of the hand
    B. Spread fingers out further   D. Form a tight fist with the fingers

42. A radiograph of an AP elbow projection demonstrates total separation between the proximal radius and ulna. What must be done to correct this positioning error on the repeat exposure?
    A. Rotate upper limb medially   C. Angle central ray 5° to 10° caudad
    B. Rotate upper limb laterally   D. Fully extend elbow

43. A radiograph of the carpal canal (inferosuperior) projection reveals that the pisiform and hamulus are superimposed. What can be done to correct this problem on the repeat exposure?
    A. Flex wrist slightly   C. Rotate wrist laterally 5° to 10°
    B. Extend wrist slightly   D. Rotate wrist medially 5° to 10°

44. A radiograph of an AP oblique-medial rotation reveals that the coronoid process is not in profile and the radial head is only partially superimposed over the ulna. What specific positioning error was involved?
    A. Insufficient medial rotation   C. Excessive extension of elbow
    B. Excessive medial rotation   D. Excessive flexion of elbow

45. A radiograph of a lateral projection of the elbow reveals that the epicondyles are not superimposed and the trochlear notch is not clearly seen. What must be done to correct this positioning error during the repeat exposure?
    A. Angle central ray 45° toward shoulder   C. Angle central ray 45° away from shoulder
    B. Place humerus/forearm in same horizontal plane   D. Extend elbow to form an 80° horizontal plane angle

46. **Situation:** A patient with a possible Barton fracture enters the emergency room. Which positioning routine should be performed to confirm the diagnosis?
    A. Elbow   C. Hand
    B. Wrist   D. Thumb

47. **Situation:** A patient with a possible Smith fracture enters the emergency room. Which positioning routine should be performed to confirm this diagnosis?
    A. Hand   C. Wrist/forearm
    B. Thumb   D. Elbow

48. **Situation:** A patient has a Colles' fracture reduced, and a large plaster cast is placed on the upper limb. The orthopedic surgeon orders a postreduction study. The original technique, used before the cast placement, involved 60 kV and 5 mAs. What new technique measurements should be used with a wet plaster cast?
    A. Same measurements   C. 65 kV and 5 mAs
    B. 75 to 78 kV and 10 mAs   D. 68 to 70 kV or 10 mAs

49. **Situation:** A pediatric patient with a possible radial head fracture is brought into the emergency room. It is too painful for the patient to extend the elbow beyond 90°or rotate the hand. What type of special (i.e., optional) projection could be performed on this patient to confirm the diagnosis without causing further discomfort?

    A. Coyle method   C. Norgaard method

    B. Modified Robert's method   D. Modified Stecher method

50. For the following critique questions, refer to the AP elbow projection radiograph shown in Fig. C5-161 in your textbook.

    A. Which positioning error(s) is (are) visible on this radiograph? (More than one answer may be selected.)

        (a) All essential anatomic structures are not demonstrated.

        (b) Central ray is centered incorrectly.

        (c) Collimation is not evident.

        (d) Exposure factors are incorrect.

        (e) No anatomic side marker is visible.

        (f) Excessive rotation in the lateral direction is evident.

        (g) Insufficient rotation in the lateral direction is evident.

        (h) Excessive flexion of the joint is evident.

    B. Which criteria error(s) identified above is (are) considered "repeatable"? _____

    C. Which of the following modifications must be made during the repeat exposure? (More than one answer may be selected.)

        (a) Increase collimation.

        (b) Center central ray correctly.

        (c) Decrease exposure factors.

        (d) Increase exposure factors.

        (e) Place anatomic side marker on IR before exposure.

        (f) Rotate elbow slightly more in the medial direction.

        (g) Rotate elbow slightly more in the lateral direction.

        (h) Extend elbow completely.

51. For the following critique questions, refer to the PA wrist projection (shown in Fig. C5-162 in the textbook.)

    A. Which special wrist projection does this represent?

        (a) Ulnar deviation

        (b) Radial deviation

    B. Which positioning error(s) is (are) visible on this radiograph? (More than one answer may be selected.)

        (a) All essential anatomic structures are not demonstrated.

        (b) Central ray is centered incorrectly.

        (c) Exposure factors are incorrect.

        (d) No anatomic marker is visible.

        (e) Excessive rotation in the lateral direction is evident.

        (f) Excessive rotation in the medial direction is evident.

        (g) Excessive deviation of the joint is evident.

    C. Which criteria error(s) identified above is (are) considered "repeatable"? _____

D. Which of the following modifications must be made during the repeat exposure? (More than one answer may be selected.)

(a) Open up collimation to include all soft tissue and bony structures.

(b) Center central ray correctly to midcarpal region.

(c) Decrease exposure factors.

(d) Increase exposure factors.

(e) Place marker on IR before exposure.

(f) Pronate hand toward IR.

(g) Supinate hand away from IR.

(h) Extend wrist.

(i) Increase deviation movement.

(j) Decrease deviation movement.

6 Humerus and Shoulder Girdle

CHAPTER OBJECTIVES

After you have successfully completed the activities in this chapter, you will be able to:

_____ 1. Identify the bones and specific features of the proximal humerus and shoulder girdle.

_____ 2. On drawings and radiographs, identify specific anatomic structures of the proximal humerus and the shoulder girdle.

_____ 3. Match specific joints of the shoulder girdle to their structural classification and movement type.

_____ 4. Describe anatomic relationships of prominent structures of the proximal humerus and the shoulder girdle.

_____ 5. On radiographic images, identify rotational positions of the proximal humerus.

_____ 6. List the technical and shielding considerations commonly used for proximal humerus and shoulder girdle radiography.

_____ 7. Match specific pathologic indications of the shoulder girdle to the correct definition.

_____ 8. Match specific pathologic indications of the shoulder girdle to the correct radiographic appearance.

_____ 9. For select forms of pathologic conditions of the shoulder girdle, indicate whether manual exposure factors should be increased or decreased or remain the same.

_____ 10. List basic and special projections of the humerus and shoulder, including the type and size of IR holder, the central ray location with correct angles, and the structures best demonstrated.

_____ 11. List the various patient dose ranges for select projections of the humerus and shoulder.

_____ 12. Given various hypothetical situations, identify the correct modification of a position and/or exposure factors to improve the radiographic image.

_____ 13. Given various hypothetical situations, identify the correct position for a specific pathologic feature or condition.

_____ 14. Given radiographs of specific humerus and shoulder girdle projections, identify specific positioning and exposure factor errors.

POSITIONING AND RADIOGRAPHIC CRITIQUE

_____ 1. Using a peer, position the patient for basic and special projections of the humerus and shoulder girdle.

_____ 2. Using a shoulder radiographic phantom, produce satisfactory radiographs of the shoulder girdle (if equipment is available).

_____ 3. Critique and evaluate shoulder girdle radiographs based on the four divisions of radiographic criteria: (1) structures shown, (2) position, (3) collimation and central ray, and (4) exposure criteria.

_____ 4. Distinguish between acceptable and unacceptable shoulder girdle radiographs based on exposure factors, motion, collimation, positioning, or other errors.

LEARNING EXERCISES

Complete the following review exercises after reading the associated pages in the textbook as indicated by each exercise. Answers to each review exercise are given at the end of the review exercises.

PART I: RADIOGRAPHIC ANATOMY
Review Exercise A: Radiographic Anatomy of the Proximal Humerus and Shoulder Girdle
(see textbook pp. 172-176)

1. The shoulder girdle consists of (A) _____, (B) _____, and

   (C) _____.

2. Identify the labeled parts on Figs. 6-1 and 6-2. Include secondary terms in parentheses where indicated.

   A. _____ (_____)

   B. _____ (_____)

   C. _____

   D. _____

   E. _____ (_____)

   F. _____

   G. Which projection (internal, external, or neutral rotation) of the proximal humerus is represented by this drawing

      and radiograph? _____

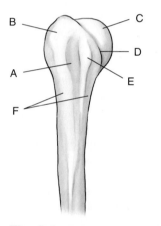

Fig. 6-1. Frontal view, proximal humerus.

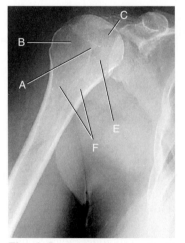

Fig. 6-2. Radiograph, proximal humerus.

3. The three aspects of the clavicle are the (A) _____, (B) _____, and

(C) _____.

4. The _____ (male or female) clavicle tends to be thicker and more curved in shape.

5. The three angles of the scapula include the (A) _____, (B) _____,

and (C) _____.

6. The anterior surface of the scapula is referred to as the _____ surface.

7. What is the anatomic name for the armpit? _____

8. What are the names of the two fossae located on the posterior scapula?

A. _____   B. _____

9. All of the joints of the shoulder girdle are classified as being _____.

10. List the movement types for the following joints:

A. Scapulohumeral: _____

B. Sternoclavicular: _____

C. Acromioclavicular: _____

11. Match each of the following anatomic structures with its correct location.

_____ 1. Greater tubercle   A. Scapula

_____ 2. Coracoid process   B. Clavicle

_____ 3. Crest of spine   C. Proximal humerus

_____ 4. Coronoid process   D. Not part of the shoulder girdle

_____ 5. Acromial extremity

_____ 6. Intertubercular groove

_____ 7. Condylar process

_____ 8. Surgical neck

12. Identify the following structures labeled on Figs. 6-3 and 6-4. Include secondary terms in parentheses where indicated.

A. _____

B. _____

(_____)

C. _____

D. _____

E. _____

F. _____

G. _____

(_____) border

H. _____

(_____) border

I. _____

(_____) surface

J. _____

(_____) surface

K. _____

L. _____

M. _____

N. _____ (_____)

O. _____

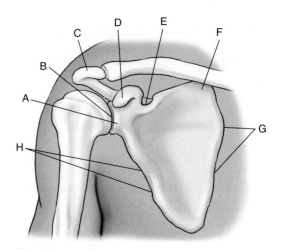

Fig. 6-3. Frontal view, scapula.

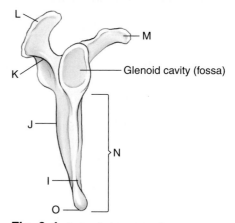

Fig. 6-4. Lateral view, scapula.

13. Identify the structures labeled on Fig. 6-5.

A. _____

B. _____ joint

C. _____

D. _____

E. _____

F. _____

G. Is this an **internal** or **external** rotation
AP projection of the proximal humerus and shoulder?

_____

H. Does Fig. 6-5 represent an **AP** or a **lateral**
projection of the proximal humerus?

_____

I. Are the epicondyles of the distal humerus **parallel** or
perpendicular to the IR on this projection?

_____

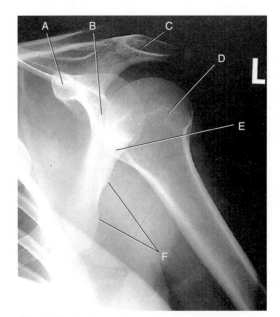

Fig. 6-5. Radiograph.

Identify the structures labeled on Fig. 6-6.

J. _____

K. _____

L. _____

M. _____

N. What is the correct term to describe the projection

shown in Fig. 6-6? _____

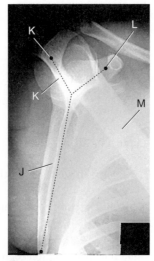

Fig. 6-6. Radiograph.

14. Identify the structures labeled on Fig. 6-7.

   A. _____

   B. _____

   C. _____

   D. _____

   E. What is the name of the projection shown in Fig. 6-7?

   _____

   F. How much (at what angle) should the affected arm be abducted from the body for this projection?

   _____

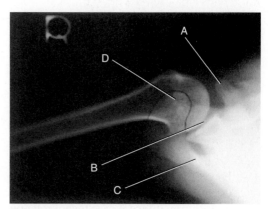

Fig. 6-7. Radiograph.

PART II: RADIOGRAPHIC POSITIONING
Review Exercise B: Positioning of the Humerus and Shoulder Girdle (see textbook pp. 177-202)

1. Identify the correct proximal humerus rotation for the each of the following.

   _____ 1. Greater tubercle profiled laterally   A. External rotation

   _____ 2. Humeral epicondyles angled 45° to image receptor (IR) B. Internal rotation

   _____ 3. Epicondyles perpendicular to IR   C. Neutral rotation

   _____ 4. Supination of hand

   _____ 5. Palm of hand against thigh

   _____ 6. Epicondyles parallel to IR

   _____ 7. Lesser tubercle profiled medially

   _____ 8. Proximal humerus in a lateral position

   _____ 9. Proximal humerus in position for an anteroposterior (AP) projection

2. Identify the proximal humerus rotation represented on the radiographs in Figs. 6-8 to 6-10.

   A. Fig. 6-8 represents _____ rotation.

   B. Fig. 6-9 represents _____ rotation.

   C. Fig. 6-10 represents _____ rotation.

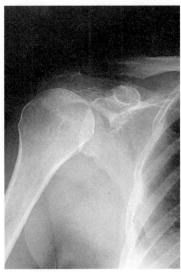

Fig. 6-8. Proximal humerus.

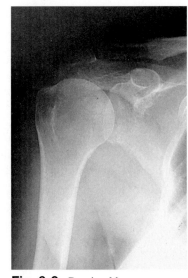

Fig. 6-9. Proximal humerus.

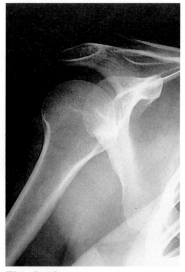

Fig. 6-10. Proximal humerus.

3. Indicate whether each of the following positioning and technical considerations is true or false for the shoulder girdle.

A. True/False: The use of a grid is not required for shoulders that measure less than 10 cm.

B. True/False: The kV range for adult shoulder projections is between 80 and 90 kV.

C. True/False: Low mA with short exposure times should be used for adult shoulder studies.

D. True/False: Large focal spot setting should be selected for most adult shoulder studies.

E. True/False: A high-speed screen-IR system is recommended for shoulder studies when using a grid.

F. True/False: A 72-inch (180-cm) source-image distance (SID) is recommended for most shoulder girdle studies.

G. True/False: The gonadal dose for most shoulder projections is 0.1 mrad or less.

H. True/False: The use of contact shields over the breast, lung, and thyroid regions is recommended for most shoulder projections.

4. Which one of the following kV ranges should be used for a shoulder series on an average adult?
   A. 70 to 80 kV   C. 80 to 90 kV
   B. 55 to 60 kV   D. 65 to 75 kV

5. If physical immobilization is required, which individual should be asked to restrain a child for a shoulder series?
   A. Parent or guardian   C. Radiography student
   B. Radiologic technologist   D. Nurse aide

6. True/False: CT arthrography of the shoulder joint requires the use of iodinated contrast media injected into the joint space.

7. True/False: Magnetic resonance imaging (MRI) is an excellent modality for demonstrating nondisplaced fractures of the shoulder girdle.

8. True/False: Nuclear medicine bone scans can demonstrate signs of osteomyelitis and cellulitis.

9. True/False: Radiography is more sensitive than nuclear medicine for demonstrating physiologic aspects of the shoulder girdle.

10. True/False: Ultrasound can provide a functional (dynamic) evaluation of joint movement that MRI cannot.

11. Match each of the following pathologic indications to its correct definition.

_____ 1. Compression between the greater tuberosity and soft tissues on the coracoacromial ligamentous and osseous arch

_____ 2. Injury of the anteroinferior glenoid labrum

_____ 3. Inflammatory condition of the tendon

_____ 4. Superior displacement of the distal clavicle

_____ 5. Compression fracture of the articular surface of the humeral head

_____ 6. Traumatic injury to one or more of the supportive muscles of the shoulder girdle

_____ 7. Atrophy of skeletal tissue

A. Acromioclavicular joint dislocation

B. Bankart lesion

C. Hill-Sachs defect

D. Impingement syndrome

E. Osteoporosis

F. Rotator cuff tear

G. Tendonitis

12. Match the following radiographic appearances to the correct pathologic indication.

_____ 1. Subacromial spurs

_____ 2. Fluid-filled joint space

_____ 3. Thin bony cortex

_____ 4. Abnormal widening of acromioclavicular joint space

_____ 5. Calcified tendons

_____ 6. Avulsion fracture of the glenoid rim

_____ 7. Narrowing of joint space

_____ 8. Closed joint space

_____ 9. Compression fracture of humeral head

A. Rheumatoid arthritis

B. Bankart lesion

C. Hill-Sachs defect

D. Osteoarthritis

E. Bursitis

F. Osteoporosis

G. Impingement syndrome

H. Acromioclavicular joint separation

I. Tendonitis

13. Which one of the following pathologic indications requires a decrease in manual exposure factors?
   A. Impingement syndrome
   B. Bursitis
   C. Bankart lesion
   D. Osteoporosis

14. Which two basic shoulder projections are routinely taken for a shoulder (with no traumatic injury) and proximal humerus?

A. _____   B. _____

15. Specifically, where is the central ray placed for an AP projection of the shoulder? _____

_____

16. Which lateral projection can be performed to demonstrate the *entire* humerus for a patient with a midhumeral fracture?

_____

17. To best demonstrate a possible Hill-Sachs defect, which additional positioning technique can be added to the infero-superior axial projection?
    A. Angle central ray 10° to 15° caudad   C. Angle central ray 3° to 5° caudad
    B. Rotate affected arm externally approximately 45°   D. Place humeral epicondyles parallel to IR

18. What type of central ray angulation is required for the inferosuperior axial projection for the shoulder?
    A. 25° to 30° medially   C. 25° anterior and 25° medially
    B. 35° to 45° medially   D. Central ray perpendicular to IR

19. The _____ projection of the shoulder produces an image of the glenoid process in profile.

This projection is also referred to as the _____ method.

20. Which one of the following projections produces a tangential projection of the intertubercular groove?
    A. Tangential projection (Fisk modification)   C. Hobbs modification
    B. Grashey method   D. Lawrence method

21. The supine version of the tangential projection for the intertubercular groove requires that the central ray be angled

_____ posteriorly from the horizontal plane.

22. Which one of the following projections would be best for demonstrating a possible dislocation of the proximal humerus?
    A. Grashey method   C. Inferosuperior axiolateral projection
    B. Tangential projection (Fisk modification)   D. Scapular Y

23. The _____ projection is the special projection of the shoulder that best demonstrates the acromiohumeral space for possible subacromial spurs, which create shoulder impingement symptoms.

This projection is also referred to as the _____ method.

24. Which of the following nontrauma projections can be performed erect to provide a lateral view of the proximal humerus in relationship to the glenohumeral joint?
    A. Tangential projection (Fisk modification)
    B. Inferosuperior axial projection (Clements modification)
    C. Superoinferior axial projection (Hobbs modification)
    D. Posterior oblique position (Grashey method)

25. How much is the CR angled for the inferosuperior axial projection (Clements modification) if the patient cannot fully abduct the arm 90°?
    A. 5° to 15°   C. 25° to 30°
    B. 45°   D. 20°

26. What CR angle is required for the AP axial projection (Alexander method) for AC joints?
    A. 25° cephalad   C. 5° to 10° caudad
    B. 45° caudad   D. 15° cephalad

27. True/False: The superoinferior axial projection (Hobbs modification) requires no CR angle.

28. True/False: The transthoracic lateral projection can be performed for possible fractures or dislocations of the proximal humerus.

29. True/False: The use of a breathing technique is recommended for the transthoracic lateral humerus projection.

30. True/False: The affected arm must be placed into external rotation for the transthoracic lateral projection.

31. True/False: A central ray angle of 10° to 15° caudad may be used for the transthoracic lateral projections if the patient is unable to elevate the uninjured arm and shoulder sufficiently.

32. True/False: The scapular Y lateral (anterior oblique) position requires the body to be rotated 45° to 60° anteriorly toward the affected side.

33. Which one of the following shoulder projections delivers the greatest skin dose to the patient?
    A. AP axial clavicle   C. Transthoracic lateral
    B. AP projection, neutral position   D. Tangential projection for intertubercular groove

34. Which of the following requires the smallest thyroid dose?
    A. AP neutral rotation shoulder   C. AP clavicle
    B. Transthoracic lateral   D. Scapular Y lateral

35. Which of the following would result in the highest thyroid dose?
    A. AP neutral rotation shoulder   C. AP clavicle
    B. Transthoracic lateral   D. Scapular Y lateral

36. Which special projection of the shoulder requires that the affected side be rotated 45° toward the cassette and uses a

    45° caudad central ray angle? _____

37. A posterior dislocation of the humerus projects the humeral head _____ (**superior** or **inferior**) to the glenoid cavity with the special projection described in the previous question.

38. A thin-shouldered patient requires _____ (more or less) CR angle for an AP axial clavicle projection than a large-shouldered patient.

39. What must be ruled out before performing the weight-bearing study for acromioclavicular joints?

    _____

40. Match each of the following projections with its corresponding method name. Method names may be used more than once.

_____ 1. Inferosuperior axial

_____ 2. AP oblique for glenoid cavity

_____ 3. Tangential for intertubercular (bicipital) groove

_____ 4. Supraspinatus outlet tangential

_____ 5. Transthoracic lateral

_____ 6. AP apical oblique axial

A. Neer method

B. Grashey method

C. Lawrence method

D. Fisk modification

E. Garth method

Review Exercise C: Problem Solving for Technical and Positioning Errors

1. The following factors were used to produce a radiograph of an AP projection of the shoulder: 85 kV, 20 mAs, high-speed screens, 40-inch (102-cm) SID, grid, and suspended respiration. The resultant radiograph demonstrated poor radiographic contrast between bony and soft tissue structures. Which of these factors can be altered during the repeat exposure to improve radiographic quality?

_____

2. A radiograph of an AP axial clavicle projection reveals that the clavicle is projected below the superior border of the scapula. What can the technologist do to correct this problem during the repeat exposure?

_____

3. A radiograph of an AP scapula reveals that the scapula is within the lung field and difficult to see. Which two things can the technologist do to improve the visibility of the scapula during the repeat exposure?

_____

4. A radiograph of an AP projection (with external rotation) of a shoulder (with no traumatic injury) reveals that neither the greater nor lesser tubercles are profiled. What must be done to correct this during the repeat exposure?

_____

5. A radiograph of a lateral scapula position reveals that it is not a true lateral projection. (Considerable separation exists between the axillary and vertebral borders.) The projection was taken using the following factors: erect position, 40-inch (102-cm) SID, 45° rotation toward cassette from posteroanterior (PA), central ray centered to midscapula, and no central ray angulation. Based on these factors, how can this position be improved during the repeat exposure?

_____

6. A radiograph of the AP oblique (Grashey method) taken as a 35° oblique projection reveals that the borders of the glenoid cavity are not superimposed. The patient had large, rounded shoulders. What must be done to get better superimposition of the cavity during the repeat exposure?

_____

7. **Situation:** A patient with a possible right shoulder dislocation enters the emergency room. The technologist attempts to perform an erect transthoracic lateral projection, but the patient is unable to raise the left arm and shoulder high enough. The resultant radiograph reveals that the shoulders are superimposed, and the right shoulder and humeral head are not well visualized. What can be done to improve this image during the repeat exposure?

_____

8. **Situation:** A patient with a possible fracture of the right proximal humerus from an automobile accident enters the emergency room. The patient has other injuries and is unable to stand or sit erect. Which positioning routine should

be used to determine the extent of the injury? _____

9. **Situation:** A patient with a clinical history of chronic shoulder dislocation comes to the radiology department. The orthopedic physician suspects that a Hill-Sachs defect may be present. Which specific position(s) may be used to best

demonstrate this pathologic feature? _____

10. **Situation:** A patient with a possible Bankart lesion comes to the radiology department. List three projections that can be performed that may demonstrate signs of this injury.

A. _____

B. _____

C. _____

11. **Situation:** A patient with a possible rotator cuff tear comes to the radiology department. Which one of the following imaging modalities would best demonstrate this injury?
   A. Arthrography
   B. MRI
   C. Nuclear medicine
   D. Radiography

12. **Situation:** A patient with a clinical history of tendon injury in the shoulder region comes to the radiology department. The orthopedic physician needs a *functional* study of the shoulder joint performed to determine the extent of the tendon injury. Which of the following modalities would best demonstrate this injury?
   A. Arthrography
   B. MRI
   C. Ultrasound
   D. Nuclear medicine

13. A radiograph of an AP projection with external rotation of the shoulder does not demonstrate either the greater or lesser tubercle in profile. What is the most likely cause for this radiographic outcome?

_____

14. A radiograph of a transthoracic lateral projection demonstrates considerable superimposition of lung markings and ribs over the region of the proximal shoulder. What can the technologist do to minimize this problem during the repeat exposure?

_____

15. **Situation:** A patient enters the ER with a definite fracture to the midhumerus. Due to other trauma the patient is unable to stand. Which lateral projection would demonstrate the entire humerus?

_____

16. **Situation:** The AP apical oblique axial projection (Garth method) is performed on a patient with a shoulder injury. The resultant radiograph demonstrates the proximal humeral head projected below the glenoid cavity. What type of trauma or pathology is indicated with this radiographic appearance?

_____

Review Exercise D: Critique Radiographs of the Humerus and Shoulder Girdle (see textbook p. 203)

The following questions relate to the radiographs found at the end of Chapter 6 of the textbook. Evaluate these radiographs for the radiographic criteria categories (1 through 5) that follow. Describe the corrections needed to improve the overall image. The major, or "repeatable," errors are specific errors that indicate the need for a repeat exposure, regardless of the nature of the other errors.

A. AP clavicle (Fig. C6-96)

Description of possible error:

    1. Structures shown: _____

    2. Part positioning: _____

    3. Collimation and central ray: _____

    4. Exposure criteria: _____

    5. Anatomic side markers: _____

Repeatable error(s): _____

B. AP shoulder—external rotation (C6-97)

Description of possible error:

    1. Structures shown: _____

    2. Part positioning: _____

    3. Collimation and central ray: _____

    4. Exposure criteria: _____

    5. Anatomic side markers: _____

Repeatable error(s): _____

C. AP scapula (Fig. C6-98)

Description of possible error:

    1. Structures shown: _____

    2. Part positioning: _____

    3. Collimation and central ray: _____

4. Exposure criteria:_____

5. Anatomic side markers:_____

Repeatable error(s):_____

D. AP humerus (Fig. C6-99)

Description of possible error:

1. Structures shown:_____

2. Part positioning:_____

3. Collimation and central ray:_____

4. Exposure criteria:_____

5. Anatomic side markers:_____

Repeatable error(s):_____

Which projection (AP, lateral, or oblique) and which rotation of the proximal humerus are evident (internal, external, or

neutral)?_____

PART III: LABORATORY EXERCISES

You must gain experience in positioning each part of the humerus and shoulder girdle before performing the following exams on actual patients. You can get experience in positioning and radiographic evaluation of these projections by performing exercises using radiographic phantoms and practicing on other students (although you will not be taking actual exposures).

The following suggested activities assume that your teaching institution has an energized lab and radiographic phantoms. If not, perform Laboratory Exercises B and C, the radiographic evaluation and the physical positioning exercises. (Check off each step and projection as you complete it.)

Laboratory Exercise A: Energized Laboratory

1. Using the thorax radiographic phantom, produce radiographs of the following basic routines:

_____ AP shoulder   _____ AP oblique (Grashey method)

_____ AP and AP axial clavicle   _____ AP and lateral scapula

Laboratory Exercise B: Radiographic Evaluation

1. Evaluate and critique the radiographs produced above, additional radiographs provided by your instructor, or both. Evaluate each radiograph for the following points:

_____ Evaluate the completeness of the study. (Are all of the pertinent anatomic structures included on the radiograph?)

_____ Evaluate for positioning or centering errors (e.g., rotation, off centering).

_____ Evaluate for correct exposure factors and possible motion. (Are the density and contrast of the images acceptable?)

_____ Determine whether markers and an acceptable degree of collimation and/or area shielding are seen on the images.

Laboratory Exercise C: Physical Positioning

On another person, simulate performing all of the following basic and special projections of the proximal humerus and shoulder girdle. Include the six steps listed below and described in the textbook. (Check off each step when completed satisfactorily.)

Step 1. Appropriate size and type of image receptor with correct markers

Step 2. Correct central ray placement and centering of part to central ray and/or IR

Step 3. Accurate collimation

Step 4. Area shielding of patient where advisable

Step 5. Use of proper immobilizing devices when needed

Step 6. Approximate correct exposure factors, breathing instructions where applicable, and "making" exposure

Projections	Step 1	Step 2	Step 3	Step 4	Step 5	Step 6
● Humerus (AP and lateral)	_____	_____	_____	_____	_____	_____
● Transthoracic lateral for humerus	_____	_____	_____	_____	_____	_____
● Shoulder series (nontrauma) (AP internal and external rotation)	_____	_____	_____	_____	_____	_____
● Inferosuperior axial (Lawrence)	_____	_____	_____	_____	_____	_____
● AP oblique (Grashey)	_____	_____	_____	_____	_____	_____
● Tangential (Fisk) for intertubercular groove	_____	_____	_____	_____	_____	_____
● Anterior oblique-Scapular Y	_____	_____	_____	_____	_____	_____
● Transthoracic lateral	_____	_____	_____	_____	_____	_____
● AP apical oblique axial (Garth)	_____	_____	_____	_____	_____	_____
● AP and AP axial clavicle	_____	_____	_____	_____	_____	_____
● AP and lateral scapula	_____	_____	_____	_____	_____	_____
● Acromioclavicular joints (with and without weights)	_____	_____	_____	_____	_____	_____

This self-test should be taken only after completing all of the readings, review exercises, and laboratory activities for a particular section. The purpose of this test is not only to provide a good learning exercise but also to serve as a strong indicator of what your final unit evaluation exam will cover. It is strongly suggested that if you do not get at least a 90% to 95% grade on each self-test that you review those areas in which you missed questions before going to your instructor for the final unit evaluation exam.

1. Select the term(s) that correctly describes the shoulder joint.
   A. Humeroscapular
   B. Scapulohumeral
   C. Glenohumeral
   D. B and C

2. Which specific joint is found on the lateral end of the clavicle?
   A. Scapulohumeral
   B. Sternoclavicular
   C. Acromioclavicular
   D. Glenohumeral

3. Which of the following is *not* an angle found on the scapula?
   A. Inferior angle
   B. Medial angle
   C. Lateral angle
   D. Superior angle

4. Which one of the following structures of the scapula extends most anteriorly?
   A. Glenoid cavity
   B. Acromion
   C. Scapular spine
   D. Coracoid process

5. True/False: The male clavicle is shorter and less curved than the female clavicle.

6. Which bony structure separates the supraspinous and infraspinous fossae?
   A. Scapular spine
   B. Glenoid cavity
   C. Acromion
   D. Superior border of scapula

7. Which one of the following structures is considered to be the most posterior?
   A. Scapular notch
   B. Coracoid process
   C. Acromion
   D. Glenoid process

8. What is the type of joint movement for the scapulohumeral joint?
   A. Plane
   B. Spheroidal
   C. Ellipsoidal
   D. Trochoidal

9. Identify the labeled structures on Fig. 6-11 (terms may be used more than once).

_____ A.

_____ B.

_____ C.

_____ D.

_____ E.

_____ F.

_____ G.

_____ H.

_____ I.

_____ J.

1. Spine of scapula

2. Lesser tubercle

3. Coracoid process

4. Lateral (axillary) border of scapula

5. Scapulohumeral joint

6. Clavicle

7. Intertubercular groove

8. Acromion of scapula

9. Neck of scapula

10. Greater tubercle

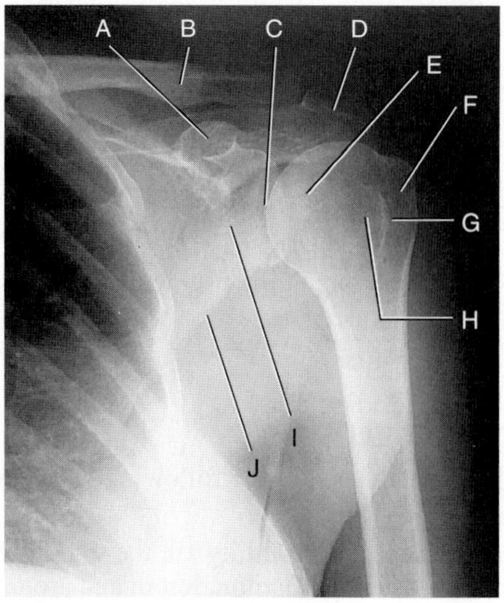

Fig. 6-11. Shoulder projection.

K. Does Fig. 6-11 represent an AP projection with: (A) an internal, (B) an external, or (C) a neutral rotation of the humerus? _____

Identify the labeled structures on Fig. 6-12 (terms may be used more than once).

_____ L.

_____ M.

_____ N.

_____ O.

_____ P.

_____ Q.

_____ R.

11. Lateral extremity of clavicle

12. Head of humerus

13. Glenoid cavity

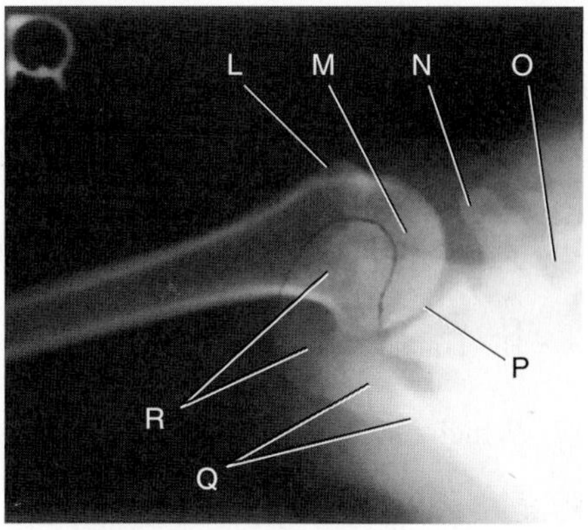

Fig. 6-12. Shoulder projection.

S. What is the correct term and method for the projection seen on Fig. 6-12?
   A. Inferosuperior axial projection
   B. Transthoracic lateral—Lawrence method
   C. Posterior oblique—Grashey method
   D. Superoinferior axial projection—Hobbs modification

10. Which one of the following technical considerations does not apply for adult shoulder radiography?
   A. Center and right automatic exposure control (AEC) chambers activated
   B. High-speed IR
   C. 40- to 44-in (100- to 110-cm) SID
   D. 70- to 80-kV (with grid)

11. True/False: Even though the amount of radiation exposure is minimal for most shoulder projections, gonadal shielding should be used for children and adults of childbearing age.

12. True/False: The greatest technical concern during a pediatric shoulder study is voluntary motion.

13. Which one of the following imaging modalities or procedures best demonstrates osteomyelitis?
    A. Ultrasound
    B. MRI
    C. CT arthrography
    D. Nuclear medicine

14. Which one of the following imaging modalities or procedures provides a functional, or dynamic, study of the shoulder joint?
    A. Ultrasound
    B. Radiography
    C. Nuclear medicine
    D. MRI

15. Match each of the following pathologic indications to its correct definition.

    _____ 1. Disability of the shoulder joint caused by chronic inflammation in and around the joint

    _____ 2. Injury to the anteroinferior glenoid labrum

    _____ 3. Chronic systemic disease with arthritic inflammatory changes throughout the body

    _____ 4. Superior displacement of distal clavicle

    _____ 5. Compression fracture of humeral head

    _____ 6. Traumatic injury to one or more muscles of the shoulder joint

    _____ 7. Reduction in the quantity of bone

    A. Rotator cuff tear

    B. Osteoporosis

    C. Rheumatoid arthritis

    D. Idiopathic chronic adhesive capsulitis

    E. Bankart lesion

    F. Acromioclavicular joint dislocation

    G. Hill-Sachs defect

16. Which one of the following projections and/or positions best demonstrates signs of impingement syndrome?
    A. AP and lateral shoulder
    B. Transaxillary
    C. Transaxillary with exaggerated, external rotation
    D. "Scapular Y" (Neer method)

17. Which one of the following pathologic conditions often produces narrowing of the joint space?
    A. Osteoarthritis
    B. Bursitis
    C. Osteoporosis
    D. Idiopathic chronic adhesive capsulitis

18. Which one of the following pathologic conditions may require a reduction in manual exposure factors?
    A. Bursitis
    B. Rheumatoid arthritis
    C. Rotator cuff tear
    D. Bankart lesion

19. Which basic projection of the shoulder requires that the humeral epicondyles be parallel to the IR?
    A. External rotation
    B. Neutral rotation
    C. Internal rotation
    D. Grashey method

20. Where is the central ray centered for an AP projection of the shoulder?
    A. Acromion
    B. 1 inch (2.5 cm) superior to coracoid process
    C. 1 inch (2.5 cm) inferior to coracoid process
    D. 2 inches (5 cm) inferior to acromioclavicular joint

21. Which position of the shoulder and proximal humerus projects the lesser tubercle in profile medially?
    A. External rotation   C. Internal rotation
    B. Neutral rotation   D. Exaggerated rotation

22. What central ray angle should be used for the inferosuperior axial projection for the glenohumeral joint space?
    A. 15° medially   C. 25° anteriorly and medially
    B. 25° to 30° medially   D. 35° to 45° medially

23. To best demonstrate the Hill-Sachs defect on the inferosuperior axial projection, which additional positioning maneuver must be used?
    A. Angle central ray 35° medially   C. Use exaggerated internal rotation
    B. Use exaggerated external rotation   D. Abduct arm 120° rotation from midsagittal plane (MSP)

24. How are the humeral epicondyles aligned for a rotational lateromedial projection of the humerus?
    A. 45° to IR   C. Parallel to IR
    B. Perpendicular to IR   D. 20° angle to IR

25. Which special projection of the shoulder places the glenoid cavity in profile for an "open" scapulohumeral joint?
    A. Garth method   C. Fisk modification
    B. Transthoracic lateral—Lawrence method   D. Grashey method

26. For the erect version of the tangential projection for the intertubercular groove, the patient leans forward

    _____ from vertical.
    A. 5° to 7°   C. 10° to 15°
    B. 20° to 25°   D. 35° to 45°

27. What is the major advantage of the supine, tangential version of the intertubercular groove projection over the erect version?
    A. Less radiation exposure   C. Less risk for motion
    B. Reduced OID   D. Ability to use automatic exposure control (AEC)

28. Which one of the following projections best demonstrates the supraspinatus outlet region?
    A. Scapular Y lateral (Neer method)   C. Inferosuperior axial
    B. Fisk method   D. Superoinferior axial projection (Hobbs modification)

29. With which one of the following projections is a breathing technique recommended?
    A. Grashey method   C. Scapular Y lateral
    B. Transthoracic lateral for humerus   D. Garth method

30. What central ray angulation is required for the supraspinatus outlet tangential projection (Neer method)?
    A. 10° to 15° caudad   C. 25° anteriorly and medially
    B. 45° caudad   D. None; central ray is perpendicular

31. Which pathologic feature is best demonstrated with the Garth method?
    A. Bursitis   C. Scapulohumeral dislocations
    B. Rheumatoid arthritis   D. Signs of shoulder impingement

32. Which anatomy of the shoulder is best demonstrated with a superoinferior axial projection (Hobbs modification)?
    A. Scapulohumeral joint space
    B. Coracoacromial arch
    C. Coracoid process
    D. Scapula in profile

33. If the patient cannot fully abduct the affected arm 90° for the inferosuperior axial projection (Clements modification),

    the technologist can angle the CR _____° toward the axilla.
    A. 5° to 15°
    B. 20° to 25°
    C. 25° to 30°
    D. 45°

34. Which one of the following projections requires the CR to be centered 2 inches (5 cm) inferior and medial from the superolateral border of the shoulder?
    A. Tangential projection (Fisk modification)
    B. Inferosuperior axial (Clements projection)
    C. Posterior oblique (Grashey method)
    D. Scapula Y lateral projection

35. Which anatomy is best demonstrated with the Alexander method?
    A. Scapulohumeral joint
    B. Coracoid process
    C. Proximal humerus
    D. AC joints

36. Which type of injury must be ruled out before the weight-bearing phase of an AC joint study?
    A. Shoulder separation
    B. Fractured clavicle
    C. Bursitis of the scapulohumeral joint
    D. Bankart lesion

37. What is the minimum amount of weight a large adult should have strapped to each wrist for the weight-bearing phase of an AC joint study?
    A. 5 to 7 lb
    B. 8 to 10 lb
    C. 12 to 15 lb
    D. 20 to 30 lb

38. True/False: A posteroanterior (PA) axial projection of the clavicle requires a 35° to 45° caudal central ray angle.

39. True/False: A 72-inch (180-cm) SID is recommended for acromioclavicular joint studies.

40. Match each of the following dose and projection types (assuming small- to average-size adult with accurate collimation) to its correct patient dose range (dose ranges may be used more than once).

    _____ 1. Thyroid dose for AP acromioclavicular joints   A. 1000 mrad or more

    _____ 2. Breast dose for AP shoulder   B. 40 to 100 mrad

    _____ 3. Thyroid dose for AP shoulder   C. 10 mrad or less

    _____ 4. Skin dose for AP shoulder

    _____ 5. Skin dose for transthoracic lateral

    _____ 6. Breast dose for AP acromioclavicular joints (two projections)

    _____ 7. Breast dose for scapular Y lateral

    _____ 8. Breast or thyroid dose for inferosuperior axiolateral shoulder

41. A radiograph of a posterior oblique (Grashey method) reveals that the anterior and posterior glenoid rims are not superimposed. The following positioning factors were used: erect position, body rotated 35° toward the affected side, central ray perpendicular to scapulohumeral joint space, and affected arm slightly abducted in neutral rotation. Which one of the following modifications will superimpose the glenoid rims during the repeat exposure?

    A. Angle central ray 10° to 15° caudad
    B. Rotate body less toward affected side
    C. Place affected arm in external rotation position
    D. Rotate body more toward affected side

42. **Situation:** A patient with a possible shoulder dislocation enters the emergency room. A neutral, AP projection of the shoulder has been taken, confirming a dislocation. Which additional projection should be taken?

    A. Grashey method
    B. Alexander method
    C. Garth method
    D. AP, external rotation

43. A radiograph of an AP axial clavicle taken on an asthenic type patient reveals that the clavicle is projected in the lung field below the top of the shoulder. The following positioning factors were used: erect position, central ray angled 15° cephalad, 40-inch (100-cm) SID, and respiration suspended at end of expiration. Which one of the following modifications should be made during the repeat exposure?

    A. Increase central ray angulation
    B. Suspend respiration at end of inspiration
    C. Reverse central ray angulation
    D. Use 72-inch (180-cm) SID

44. **Situation:** A patient with a possible acromioclavicular separation enters the emergency room. Which one of the following routines should be used?

    A. Acromioclavicular joint series: non–weight-bearing and weight-bearing projections
    B. AP neutral projection and Garth method
    C. AP neutral and transthoracic lateral projections
    D. AP internal and external projections

45. **Situation:** A patient comes to the radiology department with a history of tendonitis of the bicep tendon. Which of the following projections will best demonstrate calcification of the tendon within the intertubercular groove?

    A. Garth method
    B. Grashey method
    C. Superoinferior axial projection (Hobbs modification)
    D. Tangential projection—Fisk modification

46. An AP apical oblique axial (Garth method) radiographic image demonstrates poor visibility of the shoulder joint. The technologist used the following factors: Patient erect, facing the x-ray tube, 45° of rotation of affected shoulder toward the IR, 45° cephalad angle, and the CR centered to the scapulohumeral joint. What of the following factors would have contributed to this poor Garth position?

    A. Wrong direction of CR angle
    B. Incorrect CR centering
    C. Position must be performed recumbent
    D. Shoulder rotated in wrong direction

47. **Situation:** A patient is referred to radiology for a nontrauma shoulder series. The routine calls for a superoinferior axial projection (Hobbs modification) be included. But the patient is unable to stand and is confined to a wheelchair. What should the technologist do at this point?

    A. Ask another technologist to hold the patient erect for the projection.
    B. Perform the projection with the patient's upper chest prone on the table.
    C. Perform a recumbent posterior oblique (Grashey method) instead.
    D. Eliminate projection from positioning routine.

48. **Situation:** A patient enters ER with a proximal and midhumeral fracture. The patient is in extreme pain. Which one of the following positioning routines would demonstrate the entire humerus without excessive movement of the limb?

    A. AP and mediolateral humerus

    B. AP and transthoracic lateral (Lawrence method)

    C. AP and transthoracic lateral of humerus

    D. AP and and scapular Y lateral

49. For the following critique questions, see Fig. C6-97, an AP clavicle radiograph, on p. 203 in your textbook.

    A. Which positioning error(s) is (are) visible on this AP left clavicle radiograph? (More than one answer may be selected.)

        (a) All essential anatomic structures are not demonstrated.

        (b) Central ray is centered incorrectly.

        (c) Collimation is not evident.

        (d) Exposure factors are incorrect.

        (e) No anatomic marker is visible on the radiograph.

        (f) Slight rotation toward the right is evident.

        (g) Slight rotation toward the left is evident.

    B. Which error(s) identified above is (are) considered "repeatable"? _____

    C. Which of the following modifications must be made during the repeat exposure? (More than one answer may be selected.)

        (a) Increase collimation.

        (b) Center central ray correctly.

        (c) Decrease exposure factors.

        (d) Increase exposure factors.

        (e) Place anatomic marker on image receptor (IR) before exposure.

        (f) Ensure that no rotation occurs to the right or left.

50. For the following critique questions, refer to the AP scapula radiograph, Fig. C6-99, on p. 203 in your textbook.

    A. Which positioning error(s) is (are) visible on this radiograph? (More than one answer may be selected.)

        (a) All essential anatomic structures are not demonstrated.

        (b) Central ray is centered incorrectly.

        (c) Collimation is not evident.

        (d) Exposure factors are incorrect.

        (e) No anatomic marker is visible on radiograph.

        (f) Excessive rotation toward the right is evident.

        (g) Excessive rotation toward the left is evident.

    B. Which error(s) identified above is (are) considered "repeatable"? _____

    C. Which of the following modifications must be made during the repeat exposure? (More than one answer may be selected.)

        (a) Increase collimation.

        (b) Center central ray more inferiorly.

        (c) Decrease exposure factors.

        (d) Increase exposure factors.

        (e) Place anatomic marker on IR before exposure.

        (f) Rotate body slightly toward the left.

        (g) Rotate elbow slightly toward the right.

7 Lower Limb

Lower Limb

CHAPTER OBJECTIVES

After you have successfully completed the activities in this chapter, you will be able to:

_____ 1. Identify the bones and specific features of the toes, foot, ankle, lower leg, knee, patella, and distal femur.

_____ 2. On drawings and radiographs, identify specific anatomic features of the foot, ankle, leg, knee, patella, and distal femur.

_____ 3. Identify specific joints of the foot, ankle, leg, and knee according to the correct classification and movement type.

_____ 4. Match specific pathologic indications of the lower limb to the correct definition.

_____ 5. Match specific pathologic indications of the lower limb to the correct radiographic appearance.

_____ 6. Describe the basic and special projections of the toes, foot, ankle, calcaneus, knee, patella, intercondylar fossa, and femur, including central ray placement and angulation, correct image receptor size and placement, part positioning, technical factors, and evaluation criteria.

_____ 7. List the various patient dose ranges for each projection of the lower limb.

_____ 8. Given various hypothetical situations, identify the correct modification of a position and/or exposure factors to improve the radiographic image.

_____ 9. Given various hypothetical situations, identify the correct position for a specific pathologic form or condition.

_____ 10. Given radiographs of specific lower limb projections, identify specific positioning and exposure factor errors.

Positioning and Radiographic Critique

_____ 1. Using a peer, perform basic and special projections of the lower limb.

_____ 2. Using foot and knee phantoms, produce satisfactory radiographs of the lower limb (if equipment is available).

_____ 3. Critique and evaluate lower limb radiographs based on the four divisions of radiographic criteria: (1) structures shown, (2) position, (3) collimation and central ray, and (4) exposure criteria.

_____ 4. Distinguish between acceptable and unacceptable lower limb radiographs based on exposure factors, motion, collimation, positioning, or other errors.

LEARNING EXERCISES

Complete the following review exercises after reading the associated pages in the textbook as indicated by each exercise. Answers to each review exercise are given at the end of the review exercises.

1. Fill in the number of bones for the following:

   A. Phalanges _____   C. Tarsals _____

   B. Metatarsals _____   D. Total _____

2. What are two differences in the phalanges of the foot as compared with the phalanges of the hand?

   A. _____

   B. _____

3. Which tuberosity of the foot is palpable and a common site of foot trauma?

   _____

4. Where are the sesamoid bones of the foot most commonly located? _____

5. What is the largest and strongest tarsal bone? _____

6. What is the name of the joint found between the talus and calcaneus? _____

7. List the three specific articular facets found in the joint described in the previous question.

   A. _____   B. _____   C. _____

8. The small opening, or space, found in the middle of the joint identify in question No. 6 is called the:

   _____.

9. Match each of the following characteristics to the correct tarsal bone (answers may be used more than once).

   _____ 1. Forms an aspect of the ankle joint   A. Calcaneus

   _____ 2. The smallest of the cuneiforms   B. Talus

   _____ 3. Found on the medial side of the foot between the talus   C. Cuboid

   _____ 4. The largest of the cuneiforms   D. Navicular

   _____ 5. Articulates with the second, third, and fourth metatarsal   E. Lateral cuneiform

   _____ 6. The most superior tarsal bone   F. Intermediate cuneiform

   _____ 7. Articulates with the first metatarsal   G. Medial cuneiform

   _____ 8. Common site for bone spurs

   _____ 9. A tarsal found anterior to the calcaneus and lateral to the lateral cuneiform

   _____ 10. The second largest tarsal bone

10. Identify the labeled structures found in Figs. 7-1 and 7-2.

A. _____

B. _____

C. _____

D. _____

E. _____

F. _____

G. _____

H. _____

I. _____

J. _____

K. _____

L. _____

M. Fig. 7-1 represents a radiograph of

which projection of the foot? _____

N. _____

O. _____

P. _____

Q. _____

R. _____

S. _____

T. Fig. 7-2 represents a radiograph of which projection?

_____

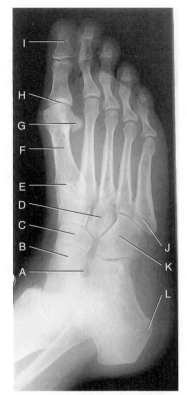

Fig. 7-1. Anatomy of the foot.

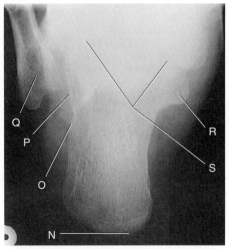

Fig. 7-2. Anatomy of the foot.

11. True/False: The cuboid articulates with the four bones of the foot.

12. The calcaneus articulates with the talus and the:
   A. Navicular
   B. Cuboid
   C. Medial cuneiform
   D. Lateral cuneiform

13. List the two arches of the foot. A. _____   B. _____

14. Which three bones make up the ankle joint?

   A. _____   B. _____   C. _____

15. The three bones of the ankle form a deep socket into which the talus fits. This socket is called the

   _____.

16. The distal tibial joint surface forming the roof of the distal ankle joint is called the:
   A. Tibial plafond
   B. Articular facet
   C. Tibial plateau
   D. Ankle mortise

17. True/False: The medial malleolus is approximately ½ inch (1 cm) posterior to the lateral malleolus.

18. The ankle joint is classified as a synovial joint with _____ type movement.

19. Identify the structures labeled on Figs. 7-3 and 7-4.

Fig. 7-3.

   A. _____

   B. _____

   C. _____

   D. _____

   E. _____

Fig. 7-4.

   F. _____

   G. _____

   H. _____

   I. _____

   J. _____

   K. _____

   L. _____

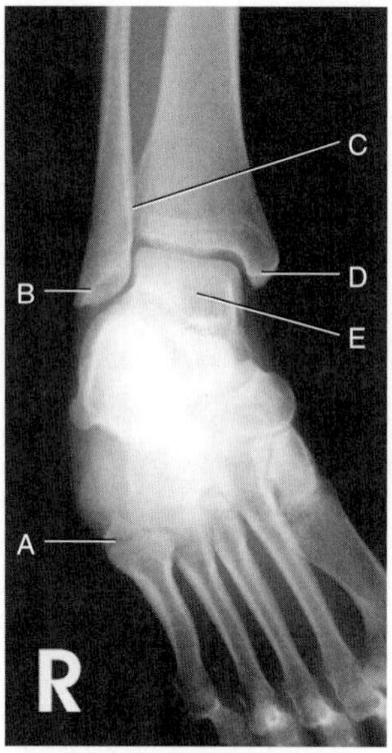

Fig. 7-3. Anatomy of the ankle.

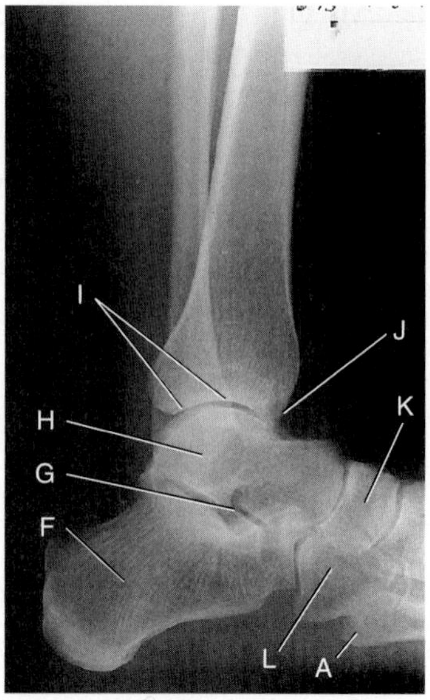

Fig. 7-4. Anatomy of the ankle.

   M. Fig. 7-3 represents a radiograph of which projection of the ankle? _____

144

Review Exercise B: Radiographic Anatomy of the Lower Leg, Knee, and Distal Femur (see textbook pp. 212-215)

1. The _____ is the weight-bearing bone of the lower leg.

2. What is the name of the large prominence located on the midanterior surface of the proximal tibia that serves as a distal attachment for the patellar tendon? _____

3. What is the name of the small prominence located on the posterolateral aspect of the medial condyle of the femur that is an identifying landmark to determine possible rotation of a lateral knee? _____

4. A small, triangular depression located on the tibia that helps form the distal tibiofibular joint is called the

   _____.

5. The articular facets of the proximal tibia are also referred to as the _____.

6. The articular facets slope _____ ° posteriorly.
   A. 25   C. 35
   B. 45   D. 10 to 15

7. The most proximal aspect of the fibula is the _____.

8. The extreme distal end of the fibula forms the _____.

9. What is the name of the largest sesamoid bone in the body? _____

10. What are two other names for the patellar surface of the femur?

    A. _____   B. _____

11. What is the name of the depression located on the posterior aspect of the distal femur? _____

12. Why must the central ray be angled 5° to 7° cephalad for a lateral knee position? _____

13. The slightly raised area located on the posterolateral aspect of the medial femoral condyle is called the:
    A. Trochlear tubercle   C. Adductor tubercle
    B. Anterior crest   D. Tibial tuberosity

14. What are the two palpable bony landmarks found on the distal femur?

    A. _____   B. _____

15. The general region of the posterior knee is called the _____.

16. True/False: Flexion of 20° of the knee forces the patella firmly against the patellar surface of the femur.

17. True/False: The patella acts like a pivot to increase the leverage of a large muscle found in the anterior thigh.

18. True/False: The posterior surface of the patella is normally rough.

19. For which large muscle does the patella serve as a pivot to increase the leverage? _____.

20. List the correct terms for the following joints:

    A. Between the patella and distal femur _____

    B. Between the two condyles of the femur and tibia _____

21. List the four major ligaments of the knee.

    A. _____   C. _____

    B. _____   D. _____

22. The crescent-shaped fibrocartilage disks that act as shock absorbers in the knee joint are called _____.

23. List the two bursae found in the knee joint.

    A. _____   B. _____

24. Match each of the following structures to the correct bone (answers may be used more than once).

    _____ 1. Tibial plafond   A. Tibia

    _____ 2. Medial malleolus   B. Fibula

    _____ 3. Lateral epicondyle   C. Distal femur

    _____ 4. Patellar surface   D. Patella

    _____ 5. Articular facets

    _____ 6. Fibular notch

    _____ 7. Styloid process

    _____ 8. Base

    _____ 9. Intercondyloid eminence

    _____ 10. Neck

25. Match each of the following articulations to the correct joint classification or movement type (answers may be used more than once).

    _____ 1. Ankle joint   A. Synarthrodial (gomphoses type)

    _____ 2. Patellofemoral   B. Ginglymus (hinge)

    _____ 3. Proximal tibiofibular   C. Sellar (saddle)

    _____ 4. Tarsometatarsal   D. Plane (gliding)

    _____ 5. Knee joint (femorotibial)   E. Amphiarthrodial (syndesmosis type)

    _____ 6. Distal tibiofibular   F. Bicondylar

26. Identify the labeled structures on Figs. 7-5 through 7-7.

Fig. 7-5.

A. _____

B. _____

C. _____

D. _____

E. _____

F. _____

G. _____

H. _____

I. _____

Fig. 7-6.

J. _____

K. _____

L. _____

M. _____

N. _____

O. _____ (degree angle)

P. _____

Q. _____

R. _____

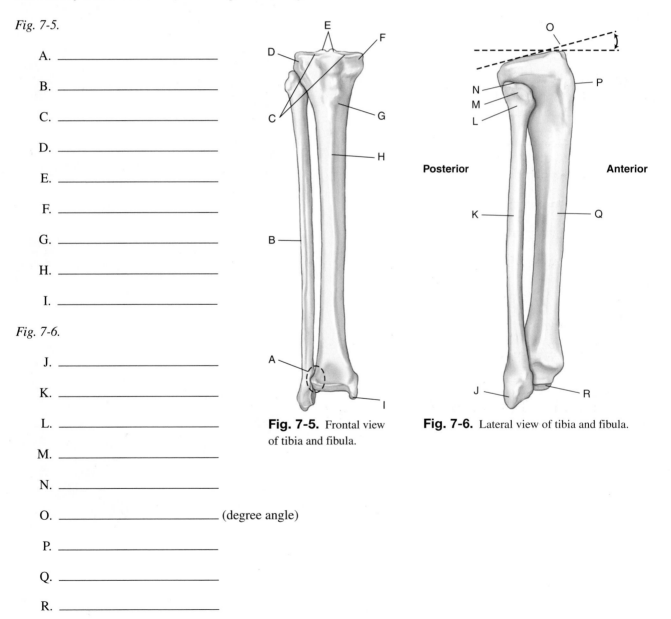

Fig. 7-5. Frontal view of tibia and fibula.

Fig. 7-6. Lateral view of tibia and fibula.

S. _____

T. _____

U. _____

V. _____

W. _____

X. Which projection does the radiograph in

Fig. 7-7 represent? _____

27. Identify the bony structures labeled on Figs. 7-8 and 7-9.

Fig. 7-8.

A. _____

B. _____

C. _____

D. _____

E. _____

F. _____

G. _____

H. _____

Fig. 7-9.

I. _____

J. _____

K. _____

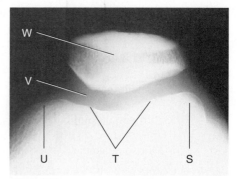

Fig. 7-7. Anatomy of the knee and patella.

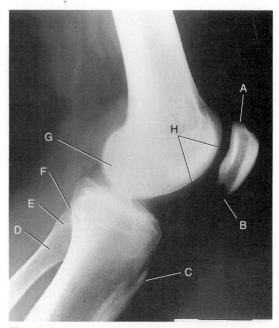

Fig. 7-8. True lateral radiograph of the knee.

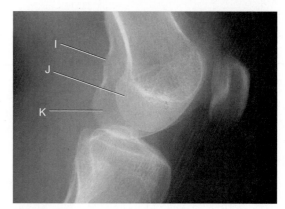

Fig. 7-9. Lateral radiograph of the knee.

28. Match the following foot and ankle movements to the correct definition.

_____ A. Inward turning or bending of ankle

_____ B. Decreasing the angle between the dorsum pedis and anterior lower leg

_____ C. Extending the ankle or pointing the foot and toe downward

_____ D. Outward turning or bending of ankle

1. Inversion (varus)

2. Plantar flexion

3. Eversion (valgus)

4. Dorsiflexion

PART II: RADIOGRAPHIC POSITIONING
Review Exercise C: Positioning of the Foot and Ankle (see textbook pp. 219-239)

1. True/False: The recommended source image receptor distance (SID) for lower limb radiography is 40 inches (100 cm).

2. True/False: To reduce scatter radiation during table top procedures, the Bucky tray should be positioned over the lower limb being radiographed.

3. True/False: With careful and close collimation, gonadal shielding does not have to be used during lower limb radiography.

4. True/False: During digital radiography, lead masking should be placed on the regions of the imaging plate, not within the collimation field.

5. True/False: A kV range between 50 and 70 should be used for film-screen lower limb radiography.

6. True/False: kV range for CR and digital radiography is typically lower as compared with film-screen ranges.

7. Match the following pathologic indications to the correct definition.

_____ A. An inflammatory condition involving the anterior, proximal tibia

_____ B. Also known as osteitis deformans

_____ C. Malignant tumor of the cartilage

_____ D. Inherited type of arthritis that commonly affects males

_____ E. Benign, neoplastic bone lesion caused by overproduction of bone at a joint

_____ F. Benign bone lesion usually developing in teens or young adults

_____ G. Most prevalent primary bone malignancy in pediatric patients

_____ H. Benign, neoplastic bone lesion filled with clear fluid

_____ I. Injury to a large ligament located between the bases of the first and second metatarsal

_____ J. Condition affecting the sacroiliac joints and lower limbs of young men, especially the posterosuperior margin of the calcaneus

1. Exostosis

2. Lisfranc joint injury

3. Bone cyst

4. Reiter's syndrome

5. Osteoid osteoma

6. Ewing's sarcoma

7. Gout

8. Paget's disease

9. Osgood-Schlatter disease

10. Chondrosarcoma

8. The formal name for "runner's knee" is _____.

9. What is another term for osteomalacia? _____

10. Match the following radiographic appearances to the correct pathologic indication.

_____ A. Asymmetric erosion of joint spaces with calcaneal erosion   1. Osteoid osteoma

_____ B. Uric acid deposits in joint spaces   2. Ewing's sarcoma

_____ C. Well-circumscribed lucency   3. Gout

_____ D. Small, round/oval density with lucent center   4. Osgood-Schlatter disease

_____ E. Narrowed, irregular joint surfaces with sclerotic articular surfaces   5. Osteoarthritis

_____ F. Fragmentation or detachment of the tibial tuberosity   6. Osteomalacia

_____ G. Ill-defined area of bone destruction with surrounding "onion peel"   7. Reiter syndrome

_____ H. Decreased bone density and bowing deformities of weight-bearing limbs   8. Bone cyst

11. Why is the central ray angled 10° to 15° toward the calcaneus for an anteroposterior (AP) projection of the toes?

_____

12. Where is the central ray centered for an AP oblique projection of the foot? _____

13. Which projection is best for demonstrating the sesamoid bones of the foot? _____

14. The foot should be dorsiflexed so that the plantar surface of the foot is _____ ° from vertical for the sesamoid projection.

15. Why should the central ray be perpendicular to the metatarsals for an AP projection of the foot?

_____

16. If a foreign body is lodged in the plantar surface of the foot, which type of central ray angle should be used for the AP projection?
   A. 10° posterior   C. 10° anterior
   B. 15° posterior   D. None; use a perpendicular central ray

17. Rotation can be determined on a radiograph of an AP foot projection by the near-equal distance between the

_____ metatarsals.

18. Which oblique projection of the foot best demonstrates the majority of the tarsal bones?

_____

19. Which oblique projection of the foot best demonstrates the navicular and the first and second cuneiforms with

minimal superimposition?_____

20. Which projection tends to place the foot into a truer lateral position: mediolateral or lateromedial?

_____

21. Which type of study should be performed to best evaluate the condition of the longitudinal arches of the foot?

_____

22. How should the central ray be angled from the long axis of the foot for the plantodorsal axial projection of the

calcaneus? _____

23. Which calcaneal structure should appear medially on a well-positioned plantodorsal projection?

_____

24. Where is the central ray placed for a lateral projection of the calcaneus? _____

25. Which joint surface of the ankle is *not* typically visualized with a correctly positioned AP projection of the ankle?
   A. Medial surface of joint   C. Lateral surface of joint
   B. Superior surface of joint   D. All of the above surfaces of the joint *are* visualized.

26. Why should AP, 45° oblique, and lateral ankle radiographs include the proximal metatarsals?

_____

27. How much (if any) should the foot and ankle be rotated for an AP mortise projection of the ankle?

_____

28. Which projection of the ankle best demonstrates a possible fracture of the lateral malleolus?

_____

29. With a true lateral projection of the ankle, the lateral malleolus is:
   A. Projected over the anterior aspect of the distal tibia
   B. Projected over the posterior aspect of the distal tibia
   C. Directly superimposed over the distal tibia
   D. Directly superimposed over the medial malleolus

30. Which projections of the ankle require forced inversion and eversion movements?

_____

Review Exercise D: Positioning of the Tibia, Fibula, Knee, and Distal Femur (see textbook pp. 240-256)

1. What is the basic positioning routine for a study of the tibia and fibula? _____

2. Why is it important to include the knee joint for an initial study of tibia trauma, even if the patient's symptoms involve the middle and distal aspect?

_____

3. To include both joints for a lateral projection of the tibia and fibula for an adult, the technologist may place the

   cassette _____ in relation to the part.
   A. Parallel   C. Diagonally
   B. Perpendicular   D. Transverse

4. What is the recommended central ray angulation for an AP projection of the knee for a patient with thick thighs and buttocks (i.e., measuring greater than 24 cm)?
   A. 3° to 5° caudad   C. Central ray perpendicular to IR
   B. 3° to 5° cephalad   D. Central ray perpendicular to patellar plane

5. Where is the central ray centered for an AP projection of the knee?
   A. ½ inch (1.25 cm) distal to apex of patella   C. Midpatella
   B. 1 inch (2½ cm) proximal to apex of patella   D. Level of tibial tuberosity

6. Which basic projection of a knee best demonstrates the proximal fibula free of superimposition?
   A. True AP   C. AP oblique, 45° medial rotation
   B. True lateral   D. AP oblique, 45° lateral rotation

7. For the AP oblique projection of the knee, the _____ rotation (medial [internal] or lateral [external]) best visualizes the lateral condyle of the tibia and the head and neck of the fibula.

8. What is the recommended central ray placement for a lateral knee position on a tall, slender male patient with a narrow pelvis?
   A. 5° to 10° caudad   C. Central ray perpendicular to IR
   B. 5° cephalad   D. Central ray perpendicular to patellar plane

9. How much flexion is recommended for a lateral projection of the knee?
   A. No flexion   C. 30° to 35°
   B. 20° to 30°   D. 45°

10. Which positioning error is present if the distal borders of the femoral condyles are not superimposed on a radiograph

    of a lateral knee? _____

11. Which positioning error is present if the posterior portions of the femoral condyles are not superimposed on a lateral

    knee radiograph? _____

12. Which anatomic structure of the femur can be used to determine which rotation error (overrotation or underrotation) is present on a slightly rotated lateral knee radiograph?

    _____

13. Which special projection of the knee best evaluates the knee joint for cartilage degeneration or deformities?

    _____

14. AP knee stress projections are performed to demonstrate:
    A. Patellar dislocation   C. Medial or collateral ligament damage
    B. Osgood-Schlatter disease   D. Osteoarthritis

15. Which one of the following special projections of the knee best demonstrates the intercondylar fossa?
    A. Holmblad   C. AP weight-bearing, bilateral projections
    B. Merchant   D. Settegast

16. How much flexion of the lower leg is required for the Camp-Coventry projection when the central ray is angled

    40°caudad? _____

17. Why is the posteroanterior (PA) axial projection for the intercondylar fossa recommended instead of an AP axial

    projection? _____

18. What type of CR angulation is required for the PA axial weight-bearing projection (Rosenberg method)?
    A. None CR is perpendicular   C. 10° cephalad
    B. 10° caudad   D. 5° to 7° cephalad

19. How much flexion of the knees is required for the PA axial weight-bearing projection (Rosenberg method)?
    A. 20° to 30°   C. 5° to 10°
    B. 35° to 40°   D. 45°

20. How much knee flexion is required for the PA axial projection (Holmblad method)?
    A. 45°   C. 60° to 70°
    B. 35°   D. None. Lower limb is fully extended

21. What type of CR angle is required for the PA axial (Holmblad method)?
    A. 10° caudad   C. 15° to 20° cephalad
    B. 10° cephalad   D. None. CR is perpendicular to IR

22. True/False: To place the interepicondylar line parallel to the image receptor for a PA projection of the patella, the lower limb must be rotated approximately 5° internally.

23. How much part flexion is recommended for a lateral projection of the patella?

    _____

24. The skin dose range for an AP knee projection is:
    A. 5 to 10 mrad   C. 50 to 60 mrad
    B. 20 to 30 mrad   D. More than 100 mrad

25. How much central ray angle from the long axis of the femora is required for a Merchant bilateral projection?

    _____

26. How much part flexion is required for the following methods?

    A. Hughston method _____

    B. Settegast method _____

27. What type of CR angle is required for the superoinferior sitting tangential method for patella?

A. 40° cephalad
C. Depends on degree of flexion
B. 5° to 10° caudad
D. None. CR is perpendicular to IR

28. Match each of the following descriptions of positioning for projections of the knee and/or patella to its correct name (using each answer only once).

_____ 1. Can be performed using a wheelchair or lowered radiographic table

_____ 2. Patient prone; requires 90° knee flexion

_____ 3. Patient prone with 40° to 50° knee flexion and with equal 40° to 50° caudad CR angle

_____ 4. IR is placed on a foot stool to minimize the OID

_____ 5. Patient prone with 45° knee flexion and 10° to 20° cephalad CR angle from long axis of lower leg.

_____ 6. Patient supine with cassette resting on midthighs

_____ 7. Patient supine with 40° knee flexion and with 30° caudad CR angle from horizontal

A. Inferosuperior axial for patellofemoral joint

B. Merchant method

C. Hughston method

D. Camp-Coventry method

E. Settegast method

F. Holmblad method (variation)

G. Superoinferior sitting tangential method

29. Which of the following special projections of the knee must be performed erect?

A. Rosenberg method
C. Settegast method
B. Camp-Coventry method
D. Hughston method

30. Which one of the following projections of the intercondylar fossa recommends using a curved cassette?

A. Rosenberg method
C. Béclere method
B. Camp-Coventry method
D. Settegast method

Review Exercise E: Problem Solving for Technical and Positioning Errors

1. **Situation:** A radiograph of an AP projection of the foot reveals that the metatarsophalangeal joints are not open and the metatarsals are somewhat foreshortened. What was the positioning error involved, and what modification should be made to improve this image on the repeat exposure?

   _____

2. **Situation:** A radiograph of an AP oblique-medial rotation projection of the foot reveals that the proximal third to fifth metatarsals are superimposed. What type of positioning error led to this radiographic outcome?

   _____

3. **Situation:** A radiograph of a plantodorsal axial projection of the calcaneus reveals considerable foreshortening of the calcaneus. What type of positioning modification is needed on the repeat exposure?

   _____

4. **Situation:** A radiograph of an AP projection of the ankle reveals that the lateral surface of the ankle joint is totally open. (It should not be open on a true AP projection.) The technologist is positive that the ankle was in the correct, true AP position with the long axis of the foot perpendicular to the IR. What else could have led to this joint space being open?

_____

5. **Situation:** A radiograph of an intended AP mortise projection reveals that the lateral malleolus is superimposed over the talus, and the distal tibiofibular joint is not well demonstrated. What is the most likely reason for this radiographic outcome?

_____

6. **Situation:** A radiograph of an AP knee projection demonstrates that the femorotibial joint space is not open at all. The patient is young and has no history of degenerative disease. What type of positioning modification may improve the outcome of this projection?

_____

7. **Situation:** A radiograph of an AP oblique with medial rotation of the knee to demonstrate the proximal fibula reveals that there is total superimposition of the proximal tibia and the fibula. What must be modified to correct this projection?

_____

8. **Situation:** A radiograph of a lateral recumbent knee reveals that the posterior border of the medial femoral condyle (identified by the adductor tubercle) is not superimposed but is slightly posterior to the lateral condyle. The fibular head is also completely superimposed by the tibia. What type of positioning error led to this radiographic outcome?

_____

9. **Situation:** A patient with trauma to the medial aspect of the foot comes to the emergency room. A heavy object was dropped on the foot near the base of the first metatarsal. Basic foot projections do not clearly demonstrate this region. What other projection of the foot could be used to better delineate this area?

_____

10. **Situation:** A radiograph of an AP and lateral tibia and fibula reveals that the ankle joint is not included on the AP projection, but both the knee and the ankle are included on the lateral projection. What should the technologist do in this situation?

_____

11. **Situation:** A radiograph obtained by using the PA axial (Camp-Coventry method) reveals that the distal femoral condyles, articular facets, and intercondylar fossa are asymmetric. What possible positioning errors may have produced this distortion of the anatomy?

_____

12. **Situation:** A radiograph of a lateral patella reveals that the patella is drawn tightly against the intercondylar sulcus. Which positioning modification should be performed to improve the quality of the image during the repeat exposure?

_____

13. **Situation:** A patient with a history of degenerative disease of the left knee joint comes to the radiology department. The orthopedic surgeon orders a radiographic study to determine the extent of damage to the joint space. Which projection(s) should be performed?

_____

14. **Situation:** A patient with a possible Lisfranc joint injury. Which radiographic position(s) would best demonstrate

this type of injury? _____

15. **Situation:** A patient with a history of pain in the feet comes to the radiology department. The referring physician orders a study to evaluate the longitudinal arches of the feet. Which positioning routine should be used?

_____

16. **Situation:** A patient with bony, loose bodies (or "joint mice") within the knee joint comes to radiology for a knee series. The AP and lateral knee projections fail to demonstrate any loose bodies. What additional knee projection can be taken to better demonstrate them?

_____

17. **Situation:** A young male patient comes to the radiology department with a clinical history of Osgood-Schlatter disease. Which single projection of the basic knee series will best demonstrate this condition?

_____

18. **Situation:** A radiograph of a mediolateral knee projection demonstrates that the medial femoral condyle is projected inferior to the lateral condyle. What can the technologist do to correct this problem during the repeat exposure?

_____

19. **Situation:** A physician orders a bilateral, tangential projection of the patella and patellofemoral joint space. But the patient is restricted to a wheelchair and can't lie on the radiographic table due to chronic pain. Which projection could be performed with the patient remaining in the wheelchair?

_____

20. **Situation:** A tangential (inferosuperior) projection of the patellofemoral joint space reveals that the patella is seated into the intercondylar sulcus and the joint space is not demonstrated. What possible positioning errors may have produced this radiographic outcome?

_____

Review Exercise F: Critique Radiographs of the Lower Limbs (see textbook p. 257)

The following questions relate to the radiographs found at the end of Chapter 7 of the textbook. Evaluate these radiographs for the radiographic criteria categories (1 through 5) that follow. Describe the corrections needed to improve the overall image. The major, or "repeatable," errors are specific errors that indicate the need for a repeat exposure, regardless of the nature of the other errors.

Comparing these radiographs with the correctly positioned and exposed radiographs in this chapter of the textbook will help you evaluate each of them for errors.

A. Bilateral tangential patella (Fig. C7-142)

Description of possible error:

    1. Structures shown: _____

    2. Part positioning: _____

    3. Collimation and central ray: _____

    4. Exposure criteria: _____

    5. Anatomic side markers: _____

Repeatable error(s): _____

B. Lateral calcaneus (Fig. C7-143)

Description of possible error:

    1. Structures shown: _____

    2. Part positioning: _____

    3. Collimation and central ray: _____

    4. Exposure criteria: _____

    5. Anatomic side markers: _____

Repeatable error(s): _____

C. AP mortise ankle (Fig. C7-144)

Description of possible error:

    1. Structures shown: _____

    2. Part positioning: _____

    3. Collimation and central ray: _____

    4. Exposure criteria: _____

    5. Anatomic side markers: _____

Repeatable error(s): _____

D. AP lower leg (Fig. C7-145)

Description of possible error:

    1. Structures shown: _____

    2. Part positioning: _____

    3. Collimation and central ray: _____

    4. Exposure criteria: _____

    5. Anatomic side markers: _____

Repeatable error(s): _____

E. Lateral knee (Fig. C7-146)

Description of possible error:

    1. Structures shown: _____

    2. Part positioning: _____

    3. Collimation and central ray: _____

    4. Exposure criteria: _____

    5. Anatomic side markers: _____

Repeatable error(s): _____

F. Lateral knee (Fig. C7-147)

Description of possible error:

    1. Structures shown: _____

    2. Part positioning: _____

    3. Collimation and central ray: _____

    4. Exposure criteria: _____

    5. Anatomic side markers: _____

Repeatable error(s): _____

PART III: LABORATORY ACTIVITIES

You must gain experience in positioning each part of the lower limb before performing the following exams on actual patients. You can get experience in positioning and radiographic evaluation of these projections by performing exercises using radiographic phantoms and practicing on other students (although you will not be taking actual exposures).

The following suggested activities assume that your teaching institution has an energized lab and radiographic phantoms. If not, perform Laboratory Exercises B and C, the radiographic evaluation and the physical positioning exercises. (Check off each step and projection as you complete it.)

Laboratory Exercise A: Energized Laboratory

1. Using the foot/ankle radiographic phantom, produce radiographs of the basic routines for the following:

   _____ Foot

   _____ Ankle

   _____ Calcaneus

2. Using the knee radiographic phantom, produce radiographs of the following basic routines:

   _____ AP

   _____ AP oblique, medial rotation

   _____ Lateral (horizontal beam lateral if flexed knee is not available)

Laboratory Exercise B: Radiographic Evaluation

1. Evaluate and critique the radiographs produced above, additional radiographs provided by your instructor, or both. Evaluate each radiograph for the following points:

   _____ Evaluate the completeness of the study. (Are all of the pertinent anatomic structures included on the radiograph?)

   _____ Evaluate for positioning or centering errors (e.g., rotation, off centering).

   _____ Evaluate for correct exposure factors and possible motion. (Are the density and contrast of the images acceptable?)

   _____ Determine whether anatomic side markers and an acceptable degree of collimation and/or area shielding are seen on the images.

Laboratory Exercise C: Physical Positioning

1. On another person, simulate performing all basic and special projections of the lower limb as follows. Include the six steps listed below and described in the textbook. (Check off each step when completed satisfactorily.)

   Step 1. Appropriate size and type of image receptor with correct markers

   Step 2. Correct central ray placement and centering of part to central ray and/or image receptor

   Step 3. Accurate collimation

   Step 4. Area shielding of patient where advisable

   Step 5. Use of proper immobilizing devices when needed

   Step 6. Approximate correct exposure factors, breathing instructions where applicable, and "making" exposure

Projections	Step 1	Step 2	Step 3	Step 4	Step 5	Step 6
● Positioning routine for a specific toe	____	____	____	____	____	____
● Basic foot routine	____	____	____	____	____	____
● Special projection for sesamoid bones	____	____	____	____	____	____
● Basic projections of the calcaneus	____	____	____	____	____	____
● Weight-bearing foot projections	____	____	____	____	____	____
● Basic ankle routine, including mortise and 45° oblique projections	____	____	____	____	____	____
● AP and lateral tibia and fibula	____	____	____	____	____	____
● Basic knee routine	____	____	____	____	____	____
● Special projections for intercondylar fossa	____	____	____	____	____	____
● Weight-bearing AP knee projections	____	____	____	____	____	____
● Special projections for patellofemoral joint space	____	____	____	____	____	____

This self-test should be taken only after completing all of the readings, review exercises, and laboratory activities for a particular section. The purpose of this test is not only to provide a good learning exercise, but also to serve as a strong indicator of what your final evaluation exam will be. It is strongly suggested that if you do not get at least a 90% to 95% grade on this self-test that you review those areas in which you missed questions before going to your instructor for the final evaluation exam for this chapter.

1. Which of the following is not an aspect of the metatarsal?
   A. Head
   B. Tail
   C. Body
   D. Base

2. True/False: The distal portion of the fifth metatarsal is a common fracture site.

3. Where are the sesamoid bones of the foot most commonly located?
   A. Plantar surface near head of first metatarsal
   B. Plantar surface at first tarsometatarsal joint
   C. Dorsum aspect near base of first metatarsal
   D. Plantar surface near cuboid bone

4. What is the name of the tarsal bone found on the medial side of the foot between the talus and three cuneiforms?
   A. Calcaneus
   B. Lateral malleolus
   C. Cuboid
   D. Navicular

5. Which tarsal bone is considered to be the smallest?
   A. Medial cuneiform
   B. Navicular
   C. Intermediate cuneiform
   D. Lateral cuneiform

6. What is another term for the talocalcaneal joint?
   A. Tarsometatarsal joint
   B. Subtalar joint
   C. Mortise joint
   D. Tibiocalcaneal joint

7. The distal tibial joint surface is called the:
   A. Medial malleolus
   B. Tibial plafond
   C. Lateral malleolus
   D. Anterior tubercle

8. True/False: The mortise of the ankle should be totally open and visible on a correctly positioned anteroposterior (AP) projection of the ankle.

9. Match each of the following structures or characteristics to the correct bone of the foot or ankle (using each choice only once).

_____ 1. Trochlear process   A. Metatarsal

_____ 2. Lateral malleolus   B. Talus

_____ 3. The second largest tarsal bone   C. Tibia

_____ 4. Found between the navicular and base of first metatarsal   D. Calcaneus

_____ 5. Base   E. Sinus tarsi

_____ 6. Found between the calcaneus and talus cuneiform   F. Medial cuneiform

_____ 7. Anterior tubercle   G. Fibula

10. Match the structures labeled on Fig. 7-10 (using each choice only once).

_____ A.   1. Talus

_____ B.   2. First metatarsal

_____ C.   3. Lateral malleolus

_____ D.   4. Distal tibiofibular joint

_____ E.   5. Medial malleolus

F. What projection does this radiograph represent?
  A. AP mortise ankle   C. AP ankle
  B. AP stress ankle—inversion   D. AP stress ankle—eversion

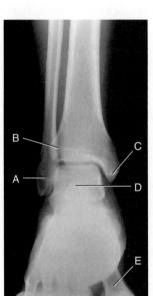

Fig. 7-10. Anatomy of the ankle.

11. Match the structures labeled on the radiographs in Figs. 7-11 through 7-13 (answers may be used more than once).

_____ A.

_____ B.

_____ C.

_____ D.

_____ E.

_____ F.

_____ G.

_____ H.

_____ I.

_____ J.

_____ K.

1. Distal phalanx, second digit

2. Proximal phalanx, first digit

3. Interphalangeal joint

4. Head of second metatarsal

5. Metatarsophalangeal joint of first digit

6. Base of first metatarsal

7. Proximal phalanx, second digit

8. Head of first metatarsal

9. Distal phalanx, first digit

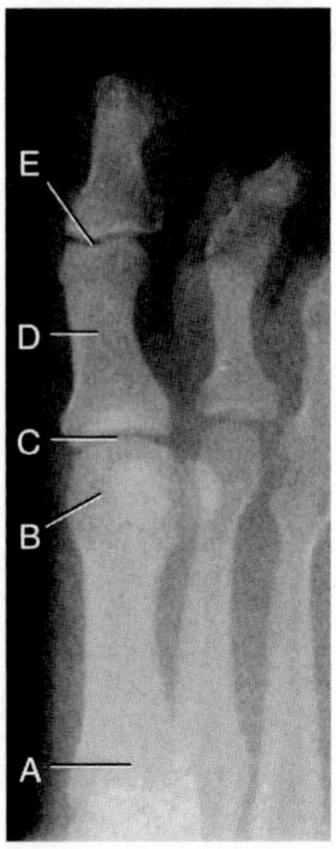

Fig. 7-11. Anatomy of the metatarsal bones and digits.

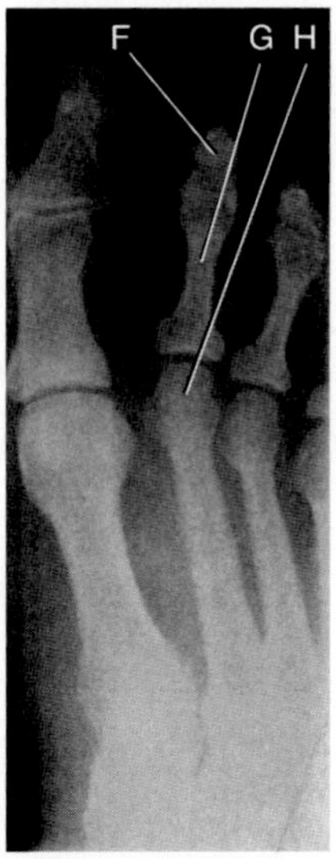

Fig. 7-12. Anatomy of the metatarsal bones and digits.

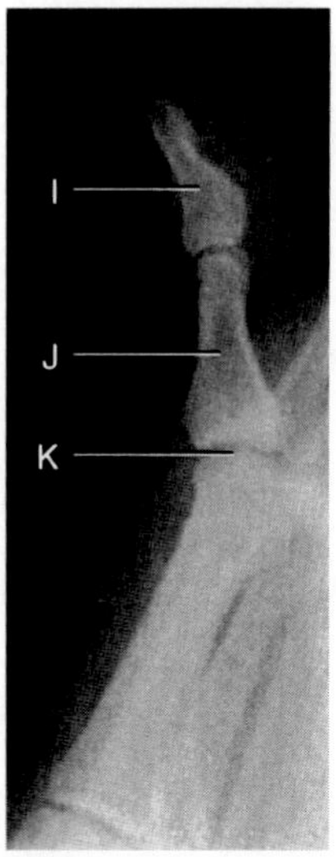

Fig. 7-13. Anatomy of the metatarsal bones and digits.

12. Which of the radiographs in the previous question represents an AP oblique projection of the toes?
    A. Fig. 7-11   C. Fig. 7-12
    B. Fig. 7-13   D. None of the above

13. What is the correct central ray centering placement for an AP projection of the toes?
    A. Affected MTP joint   C. Affected PIP joint
    B. Affected DIP joint   D. Head of affected metatarsal

14. Which type of central ray angle is required for an AP projection of the toes?
    A. None (central ray is perpendicular) C. 5° posterior
    B. 10° to 15° posterior   D. 20° to 25° posterior

15. Which of the following projections is used for the sesamoid bones of the foot?
    A. AP and lateral weight-bearing   C. Tangential
    B. Camp-Coventry   D. AP mortise

16. How much foot rotation is required for the AP oblique, medial rotation projection of the foot?
    A. 3° to 5°   C. 15° to 20°
    B. 45°   D. 30° to 40°

17. What is another term for the AP projection of the foot?
   A. Mortise projection
   B. Plantodorsal projection
   C. Weight-bearing study
   D. Dorsoplantar projection

18. What CR angle is generally required for the AP projection of the foot?
   A. 10° posterior
   B. 10° anterior
   C. 15° posterior
   D. None (central ray is perpendicular)

19. Which projection of the foot best demonstrates the cuboid?
   A. AP
   B. AP oblique—lateral rotation
   C. AP oblique—medial rotation
   D. Lateromedial

20. What is another term for the intercondyloid eminence?
   A. Tibial plateaus
   B. Intercondylar fossa
   C. Tibial tuberosity
   D. Intercondylar tubercles

21. What is the name of the deep depression found on the posterior aspect of the distal femur?
   A. Intercondylar fossa
   B. Intercondylar sulcus
   C. Patellar surface
   D. Articular facets

22. A line drawn across the most distal aspect of the medial and lateral femoral condyles would be

   _____ from being at a right angle (90°) to the long axis of the femur.
   A. 5° to 7°
   B. 3° to 5°
   C. 0°
   D. 10° to 20°

23. True/False: The angle referred to in question No. 22 would be less on a tall, slender person.

24. The upper, or superior, portion of the patella is called the:
   A. Apex
   B. Base
   C. Styloid process
   D. Patellar head

25. Which two ligaments of the knee joint help stabilize the knee from the anterior and posterior perspective?
   A. Collaterals
   B. Patellar
   C. Cruciates
   D. Quadriceps femoris

26. Which structures serve as shock absorbers within the knee joint?
   A. Articular facets
   B. Infrapatellar and suprapatellar bursae
   C. Menisci
   D. Infrapatellar fat pads

27. Match the structures labeled on Figs. 7-14 and 7-15 (using each choice only once).

_____ A.   1. Medial condyle of tibia

_____ B.   2. Neck of fibula

_____ C.   3. Head of fibula

_____ D.   4. Articular facets

_____ E.   5. Patella

_____ F.   6. Lateral condyle of femur

_____ G.   7. Proximal tibiofibular joint

_____ H.   8. Intercondyloid eminence

_____ I.   9. Femorotibial joint space

_____ J.   10. Lateral condyle of tibia

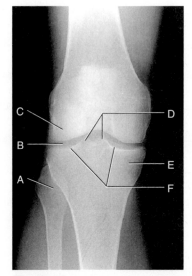

Fig. 7-14. AP radiograph of the knee.

28. Which knee projection does Fig. 7-15 represent?
   A. AP   C. AP oblique—lateral rotation
   B. AP oblique—medial rotation D. AP weight-bearing

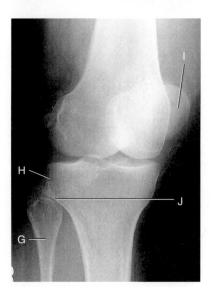

Fig. 7-15. Radiograph of the knee.

29. Match the parts labeled on Figs. 7-16 and 7-17 (answers may be used more than once).

_____ A.

_____ B.

_____ C.

_____ D.

_____ E.

_____ F.

_____ G.

_____ H.

_____ I.

_____ J.

1. Adductor tubercle

2. Head of fibula

3. Medial femoral condyle

4. Anterior aspect of medial condyle

5. Lateral femoral condyle

6. Anterior aspect of lateral femoral condyle

7. Tibial tuberosity

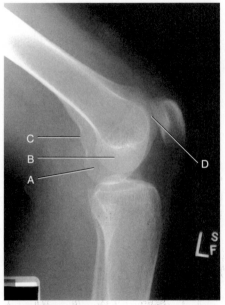

Fig. 7-16. Anatomy of the knee.

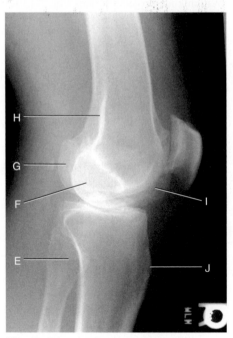

Fig. 7-17. Anatomy of the knee.

30. What is the *primary* positioning error present on Fig. 7-16 (mediolateral projection)?
    A. Overangulation of central ray
    B. Underrotation toward image receptor
    C. Overrotation of knee toward image receptor
    D. Underangulation of central ray

31. True/False: The mediolateral knee position in Fig. 7-16 is excessively flexed.

32. What is the *primary* positioning error in Fig. 7-17 (mediolateral projection)?
    A. Overangulation of central ray
    B. Underrotation toward image receptor
    C. Overrotation of knee toward image receptor
    D. Underangulation of central ray

33. Which one of the following conditions may cause the tibial tuberosity to be pulled away from the tibial shaft?
    A. Gout
    B. Reiter syndrome
    C. Osteomalacia
    D. Osgood-Schlatter disease

34. Which of the following pathologic conditions involves a ligament found in the foot?
    A. Reiter syndrome
    B. Paget's disease
    C. Exostosis
    D. Lisfranc injury

35. Which one of the following conditions may produce the radiographic appearance of a destructive lesion with irregular periosteal reaction?
    A. Osteogenic sarcoma
    B. Gout
    C. Bone cyst
    D. Osteoid osteoma

36. What is the common term for chondromalacia patellae?
    A. Brittle bone disease
    B. Runner's knee
    C. Degenerative joint disease
    D. Giant cell tumor

37. Where is the central ray placed for a plantodorsal axial projection of the calcaneus?
    A. Calcaneal tuberosity
    B. Sustentaculum tali
    C. Base of third metatarsal
    D. 1 inch (2½ cm) inferior to medial malleolus

38. Which ankle projection is best for demonstrating the mortise of the ankle?
    A. AP
    B. AP oblique (15° to 20° medial rotation)
    C. AP oblique (15° to 20° lateral rotation)
    D. Mediolateral

39. Which imaginary plane should be placed parallel to the IR for an AP projection of the knee?
    A. Intermalleolar
    B. Midcoronal
    C. Midsagittal
    D. Interepicondylar

40. Which joint space should be open or almost open for a well-positioned AP oblique knee projection with medial rotation?
    A. Both sides of knee joint
    B. Proximal tibiofibular
    C. Distal tibiofibular
    D. Patellofemoral

41. True/False: A 5° to 7° cephalad angle of the central ray for a lateral projection of the knee helps superimpose the distal borders of the medial and lateral condyles of the femur.

42. Why is a PA projection of the patella preferred to an AP projection?
    A. Less object image receptor distance (OID)
    B. Less distortion of patella
    C. Less magnification of patella
    D. All of the above

43. **Situation:** A projection is performed for the patellofemoral joint with the patient supine and the knee flexed 40°. The central ray is angled 30° caudad from horizontal. The cassette is resting on the lower legs supported by a special cassette-holding device. Which one of the following methods has been described?
    A. Camp-Coventry
    B. Settegast
    C. Hughston
    D. Bilateral Merchant

44. What is the major *disadvantage* of the Settegast method?
    A. Requires use of specialized equipment
    B. Requires AP positioning
    C. Requires overflexion of knee
    D. Requires the use of a long OID

45. **Situation:** A radiograph of an AP knee reveals that the joint spaces are not equally open and the proximal fibula is superimposed over the tibia. Which specific positioning error lead to this radiographic outcome?
    A. Underangulation of central ray
    B. Lateral rotation of lower limb
    C. Overangulation of central ray
    D. Medial rotation of lower limb

46. **Situation:** A radiograph of the Camp-Coventry method was produced, but the intercondylar fossa is not open and is foreshortened. The following positioning factors were used: prone position, lower leg flexed 45°, and central ray angled 30° caudad and centered to the popliteal crease. Which of the following should be done during the repeat exposure to produce a more diagnostic image?
    A. Decrease lower leg flexion to 30°
    B. Rotate lower limb 5° internally
    C. Increase CR angle to 45° caudad
    D. Increase flexion of lower limb to 50° to 60°

47. **Situation:** A radiograph of a plantodorsal axial projection of the calcaneus reveals that the calcaneus is foreshortened. The following positioning factors were used: supine position, foot dorsiflexed perpendicular to image receptor, and central ray angled 30° cephalad and centered to base of third metatarsal. Which of the following should be done during the repeat exposure to produce a more diagnostic image?
    A. Increase central ray angulation to 40°
    B. Reverse direction of central ray angulation
    C. Reduce dorsiflexion of foot
    D. Center central ray to sustentaculum tali

48. **Situation:** A bilateral patellofemoral joint space study is ordered. The patient is parapelgic and can't stand. Which of the following projections would be best suited for this patient?
    A. Superoinferior (sitting) tangential
    B. Bilateral inferosuperior
    C. Bilateral Merchant method
    D. Bilateral Settegast method

49. **Situation:** A radiograph of an AP mortise projection of the ankle reveals that the lateral joint space is not open, but the distal tibiofibular joint space is open. What positioning error lead to this outcome?
    A. Insufficient medial rotation
    B. Excessive medial rotation
    C. Excessive dorsiflexsion of the foot
    D. Excessive plantar flexion of the foot

50. **Situation:** A patient is referred to radiology for a possible Lisfranc injury. Which of the following positioning routines would best demonstrate this condition?
    A. Weight-bearing knee study
    B. AP and lateral lower leg
    C. Knee routine to include intercondylar fossa projection
    D. Weight-bearing foot study

8 Femur and Pelvic Girdle

CHAPTER OBJECTIVES

After you have successfully completed the activities in this chapter, you will be able to:

_____ 1. Identify the bones and specific features of the femur and pelvic girdle on drawings and radiographs.

_____ 2. Identify the location of the major landmarks of the pelvis and hip and describe two methods of locating the femoral head and neck on an anteroposterior (AP) hip and pelvis radiograph.

_____ 3. List the structural and functional differences of the greater and lesser pelvis and the structural difference between the male and female pelvis.

_____ 4. List the correct classification and movement type for the pelvic joints.

_____ 5. Identify the specific pediatric and geriatric applications for pelvis and hip radiographic examinations as described in the textbook.

_____ 6. Match specific pathologic indications of the pelvic girdle to the correct definition.

_____ 7. Match specific pathologic indications of the pelvic girdle to the correct radiographic appearance.

_____ 8. Determine whether a pelvis or hip is in a true AP position based on the established radiographic criteria.

_____ 9. List the patient dose ranges for each projection of the hip and pelvis and know the approximate difference among patient doses when using a higher kV, lower mA seconds manual technique.

_____ 10. Given various hypothetical clinical situations, identify the correct modification of a position and/or exposure factors to improve the radiographic image.

_____ 11. Given radiographs of specific femur, hip and pelvis projections, identify positioning and exposure factor errors.

POSITIONING AND RADIOGRAPHIC CRITIQUE

_____ 1. Using a peer, position for the basic and special projections of the femur and pelvic girdle.

_____ 2. Using a pelvic radiographic phantom, produce satisfactory radiographs of specific positions (if equipment is available).

_____ 3. Critique and evaluate pelvic girdle radiographs based on the four divisions of radiographic criteria: (1) structures shown, (2) position, (3) collimation and central ray, and (4) exposure criteria.

_____ 4. Distinguish between acceptable and unacceptable pelvic girdle radiographs based on exposure factors, motion, collimation, positioning, or other errors.

LEARNING EXERCISES

Complete the following review exercises after reading the associated pages in the textbook as indicated by each exercise. Answers to each review exercise are given at the end of the review exercises.

PART I: RADIOGRAPHIC ANATOMY
Review Exercise A: Radiographic Anatomy of the Femur, Hips and Pelvis (see textbook pp. 260-266)

1. The largest and strongest bone of the body is the _____.

2. A small depression located in the center of the femoral head is the _____.

3. The lesser trochanter is located on the _____ (medial or lateral) aspect of the proximal femur.

   It projects _____ (anteriorly or posteriorly) from the junction between the neck and shaft.

4. Because of the alignment between the femoral head and pelvis, the lower limb must be rotated

   _____° internally to place the femoral neck parallel to the plane of the image receptor to achieve a true anteroposterior (AP) projection.

5. True/False: According to Grey's Anatomy reference textbook, the terms pelvis and pelvic girdle are not synonymous.

   A. List the four bones comprising the pelvis._____

   B. List the two bones comprising the pelvic girdle. _____

   C. List two additional terms used for the bones identified in B.

   1. _____

   2. _____

6. List the three divisions of the hip bone.

   A. _____   B. _____   C. _____

7. All three divisions of the hip bone eventually fuse at the _____ at the age of

   _____.

8. What are the two important radiographic landmarks found on the ilium?

   A. _____   B. _____

9. Which bony landmark is found on the most inferior aspect of the posterior pelvis? _____

10. What is the name of the joint found between the superior rami of the pubic bones? _____

11. The _____ of the pelvis is the largest foramen in the skeletal system.

12. The upper margin of the greater trochanter is approximately (A) _____ above the level of the superior border of the symphysis pubis, and the ischial tuberosity is about (B)_____. below.

13. An imaginary plane that divides the pelvic region into the greater and lesser pelvis is called the

_____.

14. List the alternate terms for the greater and lesser pelvis.

   A. Greater pelvis _____   B. Lesser pelvis _____

15. List the major function of the greater pelvis and the lesser pelvis.

   A. Greater pelvis _____   B. Lesser pelvis _____

16. List the three aspects of the lesser pelvis, which also describe the birth route during the delivery process.

   A. _____   B. _____   C. _____

17. Match the following structures or characteristics to the correct hip bone (answers may be used more than once).

   _____ 1. Possesses a large tuberosity found at the most   A. Ilium
              inferior aspect of the pelvis
                                                                      B. Ischium
   _____ 2. Lesser sciatic notch
                                                                      C. Pubis
   _____ 3. Ala

   _____ 4. Posterior superior iliac spine (PSIS)

   _____ 5. Possesses a slightly movable joint

   _____ 6. Anterior superior iliac spine (ASIS)

   _____ 7. Forms the anterior, inferior aspect of the lower pelvic girdle

   _____ 8. Articulates with the sacrum to form the SI joints

18. In the past, which radiographic examination was performed to measure the fetal head in comparison with the

maternal pelvis to predict possible birthing problems? _____

19. What imaging modality has replaced the procedure identified in the previous question?

_____

20. Indicate whether the following radiographic characteristics apply to a male (M) or female (F) in relation to an AP projection of the pelvis.

_____ 1. Wide, more flared ilia   M. Male

_____ 2. Pubic arch angle of 110°   F. Female

_____ 3. A heart-shaped inlet

_____ 4. Narrow ilia that are less flared

_____ 5. Pubic arch angle of 75°

_____ 6. Larger and more round-shaped inlet

21. List the joint classification, mobility type, and movement type for the joints of the pelvis. Write *N/A* (not applicable) if the mobility or movement type does not apply.

	Classification	Mobility Type	Movement Type
A. Hip	_____	_____	_____
B. Sacroiliac	_____	_____	_____
C. Symphysis pubis	_____	_____	_____
D. Acetabulum (union)	_____	_____	_____

22. Identify the structures labeled on Figs. 8-1 and 8-2. Where indicated, use the following abbreviations to identify with which bone of the pelvis each labeled part is associated: *IL,* ilium; *IS,* ischium; *P,* pubis.

Structure   Bone

A. _____   ____

B. _____   ____

C. _____   ____

D. _____   ____

E. _____   ____

F. _____   ____

G. _____   ____

H. _____

I. _____   ____

J. _____   ____

K. _____   ____

L. _____   ____

M. _____   ____

N. _____   ____

O. _____   ____

P. _____   ____

Q. _____   ____

R. _____   ____

S. _____   ____

T. _____   ____

U. _____   ____

V. _____   ____

W. _____   ____

X. _____   ____

Y. _____   ____

Z. _____   ____

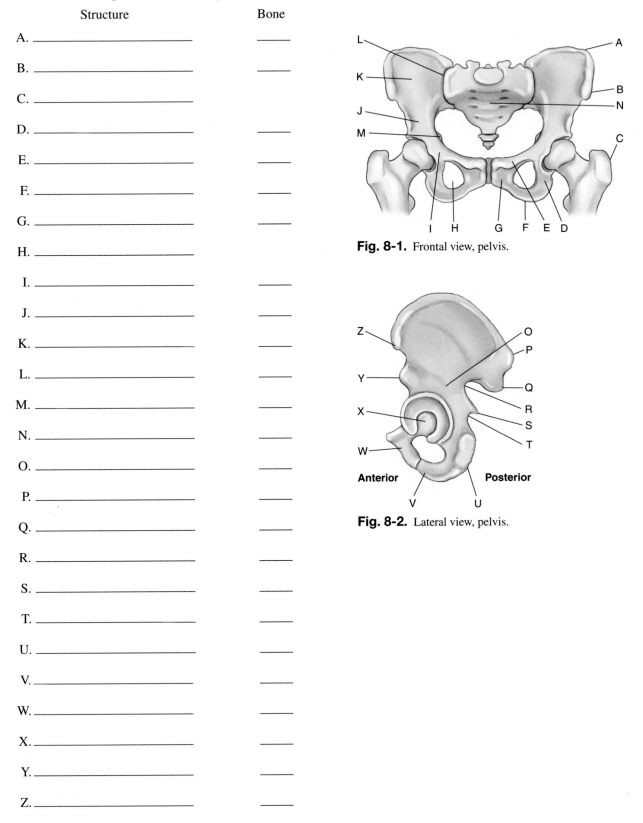

Fig. 8-1. Frontal view, pelvis.

Fig. 8-2. Lateral view, pelvis.

1. Which two bony landmarks need to be palpated for hip localization?

   A. _____   B. _____

2. From the midpoint of the imaginary line created by the two landmarks identified in the previous question, where

   would the femoral neck be located? _____

3. A second method for locating the femoral head is to palpate the _____ and go _____

   inches (_____ cm) medial at the level of the _____, which is _____ inches

   (_____ cm) distal to the original palpation point.

4. To achieve a true AP position of the proximal femur, the lower limb must be rotated _____
   internally.

5. Which structures on an AP pelvis or hip radiograph indicate whether the proximal head and neck are in position for

   a true AP projection? _____

6. Which physical sign may indicate that a patient has a hip fracture? _____

7. Which projection should be taken first and reviewed by a radiologist before attempting to rotate the hip into a lateral

   position (if trauma is suspected)? _____

8. Gonadal shielding should be used for all patients of reproductive age, unless _____.

9. Should a gonadal shield be used for a hip study on a young female? _____ If yes, describe

   how it should be placed on the patient. _____

10. Should a gonadal shield be used for a hip study on a young male? _____ If yes, describe how

    it should be placed on the patient. _____

11. What is the advantage of using 90 kV rather than 80 kV range for hip and pelvis studies on younger patients?

    _____

12. What is the disadvantage of using 90 kV for hip and pelvis studies, especially on older patients with some bone mass

    loss? _____

13. Which one of the following conditions is a common clinical indication for performing pelvic and hip examinations
    on a pediatric (newborn) patient?
    A. Osteoporosis   C. Ankylosing spondylitis
    B. Developmental dysplasia of hip (DDH)   D. Osteoarthritis

14. True/False: Geriatric patients are more prone to hip fractures because of their increased incidence of osteoporosis.

174

15. Which one of the following imaging modalities can be used on a newborn to assess hip joint stability during movement of the lower limbs?

   A. Sonography
   B. Computed tomography

   C. Magnetic resonance imaging
   D. Nuclear medicine

16. Which one of the following imaging modalities is most sensitive in diagnosing early signs of metastatic carcinoma of the pelvis?

   A. Sonography
   B. Computed tomography

   C. Magnetic resonance imaging
   D. Nuclear medicine

17. Match each of the following pathologic indications to the correct definition (using each choice only once).

   _____ A. A degenerative joint disease

   _____ B. Most common fracture in older patients because of high incidence of osteoporosis or avascular necrosis

   _____ C. A malignant tumor of the cartilage of hip

   _____ D. A disease producing extensive calcification of the longitudinal ligament of the spinal column

   _____ E. A fracture resulting from a severe blow to one side of the pelvis

   _____ F. Malignancy spread to bone via the circulatory and lymphatic systems or direct invasion

   _____ G. Now referred to as developmental dysplasia of the hip

   1. Metastatic carcinoma

   2. Ankylosing spondylitis

   3. Congenital dislocation

   4. Chondrosarcoma

   5. Proximal hip fracture

   6. Pelvic ring fracture

   7. Osteoarthritis

18. Which of the following devices will improve overall visibility of the proximal hip demonstrated on an axiolateral (inferosuperior) projection ?

   A. Small focal spot
   B. 6:1 grid

   C. Compensating filter
   D. Shadow shield

19. Which of the following modalities will best demonstrate a possible pelvic ring fracture?

   A. CT
   B. Nuclear medicine

   C. MRI
   D. Sonography

20. True/False: Both joints must be included on an AP and lateral projection of the femur even if a fracture of the proximal femur is evident.

21. Where is the central ray placed for an AP pelvis projection? _____

22. Which ionization chamber(s) should be activated when using automatic exposure control (AEC) for an AP pelvis projection?

   A. Center chamber only
   B. Upper right and left chambers

   C. Center and upper left or right chambers
   D. Upper left chamber only

23. Which specific positioning error is present when the left iliac wing is elongated on an AP pelvis radiograph?

_____

24. Which specific positioning error is present when the left obturator foramen is more open than the right side on an AP

pelvis radiograph?_____

25. Indicate whether each of the following projections is used for patients with traumatic (T) injuries or nontraumatic (NT) injuries.

_____ A. Danelius-Miller projection   T. Traumatic

_____ B. Unilateral frog-leg   NT. Not traumatic

_____ C. Modified Cleaves (bilateral frog-leg)

_____ D. Clements-Nakayama

_____ E. Anterior pelvic bones

26. Which of the following projections is recommended to demonstrate the superoposterior wall of the acetabulum?
   A. AP axial "inlet"   C. Axiolateral inferosuperior
   B. PA axial oblique   D. Modified axiolateral

27. When gonadal shielding is not used, _____ (males or females) receive a greater gonadal dose with an AP pelvis projection.

28. How many degrees are the femurs abducted (from the vertical plane) for the bilateral frog-leg projection?

_____

29. Where is the central ray placed for a unilateral frog-leg projection? _____

30. Which cassette size should be used for an adult bilateral frog-leg projection? _____

31. Where is the central ray placed for an AP bilateral frog-leg projection? _____

32. Which central ray angle is required for the "outlet" projection (Taylor method) for a female patient?
   A. 15° to 25° caudad   C. 20° to 35° cephalad
   B. 30° to 45° cephalad   D. None (central ray is perpendicular)

33. Which type of pathologic feature is best demonstrated with the Judet method?
   A. Acetabular fractures   C. Proximal femur fractures
   B. Anterior pelvic bone fractures   D. Femoral neck fractures

34. How much obliquity of the body is required for the Judet method?
   A. None (central ray is perpendicular)   C. 30°
   B. 20°   D. 45°

35. What type of CR angle is used for a PA axial oblique (Teufel) projection?
    A. 15° cephalad
    B. 15° to 20° cephalad
    C. 5° caudad
    D. 12° cephalad

36. How is the pelvis (body) positioned for a PA axial oblique (Teufel) projection?
    A. PA with 45° rotated away from affected side
    B. Prone or erect PA—no rotation
    C. PA 35° to 40° toward affected side
    D. AP with 40° away from affected side

37. True/False: Any orthopedic device or appliance of the hip should be seen in its entirety on an AP hip radiograph.

38. The axiolateral (inferosuperior) projection is designed for _____ (traumatic or nontraumatic) situations.

39. How is the unaffected leg positioned for the axiolateral hip projection? _____

40. Which one of the following factors does *not* apply to an axiolateral (inferosuperior) projection of the hip on a male patient?
    A. Cassette parallel to femoral neck
    B. 80 to 90 kV
    C. Use of gonadal shielding
    D. Use of a stationary grid

41. True/False: An AP pelvis projection using 90 kV and 8 mAs results in a patient dose of approximately 30% less than a projection using 80 kV and 12 mAs (for both males and females).

42. True/False: During an axiolateral (inferosuperior) projection of the hip, a male patient receives more than 20 times the gonadal dose than a female.

43. The modified axiolateral requires the CR to be angled _____ ° posteriorly from horizontal.

44. Which special projection of the hip demonstrates the anterior and posterior rims of the acetabulum and the ilioischial and iliopubic columns? (Include the projection name and the method name.)

    A. _____

    B. Which central ray angle (if any) is used for this projection? _____

45. What is the name of a special AP axial projection of the pelvis used to assess trauma to pubic and ischial structures?

    (Include the projection name and the method name.) _____

46. Match each of the following projections with its corresponding proper name (using each choice only once).

    _____ 1. Axiolateral (inferosuperior)   A. Judet

    _____ 2. Modified axiolateral   B. Taylor

    _____ 3. Bilateral or unilateral frog-leg   C. Clements-Nakayama

    _____ 4. PA axial oblique for acetablum   D. Danelius-Miller

    _____ 5. AP axial for pelvic "outlet" bones   E. Teufel

    _____ 6. Posterior oblique for acetabulum   F. Modified Cleaves

47. What is the optimal amount of hip abduction applied for the unilateral "frog-leg" projection to demonstrate the femoral neck without distortion?

A. 45° from vertical

C. 10° from vertical

B. 90° from vertical

D. 20° to 30° from vertical

48. True/False: The Lauenstein/Hickey method for the unilateral "frog-leg" projection will produce distoration of the femoral neck.

49. How much is the cassette tilted for the modified axiolateral projection of the hip? _____

50. True/False: Gonadal shielding can be used for males for the axiolateral (inferosuperior) projection of the hip.

Review Exercise C: Problem Solving for Technical and Positioning Errors

1. **Situation:** A radiograph of an AP pelvis projection reveals that the lesser trochanters are readily demonstrated on the medial side of the proximal femurs. The patient is ambulatory but has a history of early osteoarthritis in both hips. Which positioning modification needs to be made to prevent this positioning error?

    _____

    _____

2. **Situation:** A radiograph of an AP pelvis reveals that the right iliac wing is foreshortened as compared with the left side. Which specific positioning error has been made?

    _____

    _____

3. **Situation:** A radiograph of a unilateral frog-leg (modified Cleaves) projection reveals that the greater trochanter is superimposed over the femoral neck. Based on the AP hip projection, the radiologist suspects a nondisplaced fracture of the femoral neck. What can the technologist do to better define this region?

    _____

    _____

4. **Situation:** A radiograph of an axiolateral (inferosuperior) projection reveals that the posterior aspect of the acetabulum and femoral head were cut off of the bottom of the image. The emergency room physician requests that the position be repeated. What can be done to avoid this problem on the repeat exposure?

    _____

    _____

5. **Situation:** A radiograph of an AP axial projection for anterior pelvic bones reveals that the pubic and ischial bones are not elongated sufficiently. The following factors were used for this study: 86 kV, 7 mAs, Bucky, 20° to 30° central ray cephalad angle, and 40-inch (100-cm) source image receptor distance (SID). The female patient was placed in a supine position on the table. What must be changed to improve the quality of the image during the repeat exposure?

    _____

    _____

6. **Situation:** A patient enters ER with a pelvis injury due to a motor vehicle accident. The initial AP pelvis projection demonstrates a possible defect or fracture of the left acetabulum. No other fractures are detected and the patient is able to move comfortably. What additional projections can be taken to demonstrate a possible acetabular fracture?

_____

_____

7. **Situation:** A radiograph of an AP pelvis reveals that overall the image is underexposed (underpenetrated). The following factors were used: 80 kV, 40-inch (102-cm) SID, Bucky, and AEC with the center chamber activated. Which one of these factors should be changed to produce a darker and more diagnostic image?

_____

_____

8. **Situation:** A radiograph from a modified axiolateral projection reveals excessive grid lines on the image, which also appears underexposed. What can be done to avoid this problem during the repeat exposure?

_____

_____

9. **Situation:** A portable AP and lateral hip study is ordered for a patient who is in recovery following hip replacement surgery. The radiograph of the AP hip reveals that the upper portion of the acetabular prosthesis is slightly cut off but is included on the lateral projection. Should the technologist repeat the AP projection? Why or why not?

_____

_____

10. **Situation:** A patient with hip pain from a fall enters the emergency room. The physician orders a left hip study. When moved to the radiographic table, the patient complained loudly about the pain in the left hip. Which positioning routine should be used for this patient?

_____

_____

11. **Situation:** A patient has just been moved to his hospital room after a bilateral hip replacement surgery. The surgeon has ordered a postoperative hip routine for both hips. Which specific positioning routine should be used? (The patient can be brought to the radiology department.)

_____

_____

12. **Situation:** A patient with a possible pelvic ring fracture from a trauma enters the emergency room. The AP pelvis projection, which was taken to determine whether the right acetabulum is fractured, is inconclusive. Which other radiographic projection can be taken to better visualize the acetabulum?

_____

_____

13. **Situation:** A young patient comes to the radiology department with a chronic pain near the ASIS. She is an active athlete who injured her pelvis while running hurdles. Her physician suspects an avulsion fracture. Which position(s) may best diagnose this condition? Must the technologist increase or decrease kV for this projection to demonstrate the fracture?

_____

_____

14. **Situation:** A technologist notices that his AP pelvis projections often demonstrate a moderate degree of rotation. What positioning technique can the technologist perform to eliminate (or at least minimize) rotation on his AP pelvis projections?

_____

_____

15. **Situation:** A very young child comes to the radiology department with a clinical history of DDH. What is the most common positioning routine for this condition?

_____

_____

Review Exercise D: Critique Radiographs of the Femur and Pelvis (see textbook p. 285)

The following questions relate to the radiographs found at the end of Chapter 8 of the textbook. Evaluate these radiographs for the radiographic criteria categories (_1_ through _5_) that follow. Describe the corrections needed to improve the overall image. The major, or "repeatable," errors are specific errors that indicate the need for a repeat exposure, regardless of the nature of the other errors.

A. AP pelvis (Fig. C8-76)

Description of possible error:

1. Structures shown: _____

2. Part positioning: _____

3. Collimation and central ray: _____

4. Exposure criteria: _____

5. Markers: _____

Repeatable error(s): _____

B. AP Pelvis (Fig. C8-77)

Description of possible error:

    1. Structures shown: _____

    2. Part positioning: _____

    3. Collimation and central ray: _____

    4. Exposure criteria: _____

    5. Markers: _____

Repeatable error(s): _____

C. Unilateral "frog-leg" projection (performed cystography) (Fig. C8-78)

Description of possible error:

    1. Structures shown: _____

    2. Part positioning: _____

    3. Collimation and central ray: _____

    4. Exposure criteria: _____

    5. Markers: _____

Repeatable error(s): _____

D. Bilateral frog-leg (2-year-old) (Fig. C8-79)

Description of possible error:

    1. Structures shown: _____

    2. Part positioning: _____

    3. Collimation and central ray: _____

    4. Exposure criteria: _____

    5. Markers: _____

Repeatable error(s): _____

PART III: LABORATORY EXERCISES

You must gain experience in positioning each part of the proximal femur and pelvis before performing the following exams on actual patients. You can get experience in positioning and radiographic evaluation of these projections by performing exercises using radiographic phantoms and practicing positioning on other students (although you will not be taking actual exposures).

The following suggested activities assume that your teaching institution has an energized lab and radiographic phantoms. If not, perform Laboratory Exercises B and C, the radiographic evaluation and the physical positioning exercises. (Check off each step and projection as you complete it.)

Laboratory Exercise A: Energized Laboratory

1. Using the pelvic radiographic phantom, produce radiographs of the following basic routines:

_____ AP pelvis projection

_____ Posterior oblique positions for acetabulum, Judet method

_____ AP axial projection, Taylor method

Laboratory Exercise B: Radiographic Evaluation

1. Evaluate and critique the radiographs produced above, additional radiographs provided by your instructor, or both. Evaluate each radiograph for the following points:

_____ Evaluate the completeness of the study. (Are all of the pertinent anatomic structures included on the radiograph?)

_____ Evaluate for positioning or centering errors (e.g., rotation, off centering).

_____ Evaluate for correct exposure factors and possible motion. (Are the density and contrast of the images acceptable?)

_____ Determine whether markers and an acceptable degree of collimation and/or area shielding are visible on the images.

Laboratory Exercise C: Physical Positioning

On another person, simulate performing all basic and special projections of the proximal femur and pelvic girdle as follows. Include the six steps listed below and described in the textbook. (Check off each step when completed satisfactorily.)

Step 1. Appropriate size and type of image receptor with correct markers

Step 2. Correct central ray placement and centering of part to central ray and/or image receptor

Step 3. Accurate collimation

Step 4. Area shielding of patient where advisable

Step 5. Use of proper immobilizing devices when needed

Step 6. Approximate correct exposure factors, breathing instructions when applicable, and initiating exposure

Projections	Step 1	Step 2	Step 3	Step 4	Step 5	Step 6
● AP and lateral femur	_____	_____	_____	_____	_____	_____
● AP pelvis	_____	_____	_____	_____	_____	_____
● AP hip, unilateral	_____	_____	_____	_____	_____	_____
● Unilateral frog-leg	_____	_____	_____	_____	_____	_____
● Bilateral frog-leg	_____	_____	_____	_____	_____	_____
● Axiolateral projection	_____	_____	_____	_____	_____	_____
● Modified axiolateral	_____	_____	_____	_____	_____	_____
● Anterior oblique for acetabulum	_____	_____	_____	_____	_____	_____
● AP axial for anterior pelvic bones	_____	_____	_____	_____	_____	_____

MY SCORE = _____ %

This self-test should be taken only after completing all of the readings, review exercises, and laboratory activities for a particular section. The purpose of this test is not only to provide a good learning exercise but also to serve as a strong indicator of what your final evaluation exam for this chapter will cover. It is strongly suggested that if you do not get at least a 90% to 95% grade on each self-test that you review those areas in which you missed questions before going to your instructor for the final evaluation exam.

1. List the four bones of the pelvis.

   A. _____   C. _____

   B. _____   D. _____

2. List the three divisions of the hip bone.

   A. _____   B. _____   C. _____

3. *Innominate bone* is another name for:
   A. One half of pelvic girdle   C. Ossa coxae
   B. Hip bone   D. All of the above

4. What is the largest foramen in the body? _____

5. Which one of the following landmarks is not a palpable bony landmark?
   A. Greater trochanter   C. Ischial tuberosity
   B. Lesser trochanter   D. Anterior superior iliac spine (ASIS)

6. What are the two aspects of the ischium?

   A. _____   B. _____

7. What is the name of the imaginary plane that separates the false from the true pelvis? _____

8. Match the following structures or characteristics to the correct division of the pelvis.

   _____ 1. Lesser pelvis   A. False pelvis

   _____ 2. Supports the lower abdominal organs   B. True pelvis

   _____ 3. Formed primarily by the ala of the ilium

   _____ 4. Cavity

   _____ 5. Greater pelvis

   _____ 6. Forms the actual birth canal

   _____ 7. Found below the pelvic brim

9. The pubic arch angle on an average male pelvis is an _____ (acute or obtuse) angle that is

_____ (greater than or less than) 90°.

10. Identify the labeled structures found on the following radiographs.

A. _____

B. _____

C. _____

D. _____

E. _____

F. _____

G. _____

H. _____

I. _____

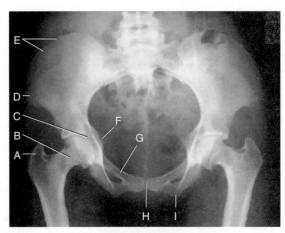

Fig. 8-3. AP pelvis radiograph.

J. Is this a male or female pelvis? _____

K. _____

L. _____

M. _____

N. _____

O. Which projection of the hip is represented

on this radiograph? _____

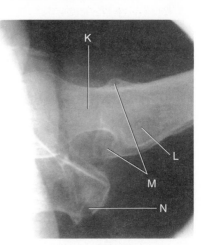

Fig. 8-4. Lateral hip radiograph.

P. _____

Q. _____

R. _____

S. _____

T. _____

U. _____

V. _____

W. Which projection of the hips is represented

on this radiograph? _____

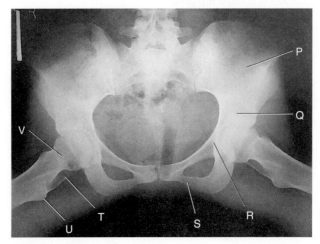

Fig. 8-5. Bilateral hip radiograph.

11. Indicate whether the following radiographic characteristics are those of a male (M) or female (F) pelvis.

_____ 1. Heart-shaped (oval) inlet

_____ 2. Acute pubic arch (less than 90°)

_____ 3. Iliac wings that are more flared

_____ 4. Obtuse pubic arch (greater than 90°)

_____ 5. Larger and more rounded inlet

_____ 6. Iliac wings that are less flared

F. Female

M. Male

12. Which one of the following structures is considered to be the most posterior?
   A. Ischial spines
   B. ASIS
   C. Symphysis pubis
   D. Acetabulum

13. The small depression near the center of the femoral head where a ligament is attached is called the

_____.

14. Which of the following joints are a synovial joint but with amphiarthrodial mobility?
   A. Union of acetabula
   B. Hip joint
   C. Sacroiliac joints
   D. Symphysis pubis

15. Which of the following devices should be used for an axiolateral (inferosuperior) projection of the hip to equalize density of the hip region?
   A. Grid
   B. High-speed IR
   C. Small focal spot
   D. Compensating filter

16. Which of the following modalities is used to assess joint stability during movement of the lower limbs on infants?
   A. Sonography
   B. MR
   C. CT
   D. Weight-bearing pelvis radiographic projections

17. A geriatric patient with an externally rotated lower limb may have:
   A. A normal hip joint
   B. Osteoarthritis
   C. Fractured proximal femur
   D. Slipped capital femoral epiphyses (SCFE)

18. Which one of the following pathologic indications may result in the early fusion of the sacroiliac (SI) joints?
   A. Chondrosarcoma
   B. Metastatic carcinoma
   C. Developmental dysplasia of the hip
   D. Ankylosing spondylitis

19. Match each of the following radiographic appearances with the correct pathologic indications (using each choice only once).

    _____ 1. Usually consists of numerous small lytic lesions

    _____ 2. Increased hip joint space and misalignment

    _____ 3. Bilateral radiolucent lines across bones and misalignment of SI joints

    _____ 4. Early fusion of SI joints and "bamboo spine"

    _____ 5. Epiphyses appear shorter and epiphyseal plate wider

    _____ 6. Hallmark sign of spurring and narrowing of joint space

A. Pelvic ring fracture

B. DDH

C. Osteoarthritis

D. SCFE

E. Ankylosing spondylitis

F. Metastatic carcinoma

20. Which one of the following radiographic signs indicates that the proximal femurs are in position for a true AP projection?
    A. Appearance of the greater trochanter in profile
    B. Limited view of fovea capitis
    C. Limited view of the lesser trochanter in profile
    D. Symmetric appearance of iliac wings

21. The gonadal dose for an average-size male with a routine axiolateral (inferosuperior) trauma hip projection is in the _____ mrad range.
    A. 50 to 100
    B. 200 to 500
    C. 10 to 50
    D. 600 to 800

22. True/False: The female gonadal dose for an AP pelvis is in the 50 to 100 mrad range, which is about three times greater than the dose for a male when no gonadal shields are used.

23. Which one of the following projections or methods is often performed to evaluate a pediatric patient for congenital hip dislocation?
    A. Bilateral modified Cleaves
    B. Clements-Nakayama
    C. Taylor method
    D. Judet method

24. What type of central ray angle is required when using the Taylor method for a male patient?
    A. None (central ray is perpendicular)
    B. 10° to 15° caudad
    C. 20° to 35° cephalad
    D. 30° to 45° cephalad

25. How much is the pelvis and/or thorax rotated for a PA axial oblique (Teufel method) for acetabulum?
    A. 15° toward affected side
    B. 30° to 35° away from affected side
    C. 20° away from from affected side
    D. 35° to 40° toward affected side

26. What type of CR angle is required for the PA axial oblique (Teufel method) for acetabulum?
    A. 12° cephalad
    B. 20° caudad
    C. 15° cephalad
    D. 25° cephalad

27. True/False: The unilateral frog-leg projection (modified Cleaves method) is intended for nontraumatic hip situations.

28. True/False: Centering for the AP pelvis projection is 1 inch, or 2½ cm, superior to the symphysis pubis.

29. True/False: The modified axiolateral (Clements-Nakayama method) is classified as a nontraumatic lateral hip projection.

30. What type of CR angle is required for the Judet method?
   A. 12° cephalad
   B. 5° to 10° caudad
   C. 15° cephalad
   D. None. CR is perpendicular

31. Which one of the following projections or methods is used to evaluate the pelvic inlet (superior aperture) for possible fracture?
   A. Danelius-Miller
   B. AP axial projection
   C. Taylor
   D. Clements-Nakayama

32. **Situation:** An initial AP pelvis radiograph reveals possible fractures involving the lower anterior pelvis. The emergency room physician asks for another projection to better demonstrate this area of the pelvis. The patient is traumatized and must remain in a supine position. Which projection should be taken?

_____

33. **Situation:** A radiograph of an axiolateral (inferosuperior) projection of a hip demonstrates a soft tissue density that is visible across the affected hip and acetabulum. This artifact is obscuring the image of the proximal femur. What is the most likely cause of the artifact, and how can it be prevented from showing up on the repeat exposure?

_____

_____

34. **Situation:** A unilateral frog-leg (modified Cleaves) demonstrates foreshortening of the femoral necks. The physician is unsure if there is a defect within the anatomical neck. What can be done to minimize distortion of the neck during a repeat expsoure?

_____

_____

35. **Situation:** A radiograph of an AP hip reveals that the lesser trochanters are not visible. Should the technologist repeat

the projection? _____ If yes, what should be modified to improve the image during the repeat exposure?

_____

_____

36. **Situation:** A young patient with a clinical history of SCFE comes to the radiology department. Which projection(s) are most often taken for this condition?

_____

_____

37. **Situation:** A radiograph produced using the Taylor method demonstrates that the anterior pelvic bones of a female patient are foreshortened. The following positioning factors were used: supine position, 40-inch (100-cm) SID, and central ray angled 30° caudad and centered 1 to 2 inches (3 to 5 cm) distal to symphysis pubis. Which one of the following modifications should be made during the repeat exposure?

    A. Increase central ray angle   C. Center central ray at level of ASIS

    B. Reverse central ray angle   D. Place patient prone on table

38. **Situation:** A radiograph of an AP projection of the pelvis demonstrates that the left obturator foramen is narrowed and the right one is open. What is the specific positioning error present on this radiograph?

_____

_____

39. **Situation:** A patient enters the emergency room with a possible pelvic ring fracture. The AP pelvis projection is inclusive on the extent and location of the fracture(s). What additional pelvis projection(s) can be taken on this patient to demonstrate possible pelvic fractures? (More than one correct answer is possible.)

_____

_____

40. **Situation:** A radiograph of the Teufel method (PA axial oblique) demonstrates distortion of the acetabulum. During positioning, the patient was rotated 35° to 40° toward the affected side and CR was angled 20° cephalad. What modifications are needed during the repeat exposure?

_____

9 Cervical and Thoracic Spine

CHAPTER OBJECTIVES

After you have successfully completed the activities in this chapter, you will be able to:

_____ 1. Using drawings and radiographs, identify specific anatomic structures of the cervical and thoracic spine.

_____ 2. Identify specific features of the cervical and thoracic vertebrae that distinguish them from other aspects of the vertebral column.

_____ 3. Identify the location, angulation, classification, and type of movement for specific joints of the cervical and thoracic spine.

_____ 4. List additional terms for the first, second, and seventh cervical vertebrae.

_____ 5. Identify topographic landmarks that can be palpated to locate specific thoracic and cervical vertebrae.

_____ 6. Match specific pathologic indications of the cervical and thoracic spine to the correct definition.

_____ 7. Identify which radiographic projection and/or procedure best demonstrates specific pathologic indications.

_____ 8. Identify structures that are best demonstrated with each position of the cervical and thoracic spine.

_____ 9. List the patient dose ranges, including thyroid and female breast doses, for specific projections of the cervical and thoracic spine.

_____ 10. Identify basic and special projections of the cervical and thoracic spine and list the correct size and type of image receptor (IR) and the central ray location, direction, and angulation for each position.

_____ 11. Given various hypothetical situations, identify the correct modification of a position and/or exposure factors to improve the radiographic image.

_____ 12. Given radiographs of specific cervical and thoracic spine projections, identify positioning and exposure factor errors.

POSITIONING AND RADIOGRAPHIC CRITIQUE

_____ 1. Using a peer, position for basic and special projections of the cervical and thoracic spine.

_____ 2. Using appropriate radiographic phantoms, produce satisfactory radiographs of specific positions (if equipment is available).

_____ 3. Critique and evaluate cervical and thoracic spine radiographs based on the four divisions of radiographic criteria: (1) structures shown, (2) position, (3) collimation and central ray, and (4) exposure criteria.

_____ 4. Distinguish between acceptable and unacceptable spine radiographs based on exposure factors, motion, collimation, positioning, or other errors.

Complete the following review exercises after reading the associated pages in the textbook as indicated by each exercise. Answers to each review exercise are given at the end of the review exercises.

PART I: RADIOGRAPHIC ANATOMY
Review Exercise A: Radiographic Anatomy of the Cervical and Thoracic Spine (see textbook pp. 288-299)

1. List the number of bones found in each division in the adult vertebral column.

   A. Cervical _____   D. Sacrum _____

   B. Thoracic _____   E. Coccyx _____

   C. Lumbar _____   F. Total _____

Refer to Fig. 9-1 to answer questions 2 through 4.

2. List the two primary or posterior convex curves seen in the vertebral column.

   A. _____

   B. _____

3. Indicate which two portions of the vertebral column are classified as secondary or compensatory curves.

   A. _____

   B. _____

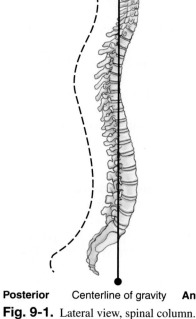

Posterior   Centerline of gravity   **Anterior**
Fig. 9-1. Lateral view, spinal column.

4. Match the correct aspect(s) of the vertebral column with the following characteristics (may be more than one answer).

   _____ 1. Convex curve (with respect to posterior)   A. Cervical spine

   _____ 2. Concave curve (with respect to posterior)   B. Thoracic spine

   _____ 3. Secondary curve   C. Lumbar spine

   _____ 4. Primary curve   D. Sacrum

   _____ 5. Develops as child learns to hold head erect

5. An abnormal, or exaggerated, "sway back" lumbar curvature is called _____.

6. An abnormal lateral curvature seen in the thoracolumbar spine is called _____.

7. The two main parts of a typical vertebra are the _____ and the _____.

8. The _____ are two bony aspects of the vertebral arch that extend posteriorly from each pedicle to join at the midline.

9. The _____ foramina are created by two small notches on the superior and inferior aspects of the pedicles.

10. The opening, or passageway, for the spinal cord is the _____.

11. The spinal cord begins with the (A) _____ of the brain and extends down to the

    (B) _____ vertebra, where it tapers and ends. This tapered ending is called the

    (C) _____ .

12. Which structures pass through the intervertebral foramina? _____

13. Identify the following structures labeled on these drawings of typical thoracic vertebrae (Fig. 9-2).

Superior view

A. _____

B. _____

C. _____

D. _____

E. _____

F. _____

Lateral view

G. _____

H. _____

I. _____

J. _____

K. _____

Lateral oblique view

L. _____

M. _____ joint

N. _____

O. _____

P. _____

Q. The joints between the ribs and vertebrae

at N are called: _____

R. The joints between the ribs and vertebrae

at P are called: _____

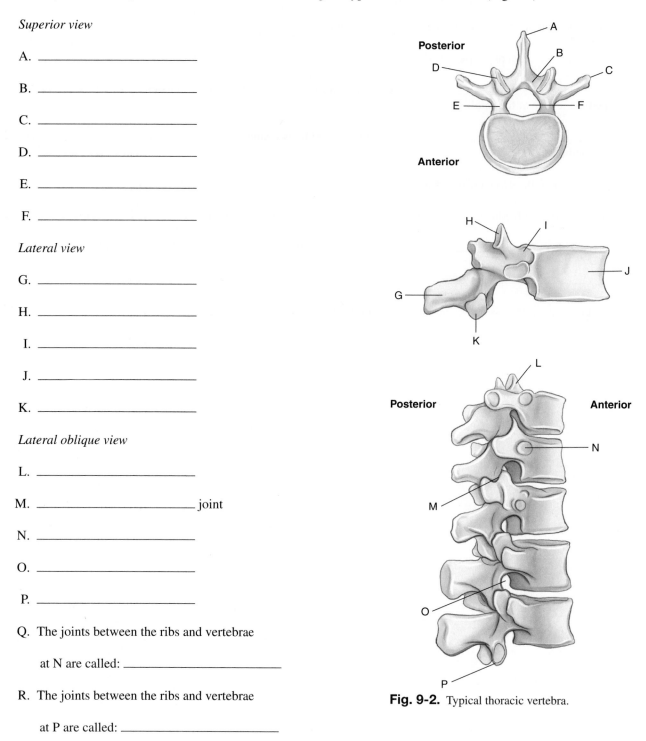

Fig. 9-2. Typical thoracic vertebra.

14. Which of the following is found between the superior and inferior articular processes?
    A. Intervertebral joints   C. Zygapophyseal joints
    B. Articular joints   D. Intervertebral facets

15. True/False: Only T1, T11, and T12 have *full* facets for articulation with ribs.

16. True/False: The zygapophyseal joints of *all* cervical vertebrae are visualized only in a true lateral position.

17. List the outer and inner aspects of the intervertebral disk.

    A. Outer aspect _____   B. Inner aspect _____

18. The condition involving a "slipped disk" is correctly referred to as _____.

19. List the alternative names for the following cervical vertebrae.

    A. C1: _____

    B. C2: _____

    C. C7: _____

20. List three features that make the cervical vertebrae unique.

    A. _____   C. _____

    B. _____

21. A short column of bone found between the superior and articular processes in a typical cervical vertebra is called

    _____.

22. What is the term for the same structure, identified in the previous question, for the C1 vertebra?

    _____

23. The zygapophyseal joints for the second through seventh cervical vertebrae are at a _____° angle

    to the midsagittal plane; the thoracic vertebrae are at a _____° angle to the midsagittal plane.

24. What is the name of the joint found between the superior articular processes of C1 and the occipital condyles of the

    skull? _____

25. The modified body of C2 is called the _____ or _____.

26. A lack of symmetry of the zygapophyseal joints between C1 and C2 may be caused by injury or may be associated

    with _____.

27. What is the unique feature of all thoracic vertebrae that distinguishes them from other vertebrae?

    _____

28. Which specific thoracic vertebrae are classified as typical thoracic vertebrae (i.e., they least resemble cervical or lumbar vertebrae)? _____

29. Identify the labeled structures on the radiographs of the cervical spine in Figs. 9-3 and 9-4. (Indicate the specific structure and the vertebra of which it is a part.)

Structure	Vertebra
A. _____	_____
B. _____	_____
C. _____	_____
D. _____	_____
E. _____	_____
F. _____	_____
G. _____	_____
H. _____	_____

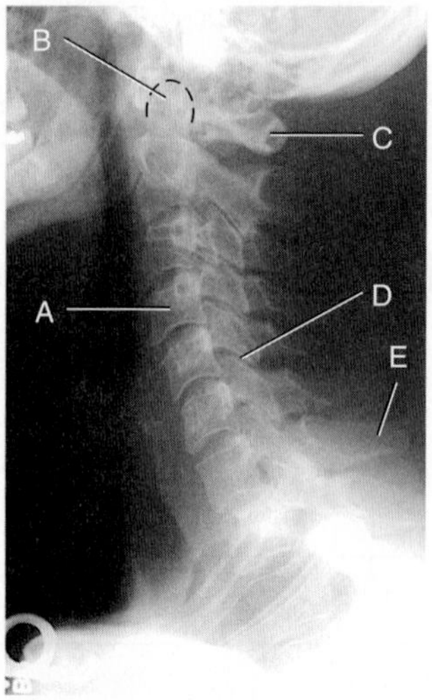

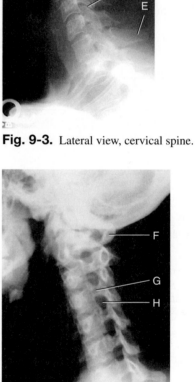

Fig. 9-3. Lateral view, cervical spine.

Fig. 9-4. 45° oblique view, cervical spine.

30. For the central ray to pass through and "open" the intervertebral spaces on a 45° posterior oblique projection of the cervical vertebrae, what central ray angle (if any) would be required? _____

1. Name the following parts of the sternum or associated topographic landmarks.

   A. Upper portion of sternum: _____

   B. Superior margin of this upper section (landmark): _____

   C. Main center portion of sternum: _____

   D. Joint between top and center portions (landmark): _____

   E. Most inferior aspect of sternum (landmark): _____

2. Match the following topographic landmarks to the correct vertebral level (using each choice only once).

   _____ 1. Gonion   A. C7-T1

   _____ 2. Xiphoid process (tip)   B. T2-3

   _____ 3. Thyroid cartilage   C. C1

   _____ 4. Jugular notch   D. T4-5

   _____ 5. Sternal angle   E. T10

   _____ 6. Mastoid tip   F. C4-C5

   _____ 7. Vertebra prominens   G. T7

   _____ 8. 3 to 4 inches (8 to 10 cm) below jugular notch H. C3

3. In addition to the gonads, which other radiosensitive organs are of greatest concern during cervical and thoracic spine radiography?

   _____

4. List the two advantages of using higher kV exposure factors for spine radiography, especially on an anteroposterior (AP) thoracic spine radiograph.

   A. _____   B. _____

5. True/False: When using digital imaging for spine radiography, it is important to use close collimation, grids, and lead masking.

6. True/False: If close collimation is used during conventional radiography of the spine, the use of lead masking is generally not required.

7. True/False: To a certain degree, magnetic resonance imaging (MRI) and computed tomography (CT) are replacing myelography as the imaging modalities of choice for the diagnosis of a ruptured intervertebral disk.

8. True/False: Nuclear medicine is often performed to diagnose bone tumors of the spine.

9. To ensure that the intervertebral joint spaces are open for lateral thoracic spine projections, it is important to:
   A. Keep the vertebral column parallel to the image receptor (IR)
   B. Use a small focal spot
   C. Use a breathing technique
   D. Angle the central ray cephalad

10. For lateral and oblique projections of the cervical spine, it is important to minimize magnification and maximize detail by (more than one answer may be used):
    A. Keeping vertebral column parallel to image receptor
    B. Using a small focal spot
    C. Increasing source image receptor distance (SID)
    D. Using a breathing technique

11. Match each of the following pathologic indications of the spine to the correct definition (using each choice only once).

    _____ A. Fracture through the pedicles and anterior arch of C2 with forward displacement upon C3

    _____ B. Inflammation of the vertebrae

    _____ C. Abnormal or exaggerated convex curvature of the thoracic spine

    _____ D. Comminuted fracture of the vertebral body with posterior fragments displaced into the spinal canal

    _____ E. Avulsion fracture of the spinous process of C7

    _____ F. Abnormal lateral curvature of the spine

    _____ G. A form of rheumatoid arthritis

    _____ H. Impact fracture from axial loading of the anterior and posterior arch of C1

    _____ I. Mild form of scoliosis and kyphosis developing during adolescence

    _____ J. Produces the "bow tie" sign

    1. Ankylosing spondylitis

    2. Clay shoveler's fracture

    3. Unilateral subluxation

    4. Kyphosis

    5. Scheuermann disease

    6. Scoliosis

    7. Jefferson fracture

    8. Teardrop burst fracture

    9. Hangman's fracture

    10. Spondylitis

12. List the conventional radiographic examination and/or projections performed for the following pathologic indications.

   A. Scoliosis: _____

   B. Teardrop burst fracture: _____

   C. Jefferson fracture: _____

   D. Scheuermann disease: _____

   E. Unilateral subluxation of cervical spine: _____

   F. HNP: _____

13. What are the major differences between spondylosis and spondylitis? _____

_____

14. True or False: Many geriatric patients have a fear of falling off the radiographic table.

15. What is the name of the radiographic procedure that requires the injection of contrast media into the subarachnoid

   space? _____

16. Which imaging modality is ideal for detecting early signs of osteomyelitis?

_____

17. Which two landmarks must be aligned for an AP "open mouth" projection? _____

18. What is the purpose of the 15° to 20° angle for the AP axial projection of the cervical spine?

_____

19. For an AP axial of the cervical spine, a plane through the tip of the mandible and _____
    should be parallel to the angled central ray.
    A. Mastoid process   C. Base of skull
    B. Gonion   D. External auditory meatus (EAM)

20. What are two important benefits of an SID longer than 40 to 44 inches (102 to 112 cm) for the lateral cervical spine
    projection?

   A. _____   B. _____

21. What central ray angulation must be used with a posterior oblique projection of the cervical spine?

_____

22. Which foramina are demonstrated with a left posterior oblique (LPO) position of the cervical spine?

_____

23. Which foramina are demonstrated with a left anterior oblique (LAO) position of the cervical spine?

_____

24. In addition to extending the chin, which additional positioning technique can be performed to ensure that the mandible is not superimposed over the upper cervical vertebrae for the oblique projections?

_____

25. What is the recommended SID for a lateral projection of the cervical spine?

_____

26. The lateral projection of the cervical spine should be taken during _____ (inspiration, expiration, or suspended respiration). Why?

_____

27. Which specific projection must be taken first if trauma to the cervical spine is suspected and the patient is in a supine position on a backboard? _____

28. The proper name of the method for performing the cervicothoracic (swimmer's lateral) projection is the

_____.

29. Where should the central ray be placed for a cervicothoracic (swimmer's lateral) projection?

_____

30. Which region of the spine must be demonstrated with a cervicothoracic (swimmer's lateral) projection?

_____

31. Which one of the following projections is considered a "functional study" of the cervical spine?
    A. AP "wagging jaw" projection   C. Fuchs or Judd method
    B. AP "open mouth" position   D. Hyperextension and flexion lateral positions

32. When should the Judd or Fuchs method be performed? _____

33. Which AP projection of the cervical spine demonstrates the entire upper cervical spine with one single projection?

_____

34. Which two things can be done to produce equal density along the entire thoracic spine for the AP projection

(especially for a patient with a thick chest)? _____

35. What is the purpose of using a breathing technique for a lateral projection of the thoracic spine?

_____

36. Which zygapophyseal joints are demonstrated in a right anterior oblique (RAO) projection of the thoracic spine?

_____

37. Which one of the following projections delivers the greatest skin dose to the patient?
    A. AP thoracic spine projection
    B. Lateral cervical spine projection
    C. Swimmer's lateral projection
    D. Fuchs or Judd method

38. Which of the following results in the lowest midline and skin doses for the patient? (Note dose relationship to mAs.)
    A. AP thoracic spine at 90 kV, 7 mAs
    B. AP thoracic spine at 80 kV, 12 mAs
    C. Lateral thoracic spine at 80 kV, 50 mAs
    D. Oblique thoracic spine at 80 kV, 20 mAs

39. True/False: The thyroid dose used during a posterior oblique cervical spine projection is more than 10 times greater than the dose used for an anterior oblique projection of the cervical spine.

40. Which one of the following structures is best demonstrated with an AP axial vertebral arch projection?
    A. Spinous processes of lumbar spine
    B. Articular pillar (lateral masses) of cervical spine
    C. Zygapophyseal joints of thoracic spine
    D. Cervicothoracic spine region

41. What central ray angle must be used with the AP axial—vertebral arch projection?
    A. 15° to 20° cephalad
    B. 5° to 10° cephalad
    C. 20° to 30° caudad
    D. None (central ray is perpendicular to IR)

42. What ancillary device should be placed behind the patient on the table top for a recumbent lateral projection of the thoracic spine when using computed radiography?

_____

43. Which skull positioning line is aligned perpendicular to the IR for a PA (Judd) projection for the odontoid process?

_____

44. Which zygapophyseal joints is best demonstrated with a LPO position of the thoracic spine?

_____

45. How much rotation of the body is required for an oblique position of the thoracic spine from a true lateral position?

_____

Review Exercise C: Problem Solving for Technical and Positioning Errors

1. A radiograph of an AP "open mouth" projection of the cervical spine reveals that the base of the skull is superimposed over the upper odontoid process. Which **specific** positioning error is present on this radiograph?

_____

2. A radiograph of an AP axial projection of the cervical spine reveals that the intervertebral disk spaces are not open. The following positioning factors were used: extension of the skull, central ray angled 10° cephalad, central ray centered to the thyroid cartilage, and no rotation or tilt of the spine. Which of these factors need(s) to be modified to produce a more diagnostic image?

_____

3. A radiograph of a right posterior oblique (RPO) cervical spine projection reveals that the lower intervertebral foramina are *not* open. The upper intervertebral foramina are well visualized. What positioning error most likely led to this radiographic outcome?

_____

4. A radiograph on a lateral projection of the cervical spine reveals that C7 is not clearly visible. The following factors were used: erect position, 44-inch (112-cm) SID, arms down by the patient's side, and exposure made during inspiration. Which two of these factors should be changed to produce a more diagnostic image during the repeat exposure?

_____

5. A radiograph of an AP "wagging jaw" (Ottonello method) projection taken at 75 kV, 20 mAs, and ½ second demonstrates that part of the image of the mandible is still visible and obscuring the upper cervical spine. Which modification needs to be made to produce a more diagnostic image during the repeat exposure?

_____

6. A radiograph of a lateral thoracic spine reveals that lung markings and ribs make it difficult to visualize the vertebral bodies. The following factors were used: recumbent position, 40-inch (102-cm) SID, short exposure time, and exposure made during full expiration. Which one of these factors needs to be modified to produce a more diagnostic image during the repeat exposure?

_____

7. A radiograph of an AP projection of the thoracic spine reveals that the upper thoracic spine is greatly overexposed but the lower vertebrae are well visualized. The head of the patient was placed at the anode end of the table. What can be modified during the repeat exposure to produce a more diagnostic image?

_____

8. A radiograph of a cervicothoracic lateral projection demonstrates superimposition of the humeral heads over the upper thoracic spine. Because of an arthritic condition, the patient is unable to rotate the shoulders any farther apart. What can the technologist do to further separate the shoulders during the repeat exposure?

_____

9. **Situation:** A patient with a possible cervical spine injury enters the emergency room. The patient is on a backboard. Which projection of the cervical spine should be taken first?

_____

10. **Situation:** A patient who has been in a motor vehicle accident (MVA) enters the emergency room. The basic projections of the cervical spine reveal no subluxation (partial dislocation) or fracture. The physician wants the spine evaluated for whiplash injury. Which additional projections would best demonstrate this type of injury?

_____

11. **Situation:** A patient comes to the radiology department for a cervical spine series. An AP "open mouth" radiograph indicates that the base of the skull and lower edge of the front incisors are superimposed, but the top of the dens is not clearly demonstrated. What should the technologist do to demonstrate the upper portion of the dens? (A horizontal beam lateral projection has ruled out a C-spine fracture or subluxation.)

_____

12. **Situation:** A patient comes to the radiology department for a routine cervical spine series. The lateral projection only demonstrates the C1 to C6 region. The radiologist wants to see C7-T1. What additional projection can be taken to demonstrate this region of the spine?

_____

13. **Situation:** A patient enters the ER with a possible cervical spine fracture, but the initial projections do not demonstrate any gross fracture or subluxation. After reviewing the initial radiographs, the ER physician suspects either a congenital defect or fracture of the lateral mass on C4. He wants an additional projection taken to better see this aspect of the vertebrae. What additional projection can be taken to demonstrate the lateral masses of C4?

_____

14. **Situation:** A patient comes to the ER with a possible Jefferson fracture. Other than a lateral projection or a CT scan, what specific radiographic projection will best demonstrate this type of fracture?

_____

15. **Situation:** A patient comes to the radiology department with a clinical history of Scheuermann disease. Which radiographic procedure is often performed for this condition?

_____

Review Exercise D: Critique Radiographs of the Cervical and Thoracic Spine (see textbook p. 320)

The following questions relate to the radiographs found at the end of Chapter 9 of the textbook. Evaluate these radiographs for the radiographic criteria categories (1 through 5) that follow. Describe the corrections needed to improve the overall image. The major, or "repeatable," errors are specific errors that indicate the need for a repeat exposure, regardless of the nature of the other errors.

A. AP open mouth (Fig. C9-91)

Description of possible error:

    1. Structures shown: _____

    2. Part positioning: _____

    3. Collimation and central ray: _____

    4. Exposure criteria: _____

    5. Anatomic side markers: _____

Repeatable error(s): _____

B. AP open mouth (Fig. C9-92)

Description of possible error:

    1. Structures shown: _____

    2. Part positioning: _____

    3. Collimation and central ray: _____

    4. Exposure criteria: _____

    5. Anatomic side markers: _____

Repeatable error(s): _____

C. AP axial projection (Fig. C9-93)

Description of possible error:

    1. Structures shown: _____

    2. Part positioning: _____

    3. Collimation and central ray: _____

    4. Exposure criteria: _____

    5. Anatomic side markers: _____

Repeatable error(s): _____

D. Right Posterior Oblique (Fig. C9-94)

Description of possible error:

    1. Structures shown: _____

    2. Part positioning: _____

    3. Collimation and central ray: _____

    4. Exposure criteria: _____

    5. Anatomic side markers: _____

Repeatable error(s): _____

E. Lateral (trauma) (Fig. C9-95)

Description of possible error:

    1. Structures shown: ＿＿＿＿＿＿＿＿＿＿＿＿＿

    2. Part positioning: ＿＿＿＿＿＿＿＿＿＿＿＿＿

    3. Collimation and central ray: ＿＿＿＿＿＿＿＿＿＿＿＿＿

    4. Exposure criteria: ＿＿＿＿＿＿＿＿＿＿＿＿＿

    5. Anatomic side markers: ＿＿＿＿＿＿＿＿＿＿＿＿＿

Repeatable error(s): ＿＿＿＿＿＿＿＿＿＿＿＿＿

F. AP for odontoid process—Fuchs Method (Fig. C9-96)

Description of possible error:

    1. Structures shown: ＿＿＿＿＿＿＿＿＿＿＿＿＿

    2. Part positioning: ＿＿＿＿＿＿＿＿＿＿＿＿＿

    3. Collimation and central ray: ＿＿＿＿＿＿＿＿＿＿＿＿＿

    4. Exposure criteria: ＿＿＿＿＿＿＿＿＿＿＿＿＿

    5. Anatomic side markers: ＿＿＿＿＿＿＿＿＿＿＿＿＿

Repeatable error(s): ＿＿＿＿＿＿＿＿＿＿＿＿＿

PART III: LABORATORY EXERCISES

You must gain experience in positioning each part of the cervical and thoracic spine before performing the following exams on actual patients. You can get experience in positioning and radiographic evaluation of these projections by performing exercises using radiographic phantoms and practicing positioning on other students (although you will not be taking actual exposures).

    The following suggested activities assume that your teaching institution has an energized lab and radiographic phantoms. If not, perform Laboratory Exercises B and C, the radiographic evaluation and the physical positioning exercises. (Check off each step and projection as you complete it.)

Laboratory Exercise A: Energized Laboratory

1. Using the radiographic phantom, produce radiographs of the following basic routines.
    A. AP, lateral, and oblique cervical spine   B. AP, lateral, and oblique thoracic spine

Laboratory Exercise B: Radiographic Evaluation

1. Evaluate and critique the radiographs produced above, additional radiographs provided by your instructor, or both. Evaluate each radiograph for the following points.

_____ Evaluate the completeness of the study. (Are all of the pertinent anatomic structures included on the radiograph?)

_____ Evaluate for positioning or centering errors (e.g., rotation, off centering).

_____ Evaluate for correct exposure factors and possible motion. (Are the density and contrast of the images acceptable?)

_____ Determine whether anatomic side markers and an acceptable degree of collimation and/or area shielding are visible on the images.

Laboratory Exercise C: Physical Positioning

On another person, simulate performing all basic and special projections of the cervical and thoracic spine as follows. Include the six steps listed below and described in the textbook. (Check off each step when completed satisfactorily.)

Step 1. Appropriate size and type of image receptor with correct markers

Step 2. Correct central ray placement and centering of part to central ray and/or image receptor

Step 3. Accurate collimation

Step 4. Area shielding of patient where advisable

Step 5. Use of proper immobilizing devices when needed

Step 6. Approximate correct exposure factors, breathing instructions where applicable, and initiating exposure

Projections	Step 1	Step 2	Step 3	Step 4	Step 5	Step 6
● Cervical spine series (AP axial, AP C1-2, oblique, lateral)	_____	_____	_____	_____	_____	_____
● Thoracic spine series (AP and lateral)	_____	_____	_____	_____	_____	_____
● Swimmer's lateral	_____	_____	_____	_____	_____	_____
● Hyperextension and flexion laterals	_____	_____	_____	_____	_____	_____
● AP "wagging jaw" projection	_____	_____	_____	_____	_____	_____
● AP (Fuchs) projection for dens	_____	_____	_____	_____	_____	_____
● PA (Judd) projection for dens	_____	_____	_____	_____	_____	_____
● Thoracic spine oblique projections	_____	_____	_____	_____	_____	_____

This self-test should be taken only after completing all of the readings, review exercises, and laboratory activities for a particular section. The purpose of this test is not only to provide a good learning exercise but also to serve as a strong indicator of what your final evaluation exam will cover. It is strongly suggested that if you do not get at least a 90% to 95% grade on each self-test that you review those areas in which you missed questions before going to your instructor for the final evaluation exam for this chapter.

1. At which vertebral level does the solid spinal cord terminate? _____

2. How many segments make up the sacrum in the neonate? _____

3. Which of the following divisions of the spine is described as possessing a primary curve? (There may be more than one correct answer.)
   A. Thoracic   C. Lumbar
   B. Cervical   D. Sacral

4. True/False: The lumbar possesses a concave posterior spinal curvature.

5. An abnormal or exaggerated thoracic spinal curvature with increased convexity is called _____.

6. An abnormal or exaggerated lateral spinal curvature is called _____.

7. What is the correct term for the condition involving a "slipped disk"? _____

8. Which foramina are created by the superior and inferior vertebral notches? _____

9. Which joints are found between the superior and inferior articular processes? _____

10. Which one of the following structures makes up the inner aspect of the intervertebral disk?
    A. Annulus fibrosus   C. Annulus pulposus
    B. Nucleus pulposus   D. Nucleus fibrosus

11. True/False: The carotid artery and certain nerves pass through the cervical transverse foramina.

12. True/False: The thoracic spine possesses facets for rib articulations and bifid spinous processes.

13. The intervertebral foramina for the cervical spine lie at a _____ ° angle to the midsagittal plane.

14. Which ligament holds the dens against the anterior arch of C1? _____

15. The large joint space between C1 and C2 is called the _____.

16. Two partial facets found on the thoracic vertebrae are called _____.

17. Which of the following thoracic vertebrae do not possess a facet for the costotransverse joint? (There may be more than one correct answer.)
    A. T1   B. T7   C. T11   D. T12

18. What are two distinctive features of all cervical vertebrae that make them different from any other vertebrae?

A. _____ B. _____

19. What is the one feature of all thoracic vertebrae that makes them different from all other vertebrae?

_____

20. Which position of the thoracic spine best demonstrates the intervertebral foramina?

_____

21. Identify the following structures labeled on Figs. 9-5, 9-6, and 9-7 (include the specific vertebra of which each structure is a part).

	Structure	*Vertebra*

Fig. 9-5

A. _____   _____

B. _____   _____

C. _____   _____

D. _____   _____

E. _____   _____

F. _____   _____

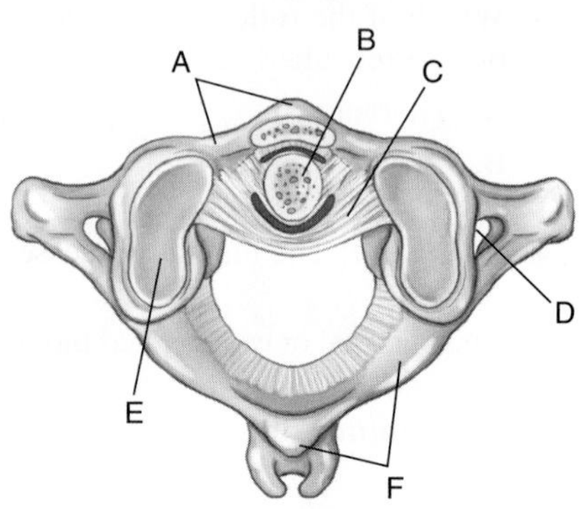

Fig. 9-5. Superior view.

Fig. 9-6

G. _____   _____

H. _____   _____

I. _____   _____

J. _____   _____

K. _____   _____

L. _____   _____

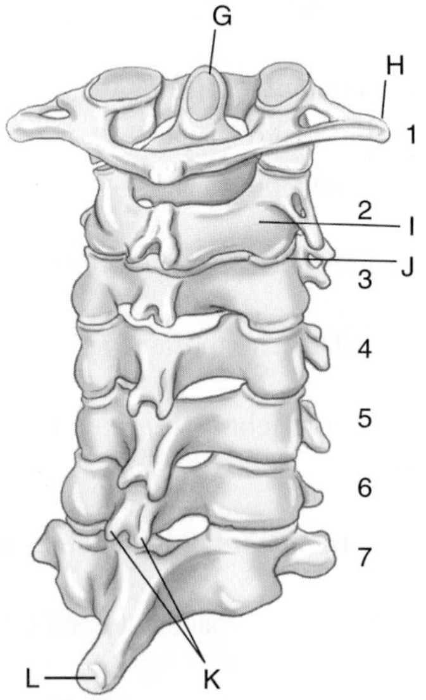

Fig. 9-6. Posterolateral view, cervical spine.

Fig. 9-7

M. _____   _____

N. _____   _____

O. _____   _____

P. _____   _____

Q. _____   _____

R. _____   _____

S. Which vertebrae are represented by this

   drawing? _____

T. How can these specific vertebrae be

   identified? _____

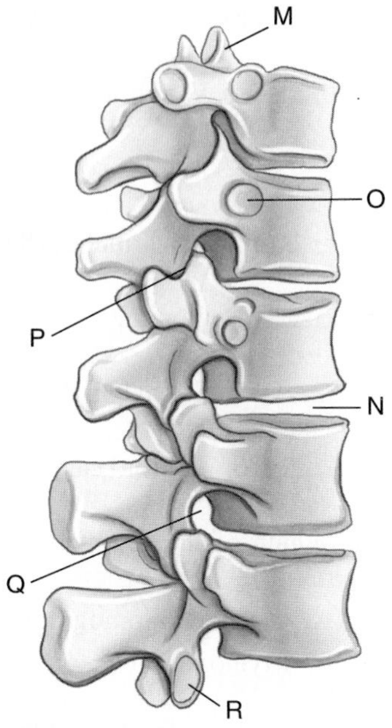

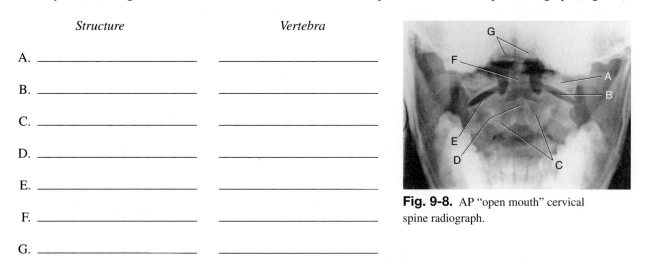

Fig. 9-7. Lateral oblique view.

22. Identify the following structures and vertebrae labeled on this AP "open mouth" cervical spine radiograph (Fig. 9-8).

Structure	*Vertebra*
A. _____	_____
B. _____	_____
C. _____	_____
D. _____	_____
E. _____	_____
F. _____	_____
G. _____	_____

Fig. 9-8. AP "open mouth" cervical spine radiograph.

23. Which position or projection of the cervical spine best demonstrates the zygapophyseal joints (between C3 to C7)?

_____

24. Which specific joint spaces are visualized with a left anterior oblique (LAO) projection of the thoracic spine?

_____

25. Match each of the following topographic landmarks to the correct vertebral level (using each choice only once).

    _____ 1. Vertebra prominens   A. T2-3

    _____ 2. Jugular notch   B. C7-T1

    _____ 3. 3 to 4 inches (8 to 10 cm) below jugular notch   C. T7

    _____ 4. Gonion   D. C3

    _____ 5. Sternal angle   E. C4-C6

    _____ 6. Thyroid cartilage   F. T4-5

26. Which of the following imaging modalities is *not* normally performed to rule out a herniated nucleus pulposus (HNP)?
A. Computed tomography (CT)   C. Magnetic resonance imaging (MRI)
B. Myelography   D. Nuclear medicine

27. An avulsion fracture of the spinous processes of C6 through T1 is called a:
A. Hangman's fracture   C. Jefferson fracture
B. Clay shoveler's fracture   D. Teardrop burst fracture

28. Scheuermann disease is a form of:
A. Scoliosis and/or kyphosis   C. Arthritis
B. Subluxation   D. Fracture

29. True/False: HNP most frequently develops at the L2-3 vertebral level.

30. Which two things can be done to minimize the effects of scatter radiation on lateral projections of the thoracic and lumbar spine?

A. _____   B. _____

31. Which position or projection best demonstrates the zygapophyseal joints between C1 and C2?

_____

32. How much and in which direction (caudad or cephalad) should the central ray be angled for each of the following projections?

A. An AP axial projection of the cervical spine: _____

B. An anterior oblique projection of the cervical spine: _____

C. A posterior oblique projection of the cervical spine: _____

33. Which one of the following projections of the cervical spine demonstrates the left intervertebral foramen?
A. Left posterior oblique (LPO)   C. Lateral projection
B. Left anterior oblique (LAO)   D. Right anterior oblique (RAO)

34. In addition to using a long SID, list the two positioning maneuvers you can use to lower the shoulders enough to visualize C7 for a lateral projection of the cervical spine.

   A. _____   B. _____

35. Which position or projection demonstrates the lower cervical and upper thoracic spine (C4 to T3) in a lateral

   perspective? (Fracture/subluxation has been ruled-out) _____

36. List the two positions or projections that will project the dens in the center of the foramen magnum.

   A. _____   B. _____

37. **Situation:** A lateral cervical spine radiograph demonstrates that the zygapophyseal joint spaces are not superimposed. Which type of positioning error(s) may lead to this radiographic outcome?

   _____

38. **Situation:** A radiograph of a lateral thoracic spine projection reveals that the intervertebral foramina and intervertebral joint spaces are not clearly demonstrated. Which type of problems can lead to this radiographic outcome?

   _____

39. **Situation:** A patient who was involved in a motor vehicle accident (MVA) 3 days ago is experiencing severe neck pain and comes to the radiology department for a cervical spine series. The patient is not wearing a cervical collar. Should the technologist take a horizontal beam lateral projection and have it cleared before proceeding with the study? Explain.

   _____

40. **Situation:** A patient with a possible Jefferson fracture enters the ER. Which specific radiographic position best demonstrates this type of fracture?

   _____

41. What dose range would be received by the breasts of a slightly larger-than-average female during a lateral thoracic spine projection taken at 80 kV and 50 mAs with proper collimation?
   A. 300 to 500 mrad   C. 100 to 200 mrad
   B. 1 to 50 mrad   D. No detectable contribution (NDC)

42. The breast dose used for a posterior oblique thoracic spine projection is approximately _____ the dose used for an anterior oblique projection.
   A. The same as   C. 2 times greater than
   B. One-half of   D. 4 times greater than

43. What skin dose range would be received by an average-size male patient during a lateral thoracic spine projection?
   A. 300 to 400 mrad   C. 1 to 2 rad
   B. 10 to 50 mrad   D. 900 to 1000 mrad

44. The thyroid dose used during a posterior oblique cervical spine projection is approximately _____ the dose used during an anterior oblique projection.
   A. The same as   C. 10 to 15 times greater than
   B. 4 times greater than   D. One quarter of the amount

45. **Situation:** A radiograph of an AP open mouth projection of the cervical spine demonstrates the upper incisors super-imposed over the top of the dens. What specific positioning error is present on this radiograph?

_____

46. **Situation:** A patient comes to the radiology department for a follow-up study for a clay shoveler's fracture. Which spine projections will best demonstrate this type of fracture?

_____

47. **Situation:** A patient comes to the radiology department for a follow-up study 6 months after having spinal fusion surgery of the lower cervical spine (C5-C6). The surgeon wants to check for anteroposterior mobility of the fused spine. Beyond the basic cervical spine projections, what additional projections can be taken to assess mobility of the spine?

_____

48. Which one of the following technical factors is most important in producing a high-quality CR image?
    A. Decrease SID whenever possible
    B. Minimize the use of grids
    C. Decrease kV as much as possible
    D. Collimate as close as possible

49. Which of the following imaging modalities is recommended for a "teardrop burst" fracture?
    A. CT
    B. MRI
    C. Nuclear medicine
    D. Sonography

50. Which cervical vertebrae may demonstrate a "cervical rib"?
    A. C1
    B. C2
    C. C6
    D. C7

10 Lumbar Spine, Sacrum, and Coccyx

CHAPTER OBJECTIVES

After you have successfully completed the activities in this chapter, you will be able to:

_____ 1. On drawings and radiographs, identify specific anatomic structures of the lumbar spine, sacrum, and coccyx.

_____ 2. Identify the anatomic structures that make up the "Scottie dog" sign.

_____ 3. Identify the classification and type of movement of the joints found in the lumbar spine.

_____ 4. List topographic landmarks that can be palpated to locate specific aspects of the lumbar spine, sacrum, and coccyx.

_____ 5. Define specific types of pathologic features of the spine as described in the textbook.

_____ 6. Identify radiographic appearances related to these specific types of pathologic spine features.

_____ 7. Identify basic and special projections of the lumbar spine, sacrum, coccyx, and sacroiliac joints, including the correct size and type of image receptor (IR), central ray location, direction, and angulation of the central ray for each projection.

_____ 8. Identify which structures are best seen with specific projections of the lumbar spine.

_____ 9. List the patient dose ranges for skin, midline, and gonadal doses for specific spine projections.

_____ 10. Identify the approximate difference in patient doses between anteroposterior (AP) compared with posteroanterior (PA) projections and anterior compared with posterior oblique positions of the lumbar spine.

_____ 11. Given various hypothetical situations, identify the correct modification of a position and/or exposure factors to improve the radiographic image.

_____ 12. Given radiographs of specific lumbosacral spine projections or positions, identify positioning and exposure factor errors.

POSITIONING AND RADIOGRAPHIC CRITIQUE

_____ 1. Using a peer, position for basic and special projections of the lumbosacral spine.

_____ 2. Using a lumbar spine radiographic phantom, produce satisfactory radiographs of specific positions (if equipment is available).

_____ 3. Critique and evaluate lumbar spine and SI joint radiographs based on the four divisions of radiographic criteria: (1) structures shown, (2) position, (3) collimation and central ray, and (4) exposure criteria.

_____ 4. Distinguish between acceptable and unacceptable lumbosacral spine radiographs based on exposure factors, motion, collimation, positioning, or other errors.

Complete the following review exercises after careful study of the associated pages in the textbook as indicated by each exercise. Answers to each review exercise are given at the end of the review exercises.

PART I: RADIOGRAPHIC ANATOMY
Review Exercise A: Anatomy of the Lumbar Spine, Sacrum, and Coccyx (see textbook pp. 321-327)

1. A portion of the lamina located between the superior and inferior articular processes is called the

   _____.

2. The superior and inferior vertebral notches join together to form the:
   A. Vertebral foramen   C. Pedicle
   B. Intervertebral foramina   D. Lamina

3. Which radiographic position best demonstrates the structure identified in the previous question?

   _____

4. Identify the parts of a typical lumbar vertebra as labeled on Fig. 10-1.

   A. _____

   B. _____

   C. _____

   D. _____

   E. _____

   F. The central ray projection labeled F in this
      drawing would best demonstrate the

      _____

      _____

   G. The central ray projection labeled G would
      best demonstrate the

      _____

      _____

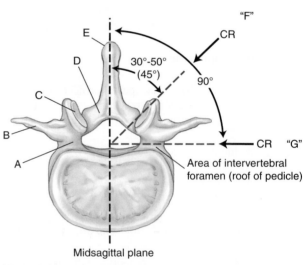

Fig. 10-1. Typical L3 vertebra.

5. Would the degree of angle to demonstrate the structures identified in F in the previous question be greater or lesser

   for the lower lumbar vertebrae as compared with the upper? _____

6. The small foramina found in the sacrum are called _____.

7. The anterior and superior aspect of the sacrum that forms the posterior wall of the pelvic inlet is called the

   _____.

8. What is another term for the sacral horns? _____

9. The sacroiliac joints lie at an oblique angle of _____° to the coronal plane.

10. What is the formal term for the "tail bone?" _____

11. What is the name for the upper broad aspect of the coccyx? _____

12. List the structure classification and movement classification and type for the following joints of the vertebrae.

	Classification	Mobility Type	Movement Type
A. Zygapophyseal	_____	_____	_____
B. Intervertebral	_____	_____	_____

13. Identify the following structures labeled on the radiographs of the lumbar spine (Figs. 10-2 and 10-3).

A. _____

B. _____

C. _____

D. _____

E. _____

F. _____ joint

G. _____

H. _____

I. _____

J. _____

K. _____

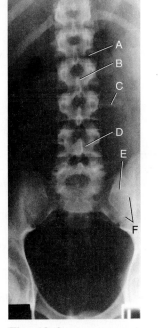

Fig. 10-2. Anteroposterior.

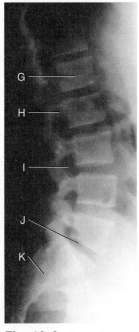

Fig. 10-3. Lateral.

Identify parts of the "Scottie dog" image, which should be visible on an oblique lumbar spine (Figs. 10-4 and 10-5).

L. _____

M. _____ joint

N. _____

O. _____

P. _____

Q. _____

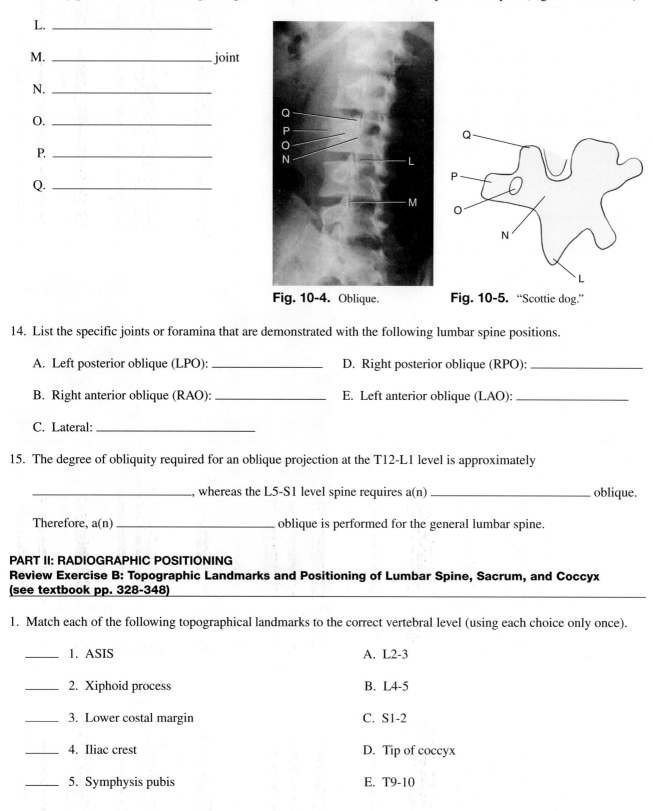

Fig. 10-4. Oblique.   **Fig. 10-5.** "Scottie dog."

14. List the specific joints or foramina that are demonstrated with the following lumbar spine positions.

A. Left posterior oblique (LPO): _____   D. Right posterior oblique (RPO): _____

B. Right anterior oblique (RAO): _____   E. Left anterior oblique (LAO): _____

C. Lateral: _____

15. The degree of obliquity required for an oblique projection at the T12-L1 level is approximately

_____, whereas the L5-S1 level spine requires a(n) _____ oblique.

Therefore, a(n) _____ oblique is performed for the general lumbar spine.

PART II: RADIOGRAPHIC POSITIONING
Review Exercise B: Topographic Landmarks and Positioning of Lumbar Spine, Sacrum, and Coccyx
(see textbook pp. 328-348)

1. Match each of the following topographical landmarks to the correct vertebral level (using each choice only once).

_____ 1. ASIS   A. L2-3

_____ 2. Xiphoid process   B. L4-5

_____ 3. Lower costal margin   C. S1-2

_____ 4. Iliac crest   D. Tip of coccyx

_____ 5. Symphysis pubis   E. T9-10

2. True/False: The use of higher kV and lower mA seconds (mAs) for lumbar spine radiography improves radiographic contrast but increases patient dose.

3. True/False: Placing a lead blocker mat behind the patient for lateral lumbar spine positions improves image quality.

4. True/False: Gonadal shielding should always be used for male and female patients for studies of the lumbar spine, sacrum, and coccyx.

5. True/False: The anteroposterior (AP) projection of the lumbar spine opens the intervertebral joint spaces better than the posteroanterior (PA) projection.

6. True/False: The knees and hips should be extended for an AP projection of the lumbar spine.

7. True/False: An increased source image receptor distance (SID) of 44 or 46 inches (112 to 117 cm) is advantageous for AP and lateral projections of the lumbar spine.

8. True/False: The lead blocker mat and close collimation must not be used when performing digital imaging of the lumbar spine.

9. Select the imaging modality that best demonstrates each of the following pathologic features or conditions (answers may be used more than once).

_____ A. Osteoporosis	1. Magnetic resonance imaging (MRI)
_____ B. Soft tissues of lumbar spine	2. Computed tomography (CT)
_____ C. Structures within subarachnoid space	3. Myelography
_____ D. Inflammatory conditions such as Paget's disease	4. Bone densitometry
_____ E. Compression fractures of the lumbar spine	5. Nuclear medicine

10. Match each of the following pathologic indications to the correct definition or statement (using each choice only once).

_____ A. Lateral curvature of the vertebral column	1. Spina bifida
_____ B. Fracture of the vertebral body caused by hyperflexion force	2. Herniated nucleus pulposus (HNP)
	3. Chance fracture
_____ C. Congenital defect in which the posterior elements of the vertebrae fail to unite	4. Spondylolisthesis
_____ D. Most common at the L4-5 level and may result in sciatica	5. Compression fracture
_____ E. Forward displacement of one vertebra onto another vertebra	6. Spondylolysis
_____ F. Inflammatory condition that is most common in males in their 30s	7. Ankylosing spondylitis
	8. Scoliosis
_____ G. Dissolution and separation of the pars interarticularis	
_____ H. A type of fracture that rarely causes neurologic deficits	

11. With a 35-x 43-cm (14- × 17-inch) IR, the central ray is centered at the level of the _____ for AP and lateral lumbar spine projections.

12. Which two structures can be evaluated to determine whether rotation is present on a radiograph of an AP projection of the lumbar spine?

   A. _____   B. _____

13. How much rotation is required to properly visualize the zygapophyseal joints at the L5-S1 level?

   _____

14. Which specific set of zygapophyseal joints is demonstrated with an LAO position?_____

15. The _____ , which is the eye of the "Scottie dog," should be near the center of the vertebral body on a correctly obliqued lumbar spine.

16. Which positioning error has been committed if the structures described in the previous question are projected too far

   posterior with a 45° oblique position of the lumbar spine? _____

17. Which position or projection of the lumbar spine series best demonstrates a possible compression fracture?

   _____

18. A patient with a wide pelvis and narrow thorax may require a central ray angle of _____°

   _____ (caudad or cephalad) for a lateral position of the lumbar spine.

19. How should the spine of a patient with scoliosis be positioned for a lateral position of the lumbar spine?

   _____

20. Why should the knees and hips be flexed for an AP lumbar spine projection? _____

21. True/False: The female ovarian dose used for a PA lumbar spine projection is approximately 30% less than the dose used for an AP projection.

22. Where is the central ray centered for a lateral L5-S1 projection of the lumbar spine? _____

23. What type of central ray angulation is required for an AP axial L5-S1 projection on a male patient?

   _____

24. True/False: A PA or AP projection for a scoliosis series frequently includes one erect and one recumbent position for comparison.

25. True/False: The lower margin of the cassette must include the symphysis pubis for a scoliosis series.

26. True/False: A PA projection for a scoliosis series requires only about one tenth the dose to the breasts as compared to the AP projection, even if proper collimation is used.

27. The typical skin dose range of the lateral projection of a scoliosis series on a small to average female is:
   A. 1000 to 1200 mrad
   B. 500 to 700 mrad
   C. 200 to 400 mrad
   D. Less than 100 mrad

28. Which side of the spine should be elevated for the second exposure for the Ferguson scoliosis series (by having patient stand on a block with one foot)? _____

29. During the AP (PA) right and left bending projections of the lumbar spine, the _____ must remain stationary during positioning.

30. Which projections should be taken to evaluate flexibility following spinal fusion surgery?

   _____

31. How much central ray angulation is required for an AP projection of the sacrum for a typical male patient?

   _____

32. If a patient cannot lie on the back for the AP sacrum because it is too painful, what alternate projection can be taken to achieve a similar view of the sacrum? _____

33. Where is the central ray centered for an AP projection of the coccyx? _____

34. True/False: The AP projections of the sacrum and coccyx can be taken as one single projection to decrease gonadal dose.

35. Patients should be asked to empty the urinary bladder before performing which projection(s) of the vertebral column? _____

36. In addition to good collimation, what should be done to minimize overall "fogging" on a lateral lumbar spine or lateral sacrum and coccyx radiograph? _____

37. Which sacroliliac (SI) joint is visualized with an RPO position? _____

38. How much rotation of the body is required for oblique positions of the SI joints? _____

39. What type of CR angle is recommended for the AP axial projection of the SI joints on a female patient?
   A. 20° cephalad
   B. 30° cephalad
   C. 30° caudad
   D. 35° cephalad

40. Where is the CR centered for an oblique projection of the SI joints? _____

Review Exercise C: Problem Solving for Technical and Positioning Errors

1. A radiograph of an AP projection of the lumbar spine reveals that the spinous processes are not midline to the vertebral column and distortion of the vertebral bodies is present. Which specific positioning error is present on this radiograph? _____

2. A radiograph of an LPO projection of the lumbar spine reveals that the downside pedicles and zygapophyseal joints are projected over the anterior portion of the vertebral bodies. Which specific positioning error is present on this

   radiograph? _____

3. A radiograph of a lateral projection of a female lumbar spine reveals that the mid-to-lower intervertebral joint spaces are not open. The technologist supported the midsection of the spine with sponges to straighten the spine.

   What else can be done to open the joint spaces during the repeat exposure?_____

4. A radiograph of a lateral L5-S1 projection reveals that the joint space is not open. The technologist did support the middle aspect of the spine with a sponge. What else can the technologist do to open up the joint space during

   the repeat exposure?_____

5. A radiograph of an AP axial projection of the coccyx reveals that the distal tip is superimposed over the symphysis pubis. What must the technologist do to eliminate this problem during the repeat exposure?

   _____

6. A radiograph of an oblique position of the lumbar spine reveals that the downside pedicle and zygapophyseal joint are posterior in relation to the vertebral body. What modification of the position must be made during the repeat

   exposure to produce a more diagnostic image? _____

7. **Situation:** A patient comes to the radiology department for a follow-up study for a compression fracture of L3. The radiologist requests that collimated projections be taken of L3. Which specific projections and centering would

   provide a quality study of L3 and the intervertebral joint spaces? _____

8. **Situation:** A young female patient comes to the radiology department for a scoliosis series. She has had repeated radiation exposure over a period of time and is understandably concerned about the radiation. What three things can the technologist do to minimize the dose delivered to the patient's breasts?

   A. _____

   B. _____

   C. _____

9. **Situation:** A patient with an injury to the coccyx enters the emergency room. When attempting the AP projection, the patient complains that it is too uncomfortable to lie on his back. He is unable to stand. What other options are

   available to complete the study? _____

10. **Situation:** A patient with a clinical history of spondylolisthesis at the L5-S1 level comes to the radiology department. Which specific lumbar spine position would be most diagnostic in demonstrating the extent of this condition?

    _____

11. A positioning series for sacroiliac (SI) joints is performed on a patient. The resultant radiographs do not demonstrate the inferior portion of the joints. What can be done during the repeat exposure to demonstrate this aspect of the SI

    joints? _____

12. **Situation:** A patient comes to the radiology department for a lumbar spine series. He has a clinical history of advanced spondylolysis. Which specific projection(s) of the lumbar spine series will best demonstrate this condition?

_____

13. **Situation:** A patient comes to the radiology department with a clinical history of HNP. Which of the following imaging modalities would provide the most diagnostic study for this condition?
   A. Sonography
   B. MRI
   C. Nuclear medicine
   D. Radiography

14. **Situation:** A patient comes to the radiology department for a lumbar spine study following spinal fusion surgery. Her surgeon wants a study to assess mobility of the spine at the fusion site. Which radiographic positions would provide

   this information? _____

15. **Situation:** A patient comes to the radiology department for a lumbar spine series. She has a clinical history of severe

   kyphosis. How should the lumbar spine series be modified for this patient? _____

Review Exercise D: Critique Radiographs of the Lumbar Spine, Sacrum, and Coccyx (see textbook p. 349)

The following questions relate to the radiographs found at the end of Chapter 10 of the textbook. Evaluate these radiographs for the radiographic criteria categories (*1* through *5*) that follow. Describe the corrections needed to improve the overall image. The major, or "repeatable," errors are specific errors that indicate the need for a repeat exposure, regardless of the nature of the other errors.

A. Lateral lumbar spine (Fig. C10-83)

   1. Structures shown: _____

   2. Part positioning: _____

   3. Collimation and central ray: _____

   4. Exposure criteria: _____

   5. Anatomic side markers: _____

Repeatable error(s): _____

B. Lateral lumbar spine (Fig. C10-84)

   1. Structures shown: _____

   2. Part positioning: _____

   3. Collimation and central ray: _____

   4. Exposure criteria: _____

   5. Anatomic side markers: _____

Repeatable error(s): _____

C. Lateral L5-S1 (Fig. C10-85)

    1. Structures shown: _____

    2. Part positioning: _____

    3. Collimation and central ray: _____

    4. Exposure criteria: _____

    5. Anatomic side markers: _____

Repeatable error(s): _____

D. Oblique lumbar spine (Fig. C10-86)

    1. Structures shown: _____

    2. Part positioning: _____

    3. Collimation and central ray: _____

    4. Exposure criteria: _____

    5. Anatomic side markers: _____

Repeatable error(s): _____

E. Oblique lumbar spine (Fig. C10-87)

    1. Structures shown: _____

    2. Part positioning: _____

    3. Collimation and central ray: _____

    4. Exposure criteria: _____

    5. Anatomic side markers: _____

Repeatable error(s): _____

PART III: LABORATORY EXERCISES

You must gain experience in positioning each part of the lumbar spine, sacrum, and coccyx before performing the following exams on actual patients. You can get experience in positioning and radiographic evaluation of these projections by performing exercises using radiographic phantoms and practicing on other students (although you will not be taking actual exposures).

The following suggested activities assume that your teaching institution has an energized lab and radiographic phantoms. If not, perform Laboratory Exercises B and C, the radiographic evaluation and the physical positioning exercises. (Check off each step and projection as you complete it.)

Laboratory Exercise A: Energized Laboratory

1. Using the abdomen/lumbosacral radiographic phantom, produce radiographs of the following basic routines:

_____ AP lumbar spine   _____ AP sacrum   _____ Posterior oblique lumbar spine

_____ Lateral lumbar spine   _____ AP coccyx   _____ Anterior oblique lumbar spine

_____ Lateral L5-S1   _____ Lateral sacrum   _____ AP axial L5-S1
                                  and coccyx

_____ Oblique SI joints
                                  _____ AP axial SI joints

Laboratory Exercise B: Radiographic Evaluation

1. Evaluate and critique the radiographs produced during the previous experiments, additional radiographs provided by your instructor, or both. Evaluate each radiograph for the following points.

_____ Evaluate the completeness of the study. (Are all of the pertinent anatomic structures included on the radiograph?)

_____ Evaluate for positioning or centering errors (e.g., rotation, off centering).

_____ Evaluate for correct exposure factors and possible motion. (Are the density and contrast of the images acceptable?)

_____ Determine whether markers and an acceptable degree of collimation and/or area shielding are visible on the images.

Laboratory Exercise C: Physical Positioning

On another person, simulate performing all basic and special projections of the lumbar spine, sacrum, and coccyx as follows. (Check off each when completed satisfactorily.) Include the following six steps as described in the textbook.

Step 1. Appropriate size and type of image receptor with correct markers

Step 2. Correct central ray placement and centering of part to central ray and/or IR

Step 3. Accurate collimation

Step 4. Area shielding of patient where advisable

Step 5. Use of proper immobilizing devices when needed

Step 6. Approximate correct exposure factors, breathing instructions where applicable, and initiating exposure

Projections	Step 1	Step 2	Step 3	Step 4	Step 5	Step 6
• AP lumbar spine	___	___	___	___	___	___
• Lateral lumbar spine	___	___	___	___	___	___
• Lateral L5-S1	___	___	___	___	___	___
• AP sacrum	___	___	___	___	___	___
• AP coccyx	___	___	___	___	___	___
• Lateral sacrum and coccyx	___	___	___	___	___	___
• Posterior oblique lumbar spine	___	___	___	___	___	___
• Anterior oblique lumbar spine	___	___	___	___	___	___
• AP axial L5-S1	___	___	___	___	___	___

Spinal fusion series:

• AP (PA) R and L bending	___	___	___	___	___	___
• Lateral hyperextension and hyper flexion	___	___	___	___	___	___

Scoliosis series:

• PA (AP) and lateral erect	___	___	___	___	___	___

SI joint series:

• AP axial SI joints	___	___	___	___	___	___
• RPO and LPO SI joints	___	___	___	___	___	___

This self-test should be taken only after completing all of the readings, review exercises, and laboratory activities for a particular section. The purpose of this test is not only to provide a good learning exercise but also to serve as a strong indicator of what your final evaluation exam will cover. It is strongly suggested that if you do not get at least a 90% to 95% grade on each self-test that you review those areas in which you missed questions before going to your instructor for the final evaluation exam for this chapter.

1. Compared with the spinous processes of the cervical and thoracic spine, the lumbar spinous processes are:
   A. Smaller
   B. Pointed downward more
   C. Larger and more blunt
   D. Absent

2. The anterior ridge of the upper sacrum is called the:
   A. Median sacral crest
   B. Cornua
   C. Promontory
   D. Sacral horns

3. Each sacroiliac joint is obliqued posteriorly _____°.
   A. 20
   B. 25 to 30
   C. 45
   D. 50

4. The angle of the midlumbar spine zygapophyseal joints in relation to the midsagittal plane is

   _____.

5. Where is the pars interarticularis found?
   A. Superior and inferior aspect of the pedicle
   B. Between the intervertebral disk and vertebra
   C. Between the superior and inferior articular processes
   D. Between the lamina and body spinous processes

6. Identify the labeled parts of the sacrum and coccyx on the following drawings (Figs. 10-6 and 10-7).

A. _____

B. _____

C. _____

D. _____

E. _____

F. _____

G. _____

H. _____

I. _____

J. _____

K. _____

L. _____

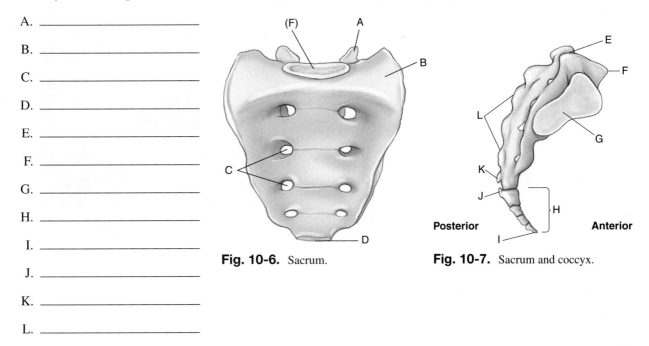

Fig. 10-6. Sacrum.

Fig. 10-7. Sacrum and coccyx.

7. Identify the labeled parts on these radiographs of individual vertebrae (Figs. 10-8 and 10-9).

A. _____

B. _____

C. _____

D. _____

E. _____

F. _____

G. _____

H. _____

I. _____

J. _____

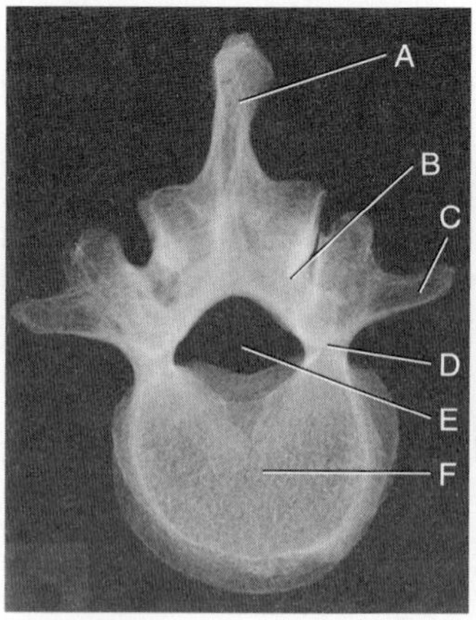

Fig. 10-8. Individual vertebra, A-F. 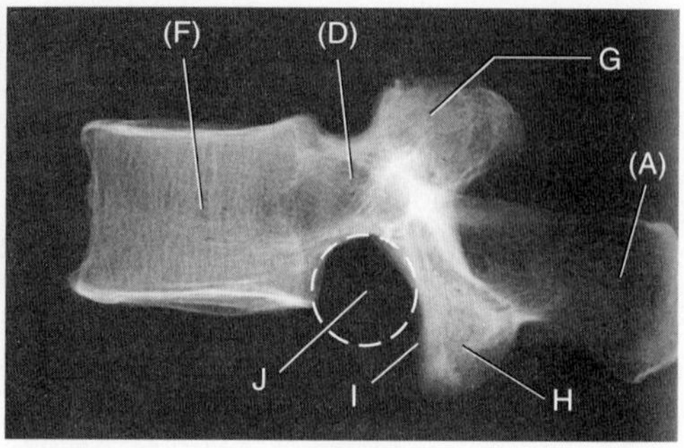 **Fig. 10-9.** Individual vertebra, G-J.

8. What are the characteristics of the vertebra in Fig. 10-9 that identify it as a lumbar vertebra rather than a thoracic?

_____

9. The zygapophyseal joints of the lumbar spine are classified as _____ joints with

_____ type of joint movement.

10. List the correct terms of the lumbar vertebra that correspond to the following labeled parts of the "Scottie dog" as seen on an oblique radiograph of the lumbar spine (Fig. 10-10).

A. _____

B. _____

C. _____

D. _____

E. _____

F. _____ joint

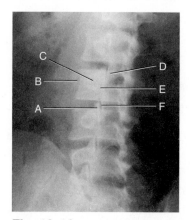

Fig. 10-10. Oblique lumbar spine.

11. The ear and front leg of the "Scottie dog" make up the _____ joint, best seen in the oblique position.

12. Which one of the following topographic landmarks corresponds to the L2-3 level?
    A. Xiphoid process
    B. Lower costal margin
    C. Iliac crest
    D. ASIS

13. True/False: It is possible to shield females for an AP projection of the sacrum or coccyx if the gonadal shields are correctly placed.

14. True/False: The female gonadal dose is approximately that of the midline dose and is almost the same for either AP or PA projections of the lumbar spine.

15. Why should the knees and hips be flexed for an AP projection of the lumbar spine? _____

16. True/False: A lead blocker mat for lateral positions of the lumbar spine should not be used with digital imaging.

17. True/False: The efficiency of CT and MRI of the spine is reducing the number of myelograms being performed.

18. Anterior wedging and loss of vertebral body height are characteristic of:
    A. Chance fracture
    B. Spina bifida
    C. Compression fracture
    D. Spondylolysis

19. Which one of the following conditions is often diagnosed by prenatal ultrasound?
    A. Scoliosis
    B. Spina bifida
    C. Spondylolisthesis
    D. Ankylosing spondylitis

20. Which one of the following conditions usually requires an increase in manual exposure factors?
    A. Ankylosing spondylitis
    B. Spondylolysis
    C. Spina bifida
    D. Spondylolisthesis

21. Where is the central ray centered for an AP projection of the lumbar spine with a 30 × 35 cm (11 × 14 inch) IR?

    _____

22. Which set of zygapophyseal joints of the lumbar spine is best demonstrated with an LAO position?

    _____

23. How much rotation of the spine is required to demonstrate the zygapophyseal joint space between L1-2?

    _____

24. Describe the body build that may require central ray angulation to open the intervertebral joint spaces with a lateral projection of the lumbar spine, even if the patient has some support under the waist.

    _____

25. What type of central ray angulation should be used for the lateral L5-S1 projection if the waist is not supported?
    A. Central ray perpendicular to IR
    B. 5° to 8° caudad
    C. 10° to 15° cephalad
    D. 3° to 5° cephalad

26. What type of central ray angulation should be used for an AP axial projection for L5-S1 on a female patient?
    A. 35° cephalad
    B. 30° cephalad
    C. 5° to 8° caudad
    D. Central ray perpendicular to IR

27. Where is the central ray centered for an AP axial projection for L5-S1?

    _____

28. True/False: The center ionization chamber should be used when using automatic exposure control (AEC) for either a lateral lumbar spine or a lateral L5-S1 projection.

29. Which projection or method is designed to demonstrate the degree of scoliosis deformity between the primary and compensatory curves as part of a scoliosis study? _____

30. Which projections are designed to measure anteroposterior movement at the site of a spinal fusion?

    _____

31. Where is the central ray centered for an AP projection of the sacrum?

    _____

32. What two things can be done to reduce the high amounts of scatter reaching the IR during a lateral projection of the sacrum and coccyx?

    A. _____   B. _____

33. Why should a single, lateral projection of the sacrum and coccyx be performed rather than separate laterals of the sacrum and coccyx? _____

34. The skin dose on a lateral sacrum and/or coccyx projection on an average-size patient is in the

    _____ range.
    A. 200 to 500 mrad
    B. 500 to 700 mrad
    C. 1000 to 1500 mrad
    D. 1500 to 2000 mrad

35. A radiograph of an AP projection of the lumbar spine reveals that the sacroiliac (SI) joints are not equidistant from the spine. The right ala of the sacrum appears larger, and the left SI joint is more open than the left. Which specific positioning error is evident on this radiograph?

    _____

36. A radiograph of an LPO projection of the lumbar spine reveals that the downside pedicles are projected toward the posterior aspect of the vertebral bodies. What must be done to correct this error during the repeat exposure?

    _____

37. An AP projection of the sacrum reveals that the sacrum is foreshortened and the foramina are not open. What

positioning error led to this radiographic outcome? _____

38. **Situation:** A patient with a possible compression fracture of L3 enters the emergency room. Which projection(s) of the lumbar spine best demonstrate(s) the extent of this injury?

_____

39. **Situation:** A patient with a clinical history of spondylolisthesis of the L5-S1 region comes to the radiology department. What basic (i.e., routine) and special (i.e., optional) projections should be included in this study? (Hint: If the obliques are included, how much spine rotation should be used?)

_____

40. **Situation:** A study of the sacroiliac joints demonstrates that the joints are not open and the upper iliac wings are nearly superimposing the joints. The technologist performed 35° RPO and LPO positions with a perpendicular CR. What can be done during the repeat exposure to open the joints ?

_____

11 Bony Thorax—Sternum and Ribs

CHAPTER OBJECTIVES

After you have successfully completed the activities in this chapter, you will be able to:

_____ 1. Using drawings and radiographs, identify specific anatomic structures of the sternum and ribs.

_____ 2. Classify ribs as either true, false, or floating ribs.

_____ 3. Classify specific joints in the bony thorax according to their structural classification, mobility classification, and movement type.

_____ 4. Define specific types of pathologic features of the bony thorax as described in the textbook.

_____ 5. Identify basic and special projections of the ribs and sternum, including the correct size and type of image receptor (IR) and the location, direction, and angulation of the central ray for each position.

_____ 6. Identify which structures are best seen with specific projections of the ribs and sternum.

_____ 7. Identify the technical considerations important in radiography of the ribs and sternum, including breathing instructions, general body position, kilovoltage range, and other imaging options.

_____ 8. Identify patient dose ranges for skin, midline, thyroid, and breast for specific projection of the ribs and sternum.

_____ 9. Given various hypothetical situations, identify the correct modification of a position and/or exposure factors to improve the radiographic image.

_____ 10. Given radiographs of specific bony thorax projections or positions, identify specific positioning and exposure factor errors.

POSITIONING AND RADIOGRAPHIC CRITIQUE

_____ 1. Using a peer, position for basic and special projections of the bony thorax.

_____ 2. Using a chest radiographic phantom, produce satisfactory radiographs of specific positions (if equipment is available).

_____ 3. Critique and evaluate cranial radiographs based on the four divisions of radiographic criteria: (1) structures shown, (2) position, (3) collimation and central ray, and (4) exposure criteria.

_____ 4. Distinguish between acceptable and unacceptable bony thorax radiographs based on exposure factors, motion, collimation, positioning, or other errors.

The following review exercises should be completed only after careful study of the associated pages in the textbook as indicated by each exercise. Answers to each review exercise are given at the end of the review exercises.

PART I: RADIOGRAPHIC ANATOMY
Review Exercise A: Anatomy of Bony Thorax, Sternum, and Ribs (see textbook pp. 352-354)

1. List the three structures that make up the bony thorax.

   A. _____   B. _____   C. _____

2. Identify the parts of the sternum and ribs labeled in Fig. 11-1.

   A. _____

   B. _____

   C. _____

   D. _____

   E. _____

   F. _____

   G. _____

   H. _____

   I. _____

   J. _____

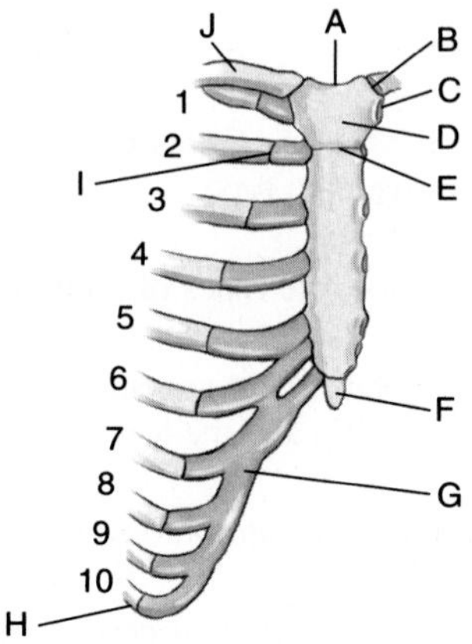

Fig. 11-1. Sternum and ribs.

3. What is the term for the long, middle aspect of the sternum? _____

4. The most distal aspect of the sternum does not ossify until a person is approximately _____ years of age.

5. The total sternum length on an average adult is about _____ inches (_____ cm).

6. A. The xiphoid end of the sternum is at the approximate level of the _____ vertebra.

   B. The sternal angle is at the level of _____.

7. What is the name of the joint that connects the upper limb to the bony thorax (the only bony connection between the

   bony thorax and upper limbs)? _____

8. What is the name of the section of cartilage that connects the anterior end of the rib to the sternum?

   _____

9. What distinguishes a true rib from a false rib? _____

10. True/False: The eleventh and twelfth ribs are classified as false and floating ribs.

11. True/False: The anterior end of the ribs is called the vertebral end.

12. Which aspect of the ribs articulates with the transverse process of the thoracic vertebrae?
    A. Head   C. Neck
    B. Costal angle   D. Tubercle

13. List the three structures found within the costal groove of each rib.

    A. _____ B. _____ C. _____

14. Answer the following questions as you study Fig. 11-2.

    A. Which end of the ribs is most superior—the posterior vertebral ends or the anterior sternal ends?

    _____

    B. Approximately how much difference in height is there between these two ends of the ribs?

    _____

    C. Which ribs articulate with the upper lateral aspect of the manubrium of the sternum?

    _____

    D. The bony thorax is widest at the lateral margins

    of which ribs? _____

    E. How many posterior ribs are shown above the diaphragm? (Hint: Recall from Chapter 3 that a minimum of 10 posterior ribs must be seen on an average inspiration posteroanterior [PA] chest projection.)

    _____

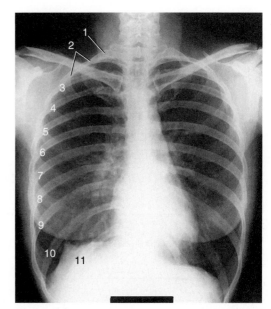

Fig. 11-2. Rib radiograph.

15. Match each of the following joints with the correct movement type.

    A. Movable—diarthrodial (plane or gliding)   B. Immovable—synarthrodial

    _____ 1. First sternocostal

    _____ 2. First through twelfth costovertebral joints

    _____ 3. First through tenth costochondral unions (between costocartilage and ribs)

    _____ 4. First through tenth costotransverse joints (between ribs and transverse processes of T vertebrae)

    _____ 5. Second through seventh sternocostal joints (between second through seventh ribs and sternum)

    _____ 6. Sixth through tenth interchondral joints (between anterior sixth through tenth costal cartilage)

16. The joints from the previous question that have diarthrodial movement are classified as _____.

17. Classify the following groups of ribs (labeled on the diagram as A, B, and C) and identify the number of the ribs in each category (Fig. 11-3).

A. _____

B. _____

C. _____

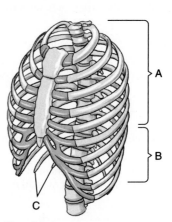

Fig. 11-3. Rib groups.

18. What is unique about the ribs in category A in the previous question?

_____

19. What is unique about the ribs in category C in the previous question?

_____

20. Identify the labeled parts of this posterior view of a typical rib (Fig. 11-4).

A. _____

B. _____

C. _____

D. _____

E. _____

F. _____

G. _____

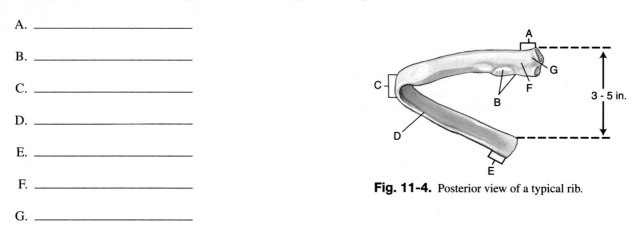

Fig. 11-4. Posterior view of a typical rib.

PART II: RADIOGRAPHIC POSITIONING
Review Exercise B: Positioning of the Ribs and Sternum (see textbook pp. 355-368)

1. True/False: It is virtually impossible to visualize the sternum with a direct PA or anteroposterior (AP) projection.

2. True/False: A large, "deep-chested" (hypersthenic) patient requires more obliquity for a frontal view of the sternum as compared with a "thin chested" (asthenic) patient.

3. How much rotation should be used for the oblique position of the sternum for a large, "deep-chested" patient?

_____

4. List the ideal ranges (high or low) for the following exposure factors as they apply to an oblique position of the sternum (breathing technique).

    A. kV range: _____

    B. mA: _____

    C. Exposure time: _____

5. What is the advantage of performing a breathing technique for radiography of the sternum?

_____

6. What is the primary reason that a source image receptor distance (SID) of less than 40 inches (100 cm) should not be used for sternum radiography? _____

7. What other imaging option is available to study the sternum if routine RAO and lateral radiographs do not provide sufficient information? _____

8. Identify the preferred positioning factors to demonstrate an injury to the ribs found below the diaphragm:

    A. General body position (erect or recumbent): _____

    B. Breathing instructions (inspiration or expiration): _____

    C. Recommended kV range: _____

9. An injury to the region of the eighth or ninth rib would require the _____ (above or below) diaphragm technique.

10. To properly elongate and visualize the axillary aspect of the ribs, the patient's spine should be rotated

_____ (toward or away from) the area of interest.

11. Which projections (AP or PA and anterior or posterior oblique) should be performed for an injury to the anterior aspect of the ribs? _____

12. Which two rib projections should be performed for an injury to the right posterior ribs?

_____

13. How can the site of injury be marked for a rib series? _____

14. If the physician suspects a pneumothorax or hemothorax has occurred as a result of a rib fracture, which additional radiographic projection(s) should be performed in addition to the routine rib projections?

_____

235

15. A flail chest is defined as a(n):
    A. Asthenic body habitus
    B. Pulmonary injury caused by blunt trauma to two or more ribs
    C. Chronic obstructive pulmonary disease (COPD; e.g., emphysema)
    D. Cardiac injury caused by blunt trauma

16. Osteolytic metastases of the ribs produce which of the following radiographic appearances?
    A. Irregular bony margins   C. Sharp lucent lines through the ribs
    B. Increased bony density of the ribs   D. Smooth lucent "holes" in the rib

17. Which of the following definitions applies to pectus excavatum?
    A. Multiple fractures of the sternum with fragments in the pericardium
    B. Abnormally prominent lower aspect of sternum
    C. Depressed sternum due to congenital defect
    D. Separation between ribs and sternum due to trauma

18. A proliferative bony lesion of increased density is generally termed:
    A. Osteoblastic   C. Osteolytic
    B. Osteoporotic   D. Osteostenotic

19. True/False: MRI provides a more diagnostic image of rib metastases as compared with a nuclear medicine scan.

20. True/False: Patients can develop osteomyelitis as a postoperative complication following open heart surgery.

21. Which is preferred for a study of the sternum: RAO or LAO? _____

    Why? _____

22. Where is the central ray centered for the oblique and lateral projections of the sternum?

    _____

23. What other position can be performed if the patient cannot assume a prone position for the RAO sternum?

    _____

24. What is the recommended SID for a lateral projection of the sternum? _____

    Why? _____

25. Which of the following criteria apply to a radiograph for an evaluation of the oblique sternum?
    A. The entire sternum should be adjacent to the spine and adjacent to the heart shadow.
    B. The entire sternum should lie over the heart shadow and be adjacent to the spine.
    C. The left sternoclavicular joint should be adjacent to the spinal column.
    D. The second rib should lie directly over the manubrium of the sternum.

26. Where is the central ray centered for a PA projection of the sternoclavicular joints?
    A. Level of T7   C. At the vertebra prominens
    B. Level of T2-3   D. Level of xiphoid process

27. What type of breathing instructions should be given to the patient for a PA projection of the sternoclavicular joints?
    A. Suspend respiration on inspiration.   C. Suspended breathing is not necessary.
    B. Use a breathing technique.

28. How much rotation of the thorax is recommended for an anterior oblique of the sternoclavicular joints?

    _____

29. Which specific oblique position best demonstrates the left sternoclavicular joint adjacent to the spine?

    _____

30. What are the three points that must be included in the patient's clinical history before a rib series?

    A. _____

    B. _____

    C. _____

31. Where is the central ray centered for an AP projection of the ribs for an injury located above the diaphragm?

    _____

32. Which two specific oblique positions can be used to elongate the left axillary portion of the ribs?

    _____

33. Which two basic projections or positions should be performed for an injury to the right anterior ribs?

    _____

34. How many degrees of rotation are needed for a oblique projection of the axillary ribs? _____

35. Both the patient thyroid dose and the breast dose for a correctly collimated PA sternoclavicular (SC) joint projection

    are in the _____ range.
    A. 1 to 5 mrad   C. 300 to 400 mrad
    B. 25 to 100 mrad   D. 500 to 1000 mrad

36. True/False: The thyroid dose for an anterior oblique rib projection is only about 5% of what it would be for a posterior oblique rib projection.

37. True/False: The breast dose for an anterior oblique rib projection is only about 5% of what it would be for a posterior oblique rib projection.

38. True/False: The amount of gonadal dose given for rib projections is less than 1 mrad.

39. To minimize patient dose for a RAO projection of the sternum, the patient's skin should be at least

    _____ below the collimator.
    A. 40" (100 cm)   C. 38 inches (15 cm)
    B. 72" (180 cm)   D. 2" (5 cm)

40. Which one of the following conditions may require a chest routine be included along with a study of the ribs?

A. Pectus carinatum   C. Pectus excavatum

B. Hemothorax   D. Osteomyelitis

Review Exercise C: Problem Solving for Technical and Positioning Errors

1. A radiograph of an RAO sternum reveals that part of the sternum is superimposed over the thoracic spine. Which specific positioning error is visible on this radiograph?

_____

2. A radiograph of an RAO sternum reveals that the sternum is difficult to visualize because of excessive density. The following factors were used for this image: 75 kV, 25 mA, 3-second exposure, 40-inch (100-cm) SID, Bucky, and 100-speed screens. Which one of these factors should be modified during the repeat exposure to produce a more diagnostic image?

_____

3. A radiograph of an RAO sternum reveals that the sternum is poorly visualized because of excessive lung markings superimposed over the sternum. The following factors were used for this image: 65 kV, 200 mA, 1¼ -second exposure, 40-inch (100-cm) SID, Bucky, and 100-speed screens. Which of these factors can be altered to increase the visibility of the sternum?

_____

4. A radiograph of a lateral projection of the sternum reveals that the patient's breasts are obscuring the sternum. What can be done to minimize the breast artifact over the sternum?

_____

5. Repeat PA projections of the sternoclavicular joints do not clearly demonstrate them. What other imaging modality may produce a more diagnostic image of these joints?

_____

6. **Situation:** A patient with trauma to the sternum and the left sternoclavicular joint region enters the emergency room. In addition to the sternum routine, the ER physician asks for a specific projection to better demonstrate the left sternoclavicular joint. Describe the positioning routine, including the breathing instructions that you would use. (HINT: Three projections are required.)

_____

_____

7. A radiograph of the upper ribs demonstrates that the diaphragm is superimposed over the eighth ribs, which is in the area of interest. The following factors were used for the initial exposure: 65 kV, 400 mA, ¼₀ second, 400-speed screens, grid, suspended respiration on expiration, erect position, 40-inch (102-cm) SID. Which one of these factors can be modified to increase the visibility of the area of interest?

_____

8. **Situation:** A patient enters the emergency room on a backboard after being involved in a motor vehicle accident. Because of the condition of the patient, the physician orders a portable study of the sternum in the ER. Which two projections of the sternum would be most diagnostic yet minimize movement of the patient? (See Chapter 18 in the textbook for a demonstration.)

9. **Situation:** A patient with trauma to the right upper anterior ribs enters the ER. He is able to sit in an erect position. Which positioning routine of the ribs should be performed? (Include general body position, breathing instructions, and specific projections or positions performed.)

10. **Situation:** A patient with trauma to the left lower anterior ribs enters the ER. Which positioning routine of the ribs should be performed? (Include general body position, breathing instructions, and specific positions performed.)

11. **Situation:** An elderly patient comes to the radiology department for a complete rib series with an emphasis on the posterior ribs. She has advanced osteoporosis and has difficulty moving and lying down. Her physician wants both upper and lower ribs examined. What type of positions should be performed? How would you adjust technical factors for this patient?

12. **Situation:** A patient enters the ER with blunt trauma to the chest. He is restricted on a backboard. The ER physician suspects a flail chest. Beyond the initial chest projections, what positioning routine would confirm the diagnosis of flail chest?

Review Exercise D: Critique Radiographs of the Bony Thorax (see textbook p. 369)

The following questions relate to the radiographs found at the end of Chapter 11 of the textbook. Evaluate these radiographs for the radiographic criteria categories (*1* through *5*) that follow. Describe the corrections needed to improve the overall image. The major, or "repeatable," errors are specific errors that indicate the need for a repeat exposure, regardless of the nature of the other errors.

A. Bilateral ribs above diaphragm (Fig. C11-46)

1. Structures shown: _____

2. Part positioning: _____

3. Collimation and central ray: _____

4. Exposure criteria: _____

5. Anatomic side markers: _____

Repeatable error(s): _____

B. Oblique sternum (Fig. C11-47)

    1. Structures shown: _____

    2. Part positioning: _____

    3. Collimation and central ray: _____

    4. Exposure criteria: _____

    5. Anatomic side markers: _____

Repeatable error(s): _____

C. Ribs below diaphragm (Fig. C11-48)

    1. Structures shown: _____

    2. Part positioning: _____

    3. Collimation and central ray: _____

    4. Exposure criteria: _____

    5. Anatomic side markers: _____

Repeatable error(s): _____

D. Lateral sternum (Fig. C11-49)

    1. Structures shown: _____

    2. Part positioning: _____

    3. Collimation and central ray: _____

    4. Exposure criteria: _____

    5. Anatomic side markers: _____

Repeatable error(s): _____

PART III: LABORATORY ACTIVITIES

You must gain experience in positioning each part of the sternum and ribs before performing the following exams on actual patients. You can get experience in positioning and radiographic evaluation of these projections by performing exercises using radiographic phantoms and practicing on other students (although you will not be taking actual exposures).

The following suggested activities assume that your teaching institution has an energized lab and radiographic phantoms. If not, perform Laboratory Exercises B and C, the radiographic evaluation and the physical positioning exercises. (Check off each step and projection as you complete it.)

Laboratory Exercise A: Energized Laboratory

1. Using the chest radiographic phantom, produce radiographs of the following basic routines:

   _____ RAO sternum

   _____ PA sternoclavicular joints

   _____ AP (PA) ribs

   _____ AP (PA) ribs, above and below diaphragm

   _____ Lateral sternum

   _____ RAO (LAO) sternoclavicular joints

   _____ Posterior and anterior oblique ribs, above diaphragm

   _____ Horizontal beam lateral sternum

Laboratory Exercise B: Radiographic Evaluation

1. Evaluate and critique the radiographs produced above, additional radiographs provided by your instructor, or both. Evaluate each radiograph for the following points.

   _____ Evaluate the completeness of the study. (Are all of the pertinent anatomic structures included on the radiograph?)

   _____ Evaluate for positioning or centering errors (e.g., rotation, off centering).

   _____ Evaluate for correct exposure factors and possible motion. (Are the density and contrast of the images acceptable?)

   _____ Determine whether markers and an acceptable degree of collimation and/or area shielding are visible on the images.

Laboratory Exercise C: Physical Positioning

On another person, simulate performing all basic and special projections of the sternum and ribs as follows. Include the six steps listed below and described in the textbook. (Check off each step when completed satisfactorily.)

Step 1. Appropriate size and type of image receptor with correct markers

Step 2. Correct central ray placement and centering of part to central ray and/or image receptor

Step 3. Accurate collimation

Step 4. Area shielding of patient where advisable

Step 5. Use of proper immobilizing devices when needed

Step 6. Approximate correct exposure factors, breathing instructions where applicable, and initiating exposure

Projections	Step 1	Step 2	Step 3	Step 4	Step 5	Step 6
● RAO sternum	____	____	____	____	____	____
● Erect lateral sternum	____	____	____	____	____	____
● Recumbent left posterior oblique (LPO) sternum	____	____	____	____	____	____
● Horizontal beam lateral sternum	____	____	____	____	____	____
● PA sternoclavicular joints	____	____	____	____	____	____
● Oblique sternoclavicular joints	____	____	____	____	____	____
● Rib routine for injury to right upper anterior ribs	____	____	____	____	____	____
● Rib routine for injury to left lower posterior ribs	____	____	____	____	____	____

Optional exercise if the school or hospital has a tomography unit.

● Linear tomogram of the sternum	____	____	____	____	____	____

This self-test should be taken only after completing all of the readings, review exercises, and laboratory activities for a particular section. The purpose of this test is not only to provide a good learning exercise but also to serve as a strong indicator of what your final evaluation exam will cover. It is strongly suggested that if you do not get at least a 90% to 95% grade on each self-test that you review those areas in which you missed questions before going to your instructor for the final evaluation exam for this chapter.

1. List the three parts of the sternum.

    A. _____

    B. _____

    C. _____

2. What is the most distal aspect of the sternum? _____

3. What is the name of the palpable junction between the upper and midportion of the sternum?

    _____

4. Which aspect of the sternum possesses the jugular notch?
    A. Body
    B. Sternal angle
    C. Xiphoid process
    D. Manubrium

5. What distinguishes a true rib from a false rib?
    A. A true rib attaches directly to the sternum with it own costocartilage.
    B. A true rib possesses a costovertebral and a costotransverse joint.
    C. A false rib does not possess a head.
    D. A false rib is primarily composed of cartilage.

6. What distinguishes a floating rib from a false rib?
    A. A floating rib is found only at the T1, T10, and T11 levels.
    B. A floating rib does not possess a head.
    C. A floating rib has no costal groove.
    D. A floating rib does not possess costocartilage.

7. The fifth rib is an example of a _____ (true rib or false rib).

8. Which part of the sternum do the second ribs articulate?
    A. Midbody
    B. Upper manubrium
    C. Middle manubrium
    D. Sternal angle

9. Which of the following structures is (are) found in the costal groove of each rib?
    A. Nerve
    B. Artery
    C. Vein
    D. All of the above

10. Match each of the following joints with the correct type of movement.

_____ 1. Sternoclavicular   A. Plane (gliding)—diarthrodial

_____ 2. Costovertebral joint   B. Immovable—synarthrodial

_____ 3. First sternocostal joint

_____ 4. Eighth interchondral joint

_____ 5. Third costochondral union

11. Identify the structures labeled on the following radiographs of the sternum (Figs. 11-5 and 11-6).

Fig. 11-5

A. _____

B. _____ (joint)

C. _____

D. _____

E. _____

F. _____

G. _____

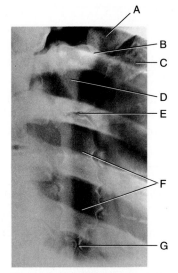

Fig. 11-5. The sternum, A-G.

Fig. 11-6

H. _____

I. _____

J. _____

K. _____

L. _____

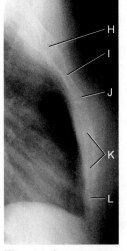

Fig. 11-6. The sternum, H-L.

12. List the correct positioning considerations for a study of the ribs above the diaphragm.

   A. Breathing instructions: _____

   B. kV range: _____

   C. General body position: _____

13. What is the minimum SID for radiography of the sternum? (Note: This is a radiation safety concern.)

   _____

14. Which one of the following breathing instructions should be employed for an RAO position of the sternum to maximize visibility of it?
   A. Suspended inspiration   C. Suspended expiration
   B. Breathing technique   D. Valsalva maneuver

15. List the two factors to be considered when determining which specific projections to include in the rib routine as described in the textbook.

   A. _____

   B. _____

16. List two chest pathologic conditions that may result from a rib injury and may require a PA and lateral chest projections to be included with the rib routine.

   A. _____   B. _____

17. A. What is the average degree of rotation for an RAO position of the sternum?

   _____

   B. Does an asthenic patient require a little more or a little less obliquity than a hypersthenic patient?

   _____

18. For which of the following conditions of the bony thorax are nuclear medicine bone scans not normally performed?
   A. Possible fractures   C. History of multiple myeloma
   B. Osteoporosis   D. Osteomyelitis

19. Pathology of the sternum is most commonly due to:
   A. Metastases   C. Infection
   B. Osteoporosis   D. Blunt trauma

20. What is the average breast dose range for each of the following projections?

   A. A posterior oblique rib projection: _____

   B. An anterior oblique rib projection: _____

21. What other position can be used for the sternum if the patient cannot assume the recumbent RAO position?
    A. LAO
    B. RPO
    C. LPO
    D. Left lateral decubitus

22. How should the arms be positioned for an erect lateral projection of the sternum?
    A. Raised over the head
    B. Drawn back
    C. Depressed by holding 5 to 10 lb in each hand
    D. Extended in front of the thorax

23. Which radiographic sign can be evaluated to determine whether rotation is present on a PA projection of the sternoclavicular joints? _____

24. How much rotation of the thorax is required for the anterior oblique projection of the sternoclavicular joints?

    _____

25. Where is the central ray centered for an AP projection of the ribs below the diaphragm?

    _____

26. What range of kV should be used for ribs above the diaphragm?
    A. 55 to 65 kV
    B. 65 to 70 kV
    C. 80 to 90 kV
    D. 90 to 100 kV

27. Which one of the following positions or projections will best demonstrate the right axillary ribs?
    A. LAO
    B. LPO
    C. RAO
    D. PA

28. A radiograph of an RAO projection of the sternum reveals that the width of the sternum is foreshortened and the sternum is shifted away from the spine and out of the heart shadow. The patient has a large "barrel" chest. The technologist performed the RAO with 20° to 25° of rotation and used a breathing technique. Which positioning error led to this radiographic outcome?

    _____

29. A radiograph of a lateral sternum reveals that anterior ribs are superimposed over the sternum. Which specific

    positioning error led to this radiographic outcome? _____

30. **Situation:** A patient with an injury to the right lower posterior ribs comes to the emergency room. She is unable to stand. List the positioning routine that would be performed for this patient. Include breathing instructions.

    A. Positions performed: _____

    B. Breathing instructions: _____

31. **Situation:** A patient with an injury to the left upper anterior ribs comes to the ER. He is unable to stand but can lie on his abdomen. List the positioning routine that would be used for this patient. Include breathing instructions.

    A. Positions performed: _____

    B. Breathing instructions: _____

32. **Situation:** A routine chest study reveals a possible lesion near the right sternoclavicular joint. A PA projection of the sternoclavicular joints is taken, but the area of interest is superimposed over the spine. What specific position can be used to better demonstrate this region? _____

33. **Situation:** A patient is brought into the ER with multiple injuries due to an MVA. The patient can move but cannot stand or lie prone because of his injuries. A sternum study is ordered. What positions should be performed for this patient? _____

34. **Situation:** A patient comes to the ER with multiple rib fractures. The ER physician suspects a flail chest. The patient is able to stand and move. Beyond a rib series, what projections should be taken for this patient?

_____

35. **True/False:** The automatic exposure control (AEC) system is recommended for sternum and rib routines if the center chamber is used.

36. **True/False:** A breathing technique is recommended for studies of the sternoclavicular joints.

37. **Situation:** A patient comes to the ER with a right, upper, anterior rib injury. A unilateral rib study is ordered. What are the basic projections taken for this patient?

_____

38. **Situation:** A patient comes to the ER with a left, lower, posterior rib injury. A unilateral rib study is ordered. The patient is unable to stand due to multiple injuries. What are the basic projections taken for this patient?

_____

39. **Situation:** A patient comes to radiology with a clinical history of pectus excavatum. What positioning routine would best demonstrate the condition?

_____

40. **Situation:** A patient comes to radiology with widespread metastases involving the bony thorax. Beyond radiographic studies, what other imaging modality will demonstrate the extent of this condition?

_____

12 Skull and Cranial Bones

CHAPTER OBJECTIVES

After you have successfully completed the activities in this chapter, you will be able to:

_____ 1. List the eight cranial bones and describe their features, related structures, location, and function.

_____ 2. Using drawings and/or radiographs, identify specific structures of the eight cranial bones.

_____ 3. Define specific terminology, reference points, positioning lines, and topographic landmarks of the cranium.

_____ 4. Identify specific radiographic and topographic landmarks of the cranium.

_____ 5. List the location, joint classification, and related terminology for the sutures and joints of the cranium.

_____ 6. List the differences among the three shape and size (morphology) classifications of the skull and their implications for radiography of the cranium.

_____ 7. Identify alternative imaging modalities that best demonstrate specific conditions or disease processes of the cranium and brain.

_____ 8. Match specific pathologic indications of the cranium to the correct definition or statements.

_____ 9. List the three main portions of the temporal bones.

_____ 10. Identify specific structures of the external, middle, and internal ear.

_____ 11. Using drawings, identify the three divisions of the ear and the structures found in each division.

_____ 12. Match specific pathologic indications of the temporal bone to the correct definition.

_____ 13. Using radiographs, identify specific structures of the temporal bone.

_____ 14. Identify the correct size and type of image receptor and central ray location, direction, and angle for basic and special projections of the cranium.

_____ 15. Identify which structures are best seen with specific projections of the cranium.

_____ 16. List the patient dose ranges for skin, midline, and thyroid for each basic and special projection of the cranium.

_____ 17. Identify the difference in dose ranges for the thyroid region for frontal projections (anteroposterior [AP]) compared with posteroanterior (PA) projections of the cranium (such as PA axial or PA Caldwell versus AP axial projections).

_____ 18. Given various hypothetical situations, identify the correct modification of a position and/or exposure factors to improve the radiographic image.

POSITIONING AND RADIOGRAPHIC CRITIQUE

_____ 1. Using a peer, position for basic and special projections of the cranium.

_____ 2. Using a cranial radiographic phantom, produce satisfactory radiographs of specific positions (if equipment is available).

_____ 3. Critique and evaluate cranial radiographs based on the four divisions of radiographic criteria: (1) structures shown, (2) position, (3) collimation and central ray, and (4) exposure criteria.

_____ 4. Distinguish between acceptable and unacceptable cranial radiographs based on exposure factors, motion, collimation, positioning, or other errors.

LEARNING EXERCISES

The following review exercises should be completed only after careful study of the associated pages in the textbook as indicated by each exercise. Answers to each review exercise are given at the end of the review exercises.

PART I: RADIOGRAPHIC ANATOMY
Review Exercise A: Anatomy and Pathology of the Cranium (see textbook pp. 372-379)

1. Fill in the total number of bones.

   A. Cranium _____   B. Facial bones _____

2. List the four cranial bones that form the calvaria (skull cap).

   A. _____   C. _____

   B. _____   D. _____

3. List the four cranial bones that form the floor of the cranium.

   A. _____   C. _____

   B. _____   D. _____

4. Identify the cranial bones labeled on Figs. 12-1 and 12-2 (Note: All eight cranial bones, including each paired bone, are visible in at least one of the following drawings).

A. _____

B. _____

C. _____

D. _____

E. _____

F. _____

G. _____

H. _____

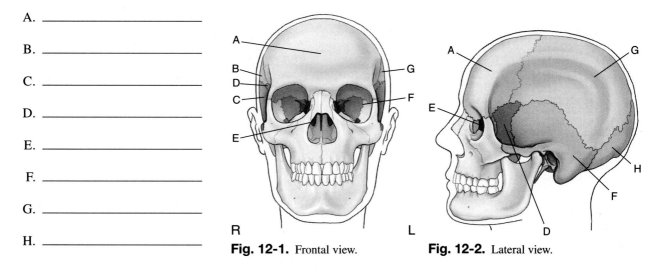

Fig. 12-1. Frontal view.   **Fig. 12-2.** Lateral view.

5. Identify all eight cranial bones on the two superior-view drawings (Figs. 12-3 and 12-4).

A. _____

B. _____

C. _____

D. _____

E. _____

F. _____

G. _____

H. _____

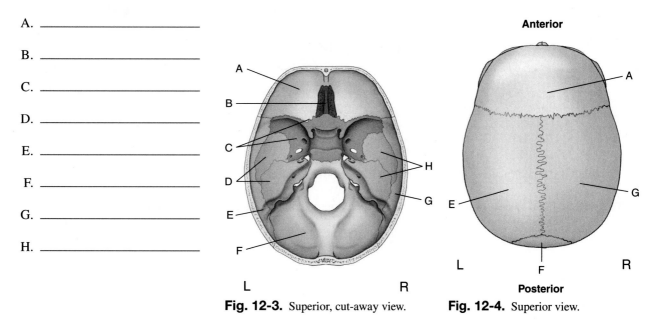

Fig. 12-3. Superior, cut-away view.   **Fig. 12-4.** Superior view.

6. Identify the labeled parts on the three views of the ethmoid bone (Figs. 12-5 and 12-6).

A. _____

B. _____

C. _____

D. _____

E. _____

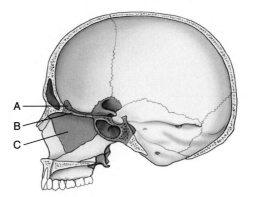

Fig. 12-5. Medial sectional view.

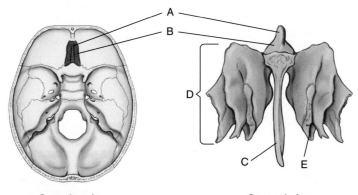

Superior view   Coronal view

Fig. 12-6. Superior (left) and coronal sectional (right) views.

7. The small horizontal plate of the ethmoid seen in the above drawings is called the _____.

8. The vertical plate of the ethmoid bone forming the upper portion of the bony nasal septum is the

_____.

9. Identify the labeled parts on the four views of the sphenoid in Figs. 12-7 through 12-10 (Note: Most of the parts are identified on more than one drawing).

A. _____

B. _____

C. _____

D. _____

E. _____

F. _____

G. _____

Foramina (H-L)

H. _____

I. _____

J. _____

K. _____

L. _____

M. _____

N. _____

O. _____

P. _____

Q. _____

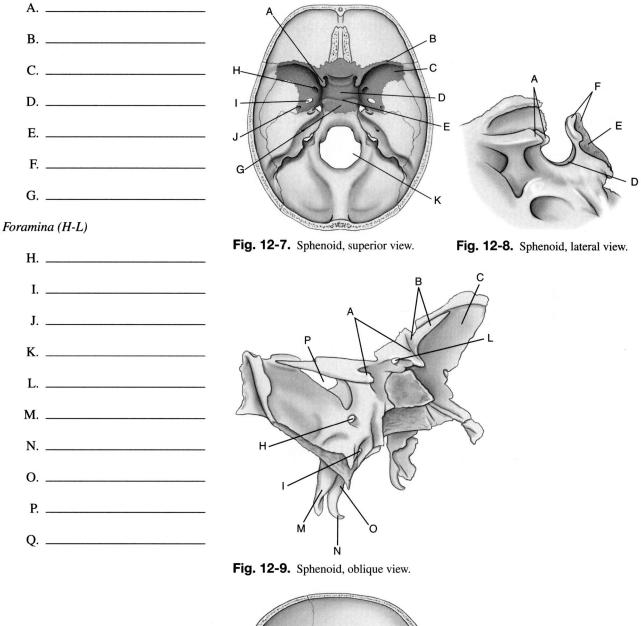

Fig. 12-7. Sphenoid, superior view.   **Fig. 12-8.** Sphenoid, lateral view.

Fig. 12-9. Sphenoid, oblique view.

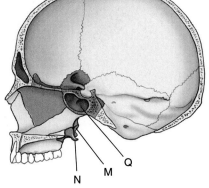

Fig. 12-10. Sphenoid, medial sectional view.

10. A structure found in the middle of the sphenoid bone that surrounds the pituitary gland is the

    _____.

11. The posterior aspect of the sella turcica is called the _____.

12. Which structure of the sphenoid bone allows for the passage of the optic nerve and is the actual opening into the

    orbit? _____

13. Which structures of the sphenoid bone help form part of the lateral walls of the nasal cavities?

    _____

14. Which radiographic cranial position best demonstrates the sella turcica? _____

15. Which aspect of the frontal bone forms the superior aspect of the orbit? _____

16. Identify the four major sutures and the six associated asterions and fontanels labeled on these drawings of an adult
    cranium and an infant cranium (Figs. 12-11 to 12-14).

Sutures

    A. _____

    B. _____

    C. _____

    D. _____

Asterions

    E. _____

    F. _____

    G. Right and left _____

    H. Right and left _____

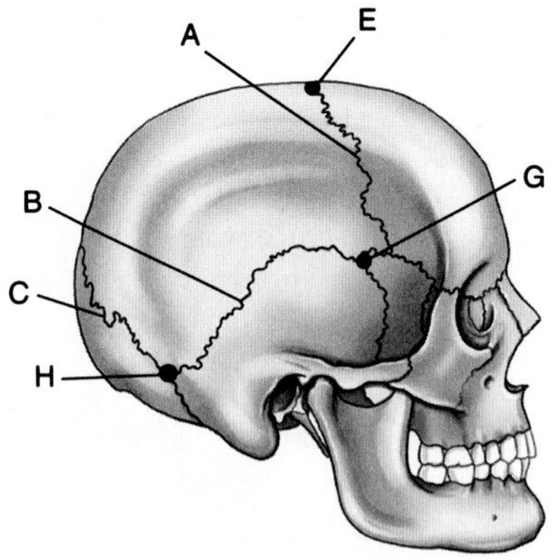

Fig. 12-11. Adult cranium, lateral view.

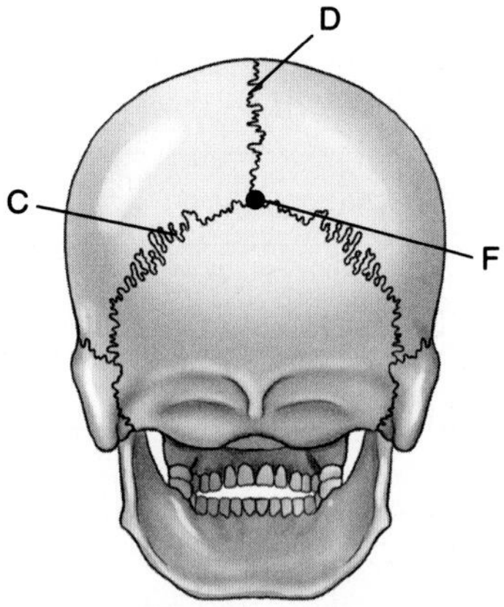

Posterior view

Fig. 12-12. Posterior view.

Fontanels: *Associated adult asterion:*

    I. _____   (_____)

    J. _____   (_____)

    K. Right and left _____   (_____)

    L. Right and left _____   (_____)

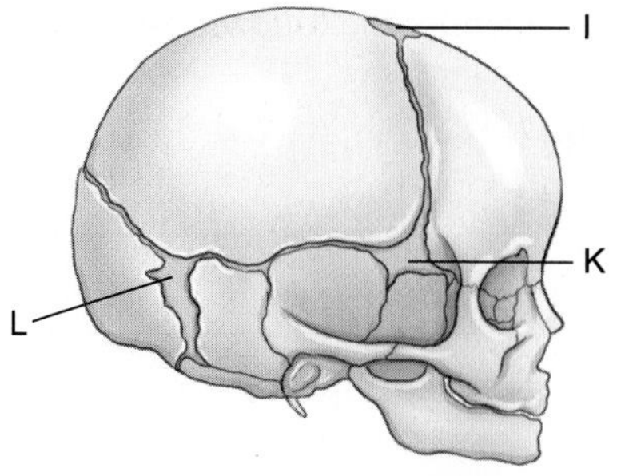

Fig. 12-13. Infant cranium, lateral view.

17. Cranial sutures are classified as being _____ joints.

18. Small irregular bones that sometimes develop in adult skull sutures are called

    _____ or _____ bones and are most

    frequently found in the _____ suture.

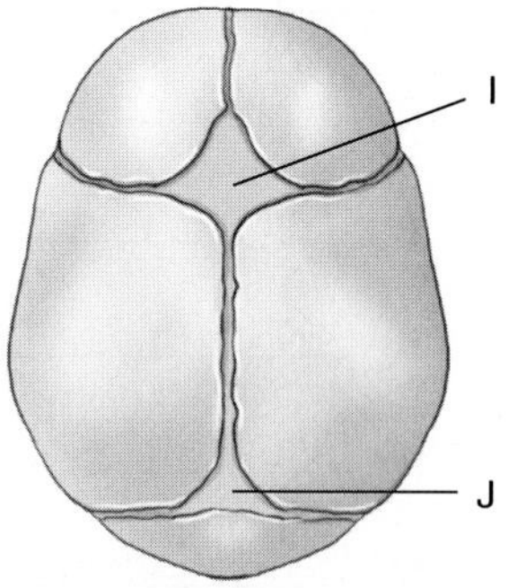

19. Which term describes the superior rim of the orbit? (Include the abbreviation also.)
    _____

20. What is the name of the notch that separates the orbital plates from each other?
    _____

Fig. 12-14. Infant cranium, superior view.

21. Which cranial bones form the upper lateral walls of the calvarium?
    _____

22. Which cranial bone contains the foramen magnum? _____

23. A small prominence located on the squamous portion of the occipital bone is called the _____.

24. What is the name of the oval processes found on the occipital bone that help form the occipito-atlantal joint?

    _____

25. List the three aspects of the temporal bones.

    A. _____   B. _____   C. _____

26. True/False: The mastoid portion of the temporal bone is the densest of the three aspects of the temporal bone.

27. Which external landmark corresponds with the level of the petrous ridge? _____

28. Which opening in the temporal bone serves as a passageway for nerves of hearing and equilibrium?

    _____

29. Identify the following cranial structures labeled on Figs. 12-15 and 12-16.

Fig. 12-15

   A. _____

   B. _____

   C. _____ (suture)

   D. _____ (suture)

   E. _____

Fig. 12-16

   A. _____

   B. _____

   C. _____

   D. _____ (suture)

   E. _____

   F. _____

   G. _____

   H. _____

   I. _____

   J. _____ (suture)

   K. _____

   L. _____

   M. _____

   N. _____

   O. _____

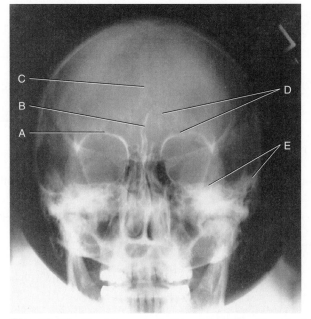

Fig. 12-15. Cranial structures, PA axial (Caldwell) projection.

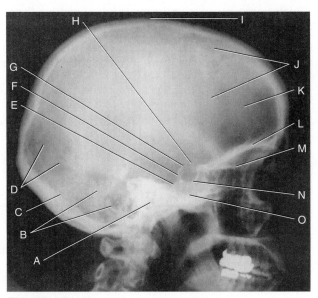

Fig. 12-16. Cranial structures, lateral projection.

Review Exercise B: Specific Anatomy and Pathology of the Temporal Bone (see textbook pp. 380-383)

1. List the three aspects of the temporal bone.

   A. _____   B. _____   C. _____

2. Which aspect of the temporal bone is considered the densest?_____

3. Which structure makes up the cartilaginous, external ear? _____

4. How long is the average external acoustic meatus (EAM)? _____

5. Which small membrane marks the beginning of the middle ear? _____

6. What is the collective term for the small bones of the middle ear? _____

7. Which structure allows for communication between the nasopharynx and middle ear? _____

8. What is the major function of the structure described in question 7? _____

9. Which structure serves as an opening between the mastoid portion of the temporal bone and the middle ear?

   _____

10. What is the name of the thin plate of bone that separates the mastoid air cells from the brain?

    _____

11. Which one of the auditory ossicles picks up sound vibrations from the tympanic membrane?

    _____

12. Which one of the auditory ossicles is considered to be the smallest? _____

13. Which one of the auditory ossicles resembles a premolar tooth? _____

14. What is the name of the small membrane that connects the middle to the inner ear? _____

15. Which two sensory functions occur within the inner ear?

    A. _____   B. _____

16. What is the name of the small membrane that will move outward to transmit impulses to the auditory nerve, thus

    creating the sense of hearing? _____

17. True/False: The cochlea is a closed system relating to the sense of hearing.

18. Identify the structures labeled on Fig. 12-17.

A. _____

B. _____

C. _____

D. _____

E. _____

F. _____

G. _____

H. _____

I. _____

J. _____

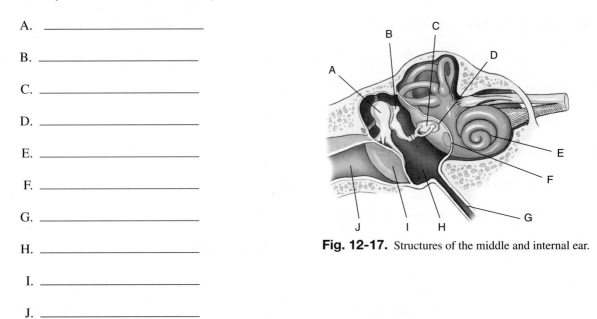

Fig. 12-17. Structures of the middle and internal ear.

19. Match each of the following pathologic indications for the temporal bone to the correct definition or description (using each choice only once).

_____ A. Neoplasia   1. Bacterial infection of the mastoid process

_____ B. Otosclerosis   2. Growth arising from a mucous membrane

_____ C. Mastoiditis   3. Hereditary disease involving excessive bone formation of middle and inner ear

_____ D. Acoustic neuroma   4. Benign, cystlike mass or tumor of the middle ear

_____ E. Polyp   5. New and abnormal growth

_____ F. Cholesteatoma   6. Benign tumor of the auditory nerve sheath

20. Which one of the following radiographic appearances pertains to an acoustic neuroma?
    A. Expansion of the internal acoustic canal   C. Increased density in the sinus
    B. Bone destruction within the middle ear   D. Sinus mucosal thickening

21. Which one of the following imaging modalities best demonstrates otosclerosis?
    A. Nuclear medicine   C. Conventional radiography
    B. CT   D. Ultrasound

PART II: RADIOGRAPHIC POSITIONING
Review Exercise C: Skull Morphology, Topography, and Positioning of the Cranium
(see textbook pp. 384-399)

1. List the three classifications of the skull; then match them with the correct shape description listed on the right.

   Classification   *Shape Description*

   A. _____   a. Width less than 75% of length

   B. _____   b. Width 80% or more than length

   C. _____   c. Width between 75% and 80% of length

2. Central ray angles and degree of rotation stated for basic skull positions are based on the _____

   (average) skull, which has an angle of _____ ° between the midsagittal plane and the long axis of the petrous bone.

3. The long, narrow-shaped skull has an angle of approximately _____ ° between the midsagittal plane and the long axis of the petrous bone.

4. True/False: Two older terms for the orbitomeatal line (OML) are Reid's base line and the anthropologic base line.

5. There is a _____ ° difference between the orbitomeatal and infraorbitomeatal lines, and

   _____ ° between the orbitomeatal and glabellomeatal lines.

6. Match each of the following cranial landmarks and positioning lines with the correct definition (using each choice only once).

_____ 1. Lateral junction of the eyelid

_____ 2. Posterior angle of the jaw

_____ 3. A line between the infraorbital margin and EAM

_____ 4. Corresponds to the highest "nuchal" line of the occipital bone

_____ 5. A line between the glabella and alveolar process of the maxilla

_____ 6. A line between the mental point and EAM

_____ 7. Located at the junction of the two nasal bones and the frontal bone

_____ 8. The small cartilaginous flap covering the ear opening

_____ 9. Corresponds to the highest level of the facial bone mass

_____ 10. A line between the midlateral orbital margin and the EAM

_____ 11. The center point of the EAM

_____ 12. A positioning line that is primarily used for the modified Waters projection

_____ 13. A line used in positioning to ensure that the skull is in a true lateral position

_____ 14. Corresponds to the level of the petrous ridge

_____ 15. A smooth, slightly depressed area between the eyebrows

A. TEA

B. Supraorbital groove

C. Interpupillary line

D. Nasion

E. Gonion

F. Tragus

G. Outer canthus

H. Glabelloalveolar line

I. OML

J. Infraorbitomeatal line (IOML)

K. Mentomeatal line

L. Lips-meatal line

M. Glabella

N. Inion

O. Auricular point

7. What is the average kV range for skull radiography? _____

8. True/False: According to HEW Report 76-8031, the patient receives no detectable gonadal exposure during skull radiography when accurate collimation is used.

9. True/False: The AP axial (Towne) skull results in about 10 times more dose to the thyroid than a PA axial (Haas) projection.

10. The thyroid dose for a submentovertex (SMV) projection of the skull is in the _____ range (which is the highest thyroid dose of any skull projection).
    A. 10 to 50 mrad
    B. 50 to 100 mrad
    C. 200 to 300 mrad
    D. 500 to 600 mrad

11. List the five most common errors made during skull radiography.

    A. _____   C. _____   E. _____

    B. _____   D. _____

12. Of the five causes listed in the previous question, which two are the most common?

    A. _____   B. _____

13. True/False: Adults with osteoporosis may require a 25% to 30% reduction in mAs during skull projections.

14. Which one of the following imaging modalities is the most common neuroimaging procedure performed for the cranium?
    A. Computed tomography (CT)   C. Magnetic resonance imaging (MRI)
    B. Ultrasound   D. Nuclear medicine

15. Which of the following imaging modalities is usually performed on neonates with a possible intracranial hemorrhage?
    A. CT   C. MRI
    B. Ultrasound   D. Nuclear medicine

16. Which of the following imaging modalities is most commonly performed to evaluate patients for Alzheimer disease?
    A. CT   C. MRI
    B. Ultrasound   D. Nuclear medicine

17. Match each of the following pathologic indications to the correct definition or statement (using each choice only once).

    _____ A. Fracture that may produce an air-fluid level in the sphenoid sinus   1. Osteoblastic neoplasm

    _____ B. Destructive lesion with irregular margins   2. Pituitary adenoma

    _____ C. Also called a "ping-pong" fracture   3. Basal skull fracture

    _____ D. Proliferative bony lesion of increased density   4. Paget's disease

    _____ E. A tumor that may produce erosion of the sella turcica   5. Osteolytic neoplasm

    _____ F. Also known as osteitis deformans   6. Depressed skull fracture

    _____ G. A bone tumor that originates in the bone marrow   7. Multiple myeloma

18. Which one of the following pathologic indications may require an increase in manual exposure factors?
    A. Paget's disease   C. Multiple myeloma
    B. Metastatic neoplasm   D. Basal skull fracture

19. Which cranial bone is best demonstrated with an AP axial (Towne method) projection of the skull?

    _____

20. When using a 30° caudad angle for the AP axial (Towne method) projection of the skull, which positioning line should be perpendicular to the image receptor?
    A. OML   C. GAL
    B. IOML   D. AML

21. A properly positioned AP axial (Towne method) projection should place the dorsum sellae into the middle aspect of the:
   A. Orbits   C. Foramen magnum
   B. Clivus   D. Anterior arch of C1

22. A lack of symmetry of the petrous ridges indicates which of the following problems with a radiograph of an AP axial projection?
   A. Tilt   C. Flexion or extension
   B. Central ray angle   D. Rotation

23. If the patient cannot flex the head adequately for the AP axial (Towne method) projection, the technologist could

   place the _____ perpendicular to the image receptor and angle the central ray

   _____ ° caudad.

24. What evidence on an AP axial (Towne method) radiograph indicates whether the correct central ray angle and

   correct head flexion were used? _____

25. What central ray angle should be used for the PA axial (Haas method) projection for the cranium?

   _____

26. Where is the central ray centered for a lateral projection of the skull? _____

27. Which specific positioning error is present if the mandibular rami are not superimposed on a lateral skull radiograph?
   A. Tilt   C. Overflexion of head and neck
   B. Rotation   D. Incorrect central ray angle

28. Where will the petrous ridges be projected with a 15° PA axial (Caldwell) projection of the cranium?

   _____

29. Which specific positioning error is present if the petrous ridges are projected higher in the orbits than expected for

   a 15° PA axial projection? _____

30. Which projection of the cranium produces an image of the frontal bone with little or no distortion?

   _____

31. With a possible trauma patient, what must be determined before performing the SMV projection of the skull?

   _____

32. Where is the central ray centered for a lateral projection of the sella turcica? _____

33. Which skull positioning line is placed parallel to the plane of the IR for the SMV projection?
   A. OML   C. AML
   B. IOML   D. GML

34. Which one of the following AP axial projections for sella turcica best visualizes the anterior clinoid processes?
    A. 30° caudal to IOML
    B. 37° caudal to IOML
    C. 30° caudal to OML
    D. 45° caudal to OML

35. Which one of the following projections best demonstrates the sella turcica in profile?
    A. AP axial
    B. SMV
    C. 15° PA axial
    D. Lateral

36. Which one of the following projections best demonstrates the foramen rotundum?
    A. SMV
    B. 25° to 30° AP axial
    C. 25° to 30° PA axial
    D. Lateral

37. Which one of the following projections best demonstrates the clivus in profile?
    A. AP axial
    B. 15° PA
    C. Lateral
    D. SMV

38. Where does the CR exit for a PA axial (Haas method) projection of the skull?
    A. 1½ inches (4 cm) superior to the nasion
    B. ¾ inch (2 cm) anterior to EAM
    C. 2½ inches (6.5 cm) above the glabella
    D. Level of nasion

39. What type of CR angle is used with the AP axial projection for sella turcica if the dorsum sellae and posterior clinoid processes are of primary interest?
    A. 25° caudad
    B. 30 ° caudad
    C. 37° caudad
    D. 25° cephalad

40. Which imaging modality is best to differentiate between an epidural and subdural hemorrhage?
    A. CT
    B. MRI
    C. Nuclear medicine
    D. PET

Review Exercise D: Problem Solving for Technical and Positioning Errors

1. A radiograph of an AP axial (Towne method) projection of the cranium reveals that the right petrous ridge is wider than the left side. Which specific positioning error is present on this radiograph?

_____

2. A radiograph of a 15° PA axial (Caldwell) projection of the cranium demonstrates that the petrous ridges are projected at the inferior orbital margin. Which positioning error(s) led to this radiographic outcome?

_____

3. A radiograph of a 15° PA axial (Caldwell) projection demonstrates that the distance between the midlateral borders of the orbit and lateral margin of the skull are not equal. Which positioning error led to this radiographic outcome?

_____

4. A radiograph of an SMV projection of the skull reveals that the mandibular condyles are within the petrous bone. Which specific positioning error led to this problem? _____

5. A radiograph of a lateral projection of the skull reveals that the orbital plates are not superimposed (one orbital plate is slightly superior to the other). Which specific positioning error led to this radiographic outcome? _____

6. A lateral skull radiograph demonstrates one mandibular ramus about 0.5 cm more anterior than the other. Which positioning error occurred? _____

7. An AP axial (Towne method) radiograph for cranium demonstrates the dorsum sellae projected above or superior to, rather than within, the foramen magnum. Which positioning error occurred? _____

8. **Situation:** A patient comes to the radiology department with a possible tumor of the pituitary gland. Which projection of the cranium best demonstrates any bony involvement of the sella turcica? _____

9. **Situation:** A patient with a possible linear fracture of the right parietal bone enters the emergency room. Which single projection of the skull best demonstrates this fracture? _____

10. **Situation:** A patient comes to the radiology department for a skull series, but the patient cannot assume the correct position for either version of the AP axial (Towne method) projection because of a very short neck and severe spinal kyphosis. What can the technologist do to demonstrate the occipital bone? _____

11. **Situation:** A patient with a possible basal skull fracture enters the emergency room. Which specific position may provide radiographic evidence of this fracture? _____

12. **Situation:** A neonate has a clinical history of craniosynostosis. Because of the age of the patient, the physician does not order a radiographic procedure of the cranium. What other imaging modality can be performed to evaluate the patient for this condition? _____

13. **Situation:** A patient with a clinical history of acoustic neuroma comes to the radiology department. Which imaging modality(ies) can be performed for this type of pathology? _____

14. A radiograph of an AP axial (Towne method) projection for cranium reveals that the anterior arch of C1 is projected within the foramen magnum. What is the positioning error? _____

15. A radiograph of an AP axial (Towne method) projection for cranium reveals that the mid- to-lower mandible is cut-off and not demonstrated. What should the technologist do? _____

Review Exercise E: Critique Radiographs of the Cranium (see textbook p. 400)

The following questions relate to the radiographs found at the end of Chapter 12 of the textbook. Evaluate these radiographs for the radiographic criteria categories (1 through 5) that follow. Describe the corrections needed to improve the overall image. The major, or "repeatable," errors are specific errors that indicate the need for a repeat exposure, regardless of the nature of the other errors.

A. Lateral skull: 4-year-old (Fig. C12-74)

    1. Structures shown: _____

    2. Part positioning: _____

    3. Collimation and central ray: _____

    4. Exposure criteria: _____

    5. Anatomic side markers: _____

Repeatable error(s): _____

B. Lateral skull: 54-year-old, posttraumatic injury (Fig. C12-75)

    1. Structures shown: _____

    2. Part positioning: _____

    3. Collimation and central ray: _____

    4. Exposure criteria: _____

    5. Anatomic side markers: _____

Repeatable error(s): _____

C. AP axial skull (Towne): (Fig. C12-76)

    1. Structures shown: _____

    2. Part positioning: _____

    3. Collimation and central ray: _____

    4. Exposure criteria: _____

    5. Anatomic side markers: _____

Repeatable error(s): _____

D. AP or PA skull (Fig. C12-77)

How can you determine whether this was a PA or an AP projection? _____

1. Structures shown: _____

2. Part positioning: _____

3. Collimation and central ray: _____

4. Exposure criteria: _____

5. Anatomic side markers: _____

Repeatable error(s): _____

E. AP or PA skull (Fig. C12-78)

Is this an AP or a PA skull? (Compare with Fig. C12-77, looking at the size of the orbits.) _____

1. Structures shown: _____

2. Part positioning: _____

3. Collimation and central ray: _____

4. Exposure criteria: _____

5. Anatomic side markers: _____

Repeatable error(s): _____

PART III: LABORATORY EXERCISES

You must gain experience in positioning each part of the cranium before performing the following exams on actual patients. You can get experience in positioning and radiographic evaluation of these projections by performing exercises using radiographic phantoms and practicing on other students (although you will not be taking actual exposures).

The following suggested activities assume that your teaching institution has an energized lab and radiographic phantoms. If not, perform Laboratory Exercises B and C, the radiographic evaluation and the physical positioning exercises. (Check off each step and projection as you complete it.)

Laboratory Exercise A: Energized Laboratory

1. Using the skull radiographic phantom, produce radiographs of the following basic routines:

_____ 15° PA axial (Caldwell) skull   _____ PA axial (Haas)   _____ AP axial sella turcica

_____ Lateral skull   _____ SMV   _____ Lateral sella turcica

_____ AP axial skull

Laboratory Exercise B: Radiographic Evaluation

1. Evaluate and critique the radiographs produced above, additional radiographs provided by your instructor, or both. Evaluate each radiograph for the following points.

_____ Evaluate the completeness of the study. (Are all of the pertinent anatomic structures included on the radiograph?)

_____ Evaluate for positioning or centering errors (e.g., rotation, off centering).

_____ Evaluate for correct exposure factors and possible motion. (Are the density and contrast of the images acceptable?)

_____ Determine whether anatomic side markers and an acceptable degree of collimation and/or area shielding are visible on the images.

Laboratory Exercise C: Physical Positioning

On another person, simulate performing all basic and special projections of the sternum and ribs as follows. Include the six steps listed below and described in the textbook. (Check off each step when completed satisfactorily.)

Step 1. Appropriate size and type of image receptor with correct markers

Step 2. Correct central ray placement and centering of part to central ray and/or image receptor

Step 3. Accurate collimation

Step 4. Area shielding of patient where advisable

Step 5. Use of proper immobilizing devices when needed

Step 6. Approximate correct exposure factors, breathing instructions where applicable, and initiating exposure

Projections	Step 1	Step 2	Step 3	Step 4	Step 5	Step 6
Skull series: basic						
● AP axial (Towne)	_____	_____	_____	_____	_____	_____
● Lateral skull	_____	_____	_____	_____	_____	_____
● PA 15° axial (Caldwell)	_____	_____	_____	_____	_____	_____
Skull series: special						
● PA axial (Haas)	_____	_____	_____	_____	_____	_____
● SMV	_____	_____	_____	_____	_____	_____
Sella turcica: basic						
● Lateral	_____	_____	_____	_____	_____	_____
● AP axial (Towne)	_____	_____	_____	_____	_____	_____

This self-test should be taken only after completing all of the readings, review exercises, and laboratory activities for a particular section. The purpose of this test is not only to provide a good learning exercise but also to serve as a strong indicator of what your final unit evaluation exam will cover. It is strongly suggested that if you do not get at least a 90% to 95% grade on each self-test that you review those areas in which you missed questions before going to your instructor for the final unit evaluation exam.

1. Which one of the following bones is not part of the floor of the cranium?
   A. Temporal   B. Ethmoid   C. Occipital   D. Sphenoid

2. Which aspect of the frontal bone is thin-walled and forms the forehead?
   A. Orbital   B. Horizontal   C. Squamous   D. Superciliary margin

3. Which four cranial bones articulate with the frontal bone?

   A. _____   C. _____

   B. _____   D. _____

4. Which structures are found at the widest aspect of the skull? _____

5. What is the name of a prominent landmark (or "bump") found on the external surface of the occipital bone?

   _____

6. List the number of individual bones that articulate with the following cranial bones.

   A. Parietal bone: _____

   B. Occipital bone: _____

   C. Temporal bone: _____

   D. Sphenoid: _____

   E. Ethmoid: _____

7. What is the thickest and densest structure in the cranium? _____

8. True/False: The hypophysis is another term for the pituitary gland.

9. True/False: The sphenoid bone articulates with all the other cranial bones.

10. The shallow depression just posterior to the base of the dorsum sellae and anterior to the foramen magnum is the

   _____.

11. What is the name of the paired collections of bone found inferior to the cribriform plate that contain numerous air cells and help form the lateral walls of the nasal cavity? _____

12. Which small section of bone is located superior to the cribriform plate? _____

13. What is the formal term for the left sphenoid fontanel in the adult? _____

14. What is the name of the cranial suture formed by the inferior junction of the parietals to the temporal bones?

_____

15. What are the two terms for the small, irregular bones found in the adult skull sutures? _____

16. Match each of the following structures to its related cranial bone.

_____ 1. Pterygoid hamulus   A. Occipital

_____ 2. Anterior clinoid processes   B. Frontal

_____ 3. Glabella   C. Sphenoid

_____ 4. Foramen ovale   D. Ethmoid

_____ 5. Perpendicular plate   E. Temporal

_____ 6. Superior nasal conchae   F. Parietal

_____ 7. Foramen magnum

_____ 8. Cribriform plate

_____ 9. Zygomatic process

_____ 10. Lateral condylar portions

_____ 11. Superciliary arch

_____ 12. EAM

_____ 13. Inion

_____ 14. Sella turcica

_____ 15. Petrous ridge

17. Identify the cranial structures, sutures, and regions labeled on the following radiographs (Figs. 12-18 and 12-19):

	Structure	*Bones(s)*
A.	_____	_____
B.	_____	_____
C.	_____	_____
D.	_____ (suture)	_____
E.	_____	_____
F.	_____	_____
G.	_____	_____
H.	_____	_____
I.	_____	_____
J.	_____	_____
K.	_____	_____
L.	_____	_____
M.	_____	_____

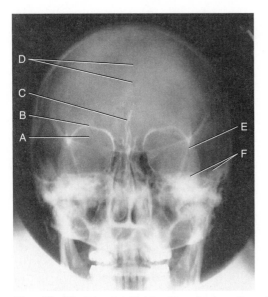

Fig. 12-18. PA axial (Caldwell) projection of cranium.

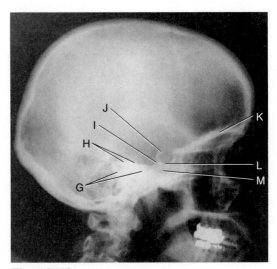

Fig. 12-19. Lateral cranium.

18. Which one of the following skull classifications applies to a skull with an angle of 54° between the midsagittal plane and the long axis of the pars petrosa?

A. Mesocephalic

C. Brachycephalic

B. Dolichocephalic

D. None of the above

19. Which of the above classifications is considered the average-shape skull? _____

20. Identify the labeled landmarks and positioning lines used in skull and facial bone positioning, as shown in Fig. 12-20 (including abbreviations).

A. _____

B. _____

C. _____

D. _____

E. _____

F. _____

G. _____

H. _____

I. _____

J. _____

K. _____

L. _____

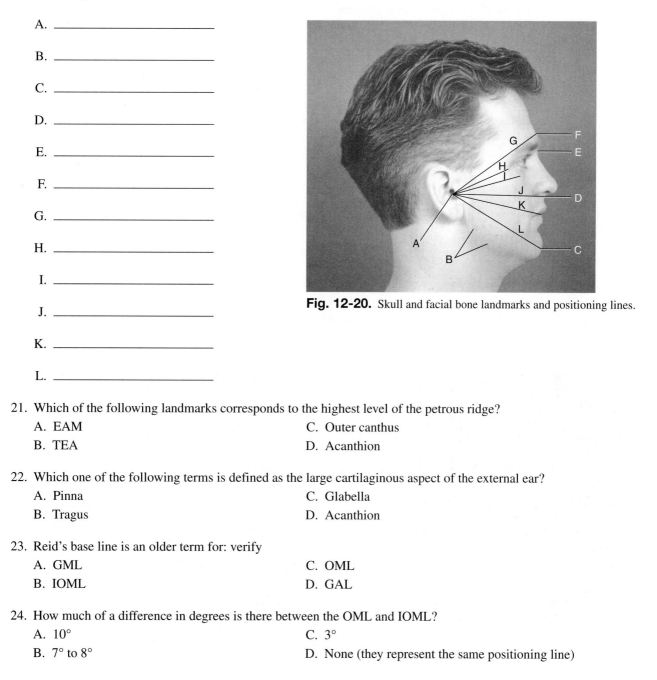

Fig. 12-20. Skull and facial bone landmarks and positioning lines.

21. Which of the following landmarks corresponds to the highest level of the petrous ridge?

A. EAM

C. Outer canthus

B. TEA

D. Acanthion

22. Which one of the following terms is defined as the large cartilaginous aspect of the external ear?

A. Pinna

C. Glabella

B. Tragus

D. Acanthion

23. Reid's base line is an older term for: verify

A. GML

C. OML

B. IOML

D. GAL

24. How much of a difference in degrees is there between the OML and IOML?

A. 10°

C. 3°

B. 7° to 8°

D. None (they represent the same positioning line)

25. Which one of the following positioning errors frequently results in a repeat exposure of a cranial position?
   A. Rotation
   B. Incorrect central ray placement
   C. Slight flexion
   D. None of the above

26. Match each of the following pathologic indications to the correct definition or description (using each choice only once).

   _____ A. Bone tumor originating in the bone marrow

   _____ B. Fracture evident by sphenoid sinus effusion

   _____ C. Condition that begins with bony destruction followed by bony repair

   _____ D. Destructive lesion with irregular margins

   _____ E. Fracture of the skull with jagged or irregular lucent line which lies at a right angle to the axis of the bone.

   _____ F. Tangential view may be helpful to determine extent or degree of this fracture

   1. Linear fracture

   2. Paget's disease

   3. Depressed fracture

   4. Osteolytic neoplasm

   5. Multiple myeloma

   6. Basal fracture

27. Which one of the following pathologic indications may require a decrease in manual exposure factors?
   A. Pituitary adenoma
   B. Linear skull fracture
   C. Paget's disease
   D. Multiple myeloma

28. Which one of the following imaging modalities may be used to examine a possible cranial bleed caused by trauma?
   A. CT
   B. MRI
   C. Ultrasound
   D. Nuclear medicine

29. Which one of the following imaging modalities provides an excellent distinction between normal and abnormal brain tissue?
   A. CT
   B. MRI
   C. Ultrasound
   D. Nuclear medicine

30. Which aspect of the temporal bone is considered to be thinnest? _____

31. Which aspect of the temporal bone contains the organs of hearing and balance? _____

32. The correct term for the eardrum is the _____.

33. Which one of the following middle ear structures is considered to be most lateral?
   A. Malleus
   B. Incus
   C. Stapes
   D. Oval window

34. Which structure helps equalize atmospheric pressure in the middle ear? _____

35. What passes through the internal acoustic meatus? _____

36. The aditus is an opening between the _____ and the _____ portion of the temporal bone.

37. An infection of the mastoid air cells, if untreated, can lead to a serious infection of the brain called

    _____.

38. Which auditory ossicle attaches to the oval window?
    A. Malleus   C. Stapes
    B. Incus   D. None

39. The internal ear is divided into the osseous or bony labyrinth and the _____ labyrinth.

40. List the three divisions of the bony labyrinth of the inner ear.

    A. _____   B. _____   C. _____

41. Identify the structures labeled on Fig. 12-21.

    A. _____

    B. _____

    C. _____

    D. _____

    E. _____

    F. _____

    G. _____

    H. _____

    I. _____

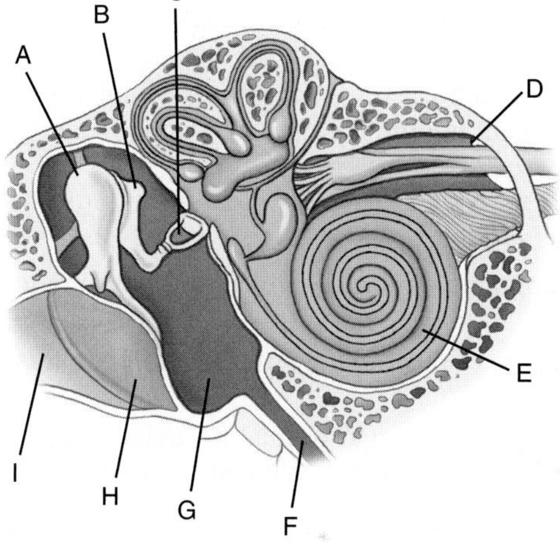

Fig. 12-21. Three divisions of the ear.

42. A benign, cystlike mass of the middle ear is a(n):
    A. Acoustic neuroma   C. Cholesteatoma
    B. Osteomyelitis   D. Acoustic sarcoma

43. True/False: Otosclerosis is a hereditary disease.

44. Which two projections of the cranium project the dorsum sellae within the foramen magnum?

    A. _____

    B. _____

45. A. What central ray angle is used for the AP axial projection (Towne method) for skull with the IOML perpendicular

    to the image receptor? _____

    B. What is the central ray angle for this same projection with a perpendicular OML? _____

46. Where is the central ray centered for a lateral projection of the cranium? _____

47. To prevent tilting of the skull for the lateral projection of the cranium, the _____ line is placed perpendicular to the image receptor.

48. Where should the petrous ridges be located (on the image) for a well-positioned, 25° caudad PA axial (Haas method)

projection? _____

49. Where is the central ray centered for an SMV projection of the skull? _____

50. A. How much is the central ray angled to the IOML for an AP axial projection of the sella turcica when the posterior

clinoid processes are of primary interest? _____

   B. How much is the central ray angled to the IOML when the anterior clinoid processes are of primary interest?

   _____

51. A radiograph of an AP axial projection for the cranium reveals that the dorsum sellae is projected just above rather than into the foramen magnum. What must be modified during the repeat exposure to correct this problem?

_____

52. A radiograph of a lateral projection of the cranium reveals that the greater wings of sphenoid are not superimposed.

What type of positioning error is present on this radiograph? _____

53. A radiograph of a 15° caudad PA axial projection of the cranium reveals that the petrous ridges are at the level of the supraorbital margin. Without changing the central ray angle, how must the head position be modified during the

repeat exposure to produce a more acceptable image? _____

54. **Situation:** A patient with a possible basilar skull fracture enters the emergency room. The physician wants a projection to demonstrate a possible sphenoid sinus effusion. Which projection of the cranium would be best for this

situation? _____

55. **Situation:** The same patient in the previous situation also requires a frontal projection of the skull. The physician wants the projection to demonstrate the frontal bone and place the petrous ridges in the lower one third of the orbits, but it has not been determined whether the patient's cervical spine has been fractured, so the patient cannot be moved

from a supine position. What should the technologist do to obtain this image? _____

56. **Situation:** A patient comes to the radiology department for a skull series. Because of the size of the patient's shoulders, he is unable to flex his neck sufficiently to place the OML perpendicular to the IR for the AP axial projection. His head cannot be raised because of possible cervical trauma. What other options does the technologist have to

obtain an acceptable AP axial projection? _____

57. A radiograph of an AP axial (Towne method) projection for cranium reveals that the anterior arch of C1 is projected within the foramen magnum. What modification is needed to correct this error present on the initial radiograph?

_____

58. A radiograph of a lateral skull demonstrates that the orbital plates (roof) of the frontal bone are not superimposed.

What is the positioning error present on this radiograph? _____

59. A radiograph of an AP axial (Towne method) for crainium reveals that the left petrous portion of the temporal bone is wider than the right. What is the specific positioning error present on this radiograph?

_____

60. A radiograph of a SMV projection of the cranium demonstrates that mandibular condyles are projected into the petrous portion (pyramids) of the temporal bone. How must the position be altered during the repeat exposure to

correct this error? _____

13 Facial Bones and Paranasal Sinuses

CHAPTER OBJECTIVES

After you have successfully completed the activities in this chapter, you will be able to:

_____ 1. List the specific features, characteristics, location, and functions of the fourteen facial bones.

_____ 2. List the seven cranial and facial bones that make up the bony orbit.

_____ 3. Using drawings and/or radiographs, identify specific structures of the facial bone region.

_____ 4. Explain the advantages of performing facial bone projections erect.

_____ 5. Identify alternative imaging modalities that best demonstrate specific facial bone and paranasal sinus pathology.

_____ 6. Identify specific types of fractures of the facial bone region.

_____ 7. List the location, function, and characteristics of the four groups of paranasal sinuses.

_____ 8. Using drawings and radiographs, identify specific paranasal sinuses.

_____ 9. Match specific pathologic indications of the paranasal sinuses to the correct definition.

_____ 10. Identify basic and special projections of the facial bones and list the correct size of image receptor, as well as the location, direction, and angulation of the central ray for each projection.

_____ 11. List which structures are best seen with basic and special projections of the facial bones.

_____ 12. Identify the basic operational and positioning considerations when performing a mandible study using the Panorex unit.

_____ 13. Identify basic and special projections of the paranasal sinuses and list the correct size and type of image receptor, as well as the location, direction, and angulation of the central ray for each position.

_____ 14. List patient dose ranges for skin, midline, and thyroid doses for specific projections of the facial bones and paranasal sinuses.

_____ 15. Given various hypothetical situations, identify the correct modification of a position and/or exposure factors to improve the radiographic image.

_____ 16. Given radiographs of specific facial and paranasal sinus projections/positions, identify specific errors in positioning and exposure factors.

POSITIONING AND RADIOGRAPHIC CRITIQUE

_____ 1. Using a peer, position for basic and special projections of the facial bones and sinuses.

_____ 2. Using a cranial radiographic phantom, produce satisfactory radiographs of specific positions (if equipment is available).

_____ 3. Critique and evaluate facial bone radiographs based on the four divisions of radiographic criteria: (1) structures shown, (2) position, (3) collimation and central ray, and (4) exposure criteria.

_____ 4. Distinguish between acceptable and unacceptable cranial radiographs resulting from exposure factors, motion, collimation, positioning, or other errors.

LEARNING EXERCISES

The following review exercises should be completed only after careful study of the associated pages in the textbook as indicated by each exercise. Answers to each review exercise are given at the end of the review exercises.

PART I: RADIOGRAPHIC ANATOMY
Review Exercise A: Radiographic Anatomy of the Facial Bones (see textbook pp. 402-407)

1. Which of the following bones is not a facial bone?
   A. Middle nasal conchae
   B. Vomer
   C. Lacrimal bone
   D. Mandible

2. What is the largest immovable bone of the face? _____

3. List the four processes of the maxilla.

   A. _____   C. _____

   B. _____   D. _____

4. Which one of the above-mentioned processes is considered most superior? _____

5. Which soft tissue landmark is found at the base of the anterior nasal spine? _____

6. Which facial bones form the posterior aspect of the hard palate? _____

7. Which two cranial bones articulate with the maxilla? _____

8. Which facial bones are sometimes called the "cheek bones"? _____

9. Which of the following bones does not articulate with the zygomatic bone?
   A. Temporal
   B. Maxilla
   C. Frontal
   D. Sphenoid

10. Which facial bone is associated with the tear ducts? _____

11. The purpose of the _____, or _____, is to divide the nasal cavity into compartments and circulate air coming into the nasal cavities. (Include both terms for these bones.)

12. True/False: The majority of the nose is formed by the right and left nasal bones.

13. A deviated nasal septum is most likely to occur at the junction between _____ and

_____.

14. Match each of the following mandibular terms to the correct definition or description (using each choice only once).

_____ A. Gonion

_____ B. Mandibular notch

_____ C. Body

_____ D. Condyloid process

_____ E. Coronoid process

_____ F. Ramus

_____ G. Mentum

_____ H. Symphysis menti

1. Vertical portion of mandible

2. The chin

3. Mandibular angle

4. The point of union between both halves of the mandible

5. Bony process located anterior to mandibular notch

6. Horizontal portion of mandible

7. Posterior process of upper ramus

8. U-shaped notch

15. Identify the labeled facial bones visible on Figs. 13-1 and 13-2.

Paired Bones

A. _____

B. _____

C. _____

D. _____

E. _____

Single Bone

F. _____

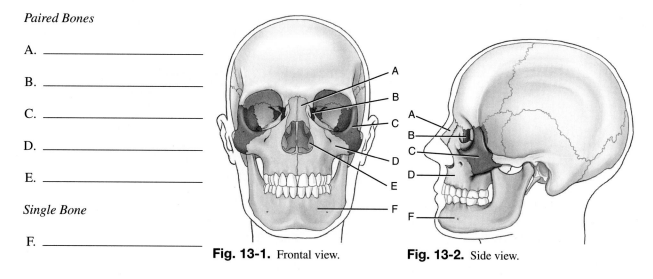

Fig. 13-1. Frontal view.   **Fig. 13-2.** Side view.

16. The one single facial bone and the one pair of facial bones not visible from the exterior and not demonstrated on

Figs. 13-1 and 13-2 are the _____ and _____, respectively. (These are demonstrated on special view drawings in the following questions.)

17. Identify the labeled structures (and the facial bones of which they are a part) on this inferior surface view of the maxillae (Fig. 13-3).

	Structure	Bone(s)
A.	_____	(_____)
B.	_____	(_____)
C.	_____	(_____)
D.	_____	(_____)

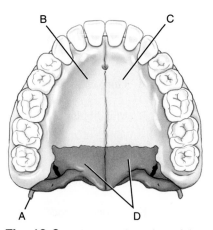

Fig. 13-3. Inferior surface view of the maxillae.

18. List the three structures that form the nasal septum as shown on Fig. 13-4.

A. _____

B. _____

C. _____

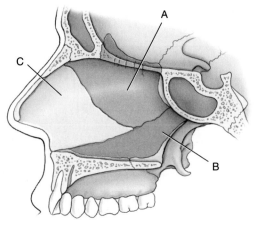

Fig. 13-4. Nasal septum.

19. Identify the parts of the mandible and skull as labeled on Figs. 13-5 and 13-6.

A. _____

B. _____

C. _____

D. _____

E. _____

F. _____

G. _____

H. _____

I. _____

J. _____

K. (Cranial bone) _____

L. (Joint) _____

M. (Key landmark) _____

N. (Landmark) _____

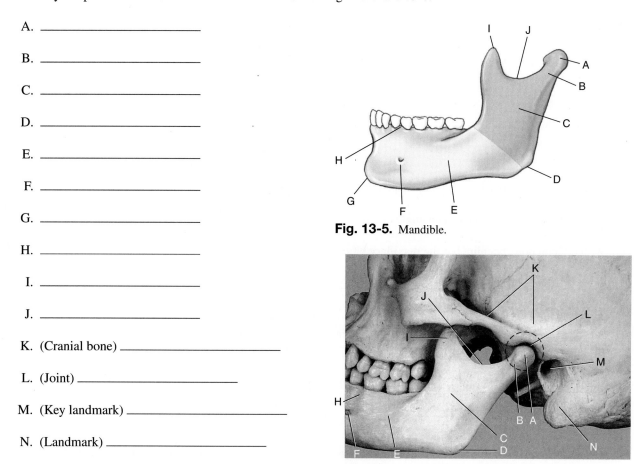

Fig. 13-5. Mandible.

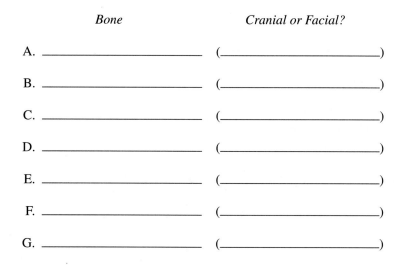

Fig. 13-6. Lateral skull and mandible.

20. Identify the seven bones that form the orbit and indicate whether they are cranial or facial bones (Fig. 13-7).

Bone	*Cranial or Facial?*
A. _____	(_____)
B. _____	(_____)
C. _____	(_____)
D. _____	(_____)
E. _____	(_____)
F. _____	(_____)
G. _____	(_____)

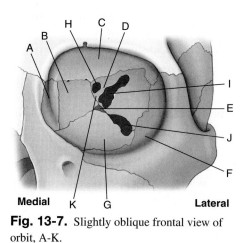

Fig. 13-7. Slightly oblique frontal view of orbit, A-K.

21. Identify the three foramina found within the orbits as labeled on Fig. 13-7.

H. _____

I. _____

J. _____

Small section of bone:

K. _____

22. From anterior to posterior, the cone-shaped orbits project upward at an angle of _____ ° and

toward the midsagittal plane at an angle of _____ °.

23. Which facial bone opening has the maxillary branch of the fifth cranial nerve passing through it?

_____

24. Which one of the facial bone openings is formed by a cleft between the greater and lesser wings of the sphenoid bone?
   A. Superior orbital fissure   C. Inferior orbital fissure
   B. Optic foramen   D. Optic canal

25. What is another term for the second cranial nerve?
   A. Olfactory nerve   C. Maxillary nerve
   B. Optic nerve   D. Trigeminal nerve

Review Exercise B: Radiographic Anatomy of the Paranasal Sinuses (see textbook pp. 408-414)

1. What is the older term for the maxillary sinuses? _____

2. An infection of the teeth may travel upward and involve the _____ sinus.

3. Specifically, where are the frontal sinuses located? _____

4. The frontal sinuses rarely become aerated before the age of _____.

5. Which specific aspect of the ethmoid bone contains the ethmoid sinuses? _____

6. The drainage pathway for the paranasal sinuses is called the:
   A. Uncinate process   C. Paranasal meatus
   B. Osteomeatal complex   D. Lateral masses

7. Which sinus will be projected through the open mouth with a PA axial transoral projection?

_____

8. Identify the sinuses, structures, or bones labeled on Fig. 13-8.

A. _____

B. _____

C. _____

D. _____

E. _____

F. _____

G. _____

H. _____

I. _____

J. _____

K. _____

L. _____

M. _____

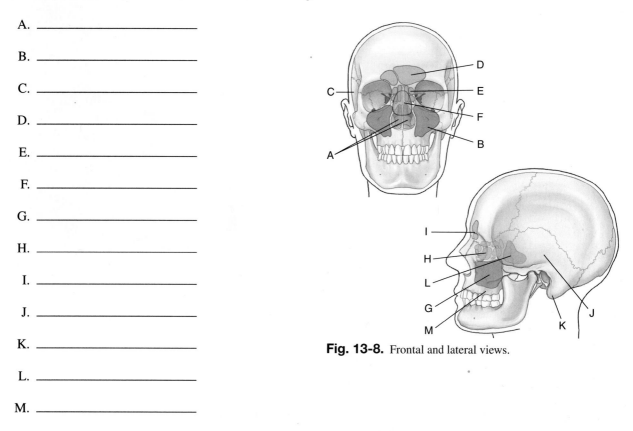

Fig. 13-8. Frontal and lateral views.

9. Identify the following paranasal sinuses labeled on Figs. 13-9 and 13-10.

Fig. 13-9

A. _____

B. _____

C. _____

D. _____

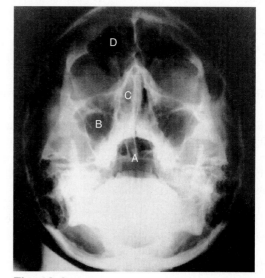

Fig. 13-9. Paranasal sinuses. PA axial transoral projection.

Fig. 13-10

E. _____

F. _____

G. _____

H. _____

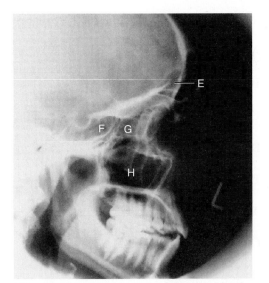

Fig. 13-10. Paranasal sinuses. Lateral projection.

10. What is the name of the passageway between the maxillary sinuses and the middle nasal meatus?

_____

11. True/False: Most CT studies of the sinuses do not require the use of contrast media.

12. Which position is most often used when performing a CT study of the sinuses?
   A. Supine
   B. Prone
   C. Erect
   D. Supine with 20° oblique of skull from AP position

PART II: RADIOGRAPHIC POSITIONING
Review Exercise C: Positioning of the Facial Bones, Nasal Bones, Zygomatic Arches, and Optic Foramina and Orbits (see textbook pp. 419-428)

1. True/False: Facial bone studies should always be performed recumbent whenever possible.

2. True/False: The common basic PA axial projection for facial bones requires a 15° caudad angle of the central ray, which projects the dense petrous ridges into the lower one-third of the orbits.

3. True/False: An increase in mAs of 25% to 30% (using manual techniques) is often required for the geriatric patient with advanced osteoporosis.

4. True/False: CT is useful for facial bone studies because it allows for visualization of bony structures as well as related soft tissues of the facial bones.

5. True/False: Nuclear medicine is not helpful in diagnosing occult facial bone fractures.

6. True/False: MRI is an excellent imaging modality for the detection of small metal foreign bodies in the eye.

7. What is the name of the fracture that results from a direct blow to the orbit leading to a disruption of the inferior

   orbital margin? _____

8. A "free-floating" zygomatic bone is the frequent result of a _____ fracture.

9. What is the major disadvantage of performing a straight PA projection for facial bones, with no CR angulation or neck extension, as compared with other PA facial bone projections?

_____

10. Where is the CR centered for a lateral position for facial bones?
    A. Outer canthus   C. Zygoma
    B. Acanthion   D. Nasion

11. What is the proper method name for the parietoacanthial projection of the facial bones? _____

12. Which facial bone structures are best seen with a parietoacanthial projection?

_____

13. What CR angle must be used to project the petrous ridges just below the orbital floor with the PA axial (Caldwell method) projection?
    A. None. CR is perpendicular.   C. 20°
    B. 30°   D. 45°

14. Which structures specifically are visualized better on the modified parietoacanthial (Waters) projection as compared

    with the basic Waters projection? _____

15. Give two reasons why projections of the facial bones are performed PA rather than AP when possible.

    A. _____   B. _____

16. What are two positioning differences between the lateral projection of the cranium and the lateral projection for the facial bones?

    A. _____

    B. _____

17. The parietoacanthial (Waters) projection for the facial bones will have the _____ line perpen-

    dicular to the image receptor, which places the orbitomeatal line (OML) at a _____ ° angle
    to the tabletop and image receptor.

18. Where does the CR exit for a parietoacanthial (Waters) projection of the facial bones?

_____

19. Where does the CR exit for a 15° PA axial (Caldwell) projection for facial bones?

_____

20. The modified parietoacanthial (modified Waters) projection requires that the _____ line is

perpendicular to the image receptor, which places the OML at a _____ ° angle to the tabletop and image receptor.

21. True/False: Lateral projections for nasal bones generally are taken bilaterally for comparison.

22. True/False: The tangential projection for a unilateral zygomatic arch requires that the skull be rotated and tilted 15° *away from* the affected side.

23. True/False: Both oblique inferosuperior (tangential) projections for the zygomatic arch are generally taken for comparison.

24. True/False: The gonadal and/or thyroid dose for all facial bone projections is NDC (no discernible contribution).

25. For a PA Waters projection, the petrous ridges should be projected directly below the _____

and projected into the lower half of the maxillary sinuses or below the _____ for a modified Waters projection.

26. For the superoinferior projection of the nasal bones, the image receptor is placed perpendicular to the

_____ line. (Include the full term and abbreviation.)

27. Which specific facial bone structures (other than the mandible) are best demonstrated with the submentovertex

(SMV) projection if the correct exposure factors are used (soft tissue technique)? _____

28. Where is the CR centered for an AP axial projection for the zygomatic arches?

_____

29. List the proper method name and the common descriptive name for the parieto-orbital oblique projection for the optic foramen.

A. _____   B. _____

30. The three aspects of the face that should be in contact with the head unit or tabletop when beginning positioning

for the parieto-orbital oblique projection are the (A) _____ , _____ ,

and _____ . The final angle between the midsagittal plane and the IR should be (B)

_____ , with the (C) _____ line perpendicular to the IR. This places

the optic foramen in the (D) _____ quadrant of the orbit.

31. Match each of the following structures to the facial bone projection that best demonstrates the structure(s) (using each choice only once).

_____ 1. Floor of orbits (blowout fractures)

_____ 2. Optic foramen

_____ 3. View of single zygomatic arch

_____ 4. Profile image of nasal bones and nasal septum

_____ 5. Bilateral zygomatic arches

_____ 6. Inferior orbital rim, maxillae, nasal septum, nasal spine, zygomatic bone and arches

A. Lateral (nasal bones)

B. Parietoacanthial projection

C. Parieto-orbital oblique projection

D. Submentovertex (SMV) projection

E. Modified Waters method

F. Oblique inferosuperior projection

Review Exercise D: Positioning of the Mandible and Temporomandibular Joints (TMJ) (see textbook pp. 429-437)

1. Which projection for the mandible results in a thyroid dose that is four or five times greater than the thyroid dose for any other projection described in this chapter? _____

2. Which projection of the mandible will project the opposite half of the mandible away from the side of interest?

   _____

3. What must be done to prevent the ramus of the mandible from being superimposed over the cervical spine with an axiolateral oblique projection of the mandible? _____

4. How much skull rotation (from the lateral skull position) toward the image receptor is required with an axiolateral oblique projection for demonstrating each of the following?

   A. Body of the mandible: _____

   B. Mentum region: _____

   C. Ramus region: _____

   D. General survey of the mandible: _____

   E. What is the maximum CR angle is needed for all of these projections? _____

5. What specific positioning error has been committed if both sides of the mandible are superimposed with an axiolateral oblique projection? _____

6. Where should the CR exit for a PA axial projection of the mandible? _____

7. Which skull positioning line is placed perpendicular to the image receptor for a PA or PA axial projection of the mandible? _____

8. True/False: For a true frontal view of the mandibular body (if this is the area of interest), the AML should be perpendicular to the image receptor.

9. True/False: The CR should be angled 20° to 25° caudad for the PA axial projection of the mandible.

10. Which aspect of the mandible is best visualized with an AP axial projection? _____

11. A. What CR angle is required for the AP axial projection of the mandible if the OML is placed perpendicular to the image receptor? _____

    B. If the infraorbitomeatal line (IOML) is perpendicular, what CR angle is needed? _____

12. Where is the CR centered for an AP axial projection of the mandible?

    _____

13. Which projection of the mandible will demonstrate the entire mandible, including the coronoid and condyloid processes? _____

14. Which imaging system provides a single, frontal perspective of the entire mandible? _____

15. What device provides inherent collimation during a Panorex procedure? _____

16. Which cranial line is placed parallel to the floor for a Panorex of the mandible? _____

17. What type of image receptor must be used with Panorex? _____

18. True/False: The modified Law method provides a bilateral and functional study of the TMJ.

19. True/False: The mandibular condyles move anteriorly as the mouth is opened.

20. Which projection of the TMJ requires that the skull be kept in a true lateral position?
    A. Modified Law   C. Axiolateral oblique projection
    B. Schuller   D. Modified Towne

21. The axiolateral (Schuller method) projection for the TMJ requires a CR angle of _____ °

    _____ (caudad or cephalad).

22. The axiolateral oblique projection of the TMJ is commonly referred to as the (A) _____ method, which requires a (B) _____ ° head rotation from lateral and a (C) _____ ° caudad CR angle.

23. If the area of interest is the temporomandibular fossae, angle the CR _____ to the OML for the AP axial (modified Towne) projection to reduce superimposition of the TM fossae and mastoid portions of the temporal bone.

24. Aligning the _____ plane perpendicular to the IR will prevent rotation of either a PA or AP axial mandible.

Review Exercise E: Positioning of the Paranasal Sinuses (see textbook pp. 438-444)

1. What kV range should be used for sinus radiography? _____

2. To demonstrate any possible air or fluid levels within the sinuses, it is important to:

   A. _____

   B. _____

3. True/False: Ultrasound exams of the maxillary sinuses to rule out sinusitis are possible.

4. True/False: Magnetic resonance imaging is the preferred modality to study soft tissue changes and masses within the sinuses.

5. True/False: Secondary osteomyelitis is often due to tumor invasion.

6. List the four most commonly performed basic or routine projections for paranasal sinuses.

   A. _____   C. _____

   B. _____   D. _____

7. Which single projection for a paranasal sinus routine provides an image of all four sinus groups?

   _____

8. If the patient cannot stand for the lateral projection of the paranasal sinuses, it should be taken with:

   _____

9. Which paranasal sinuses are best demonstrated with a PA (Caldwell) projection? _____

10. To avoid angling the CR for the erect PA Caldwell sinus projection, the head should be adjusted so that the OML is

    _____ ° from horizontal.

11. A. Which group of paranasal sinuses is best demonstrated with a parietoacanthial (Water) projection?

    _____

    B. The OML forms a _____ ° angle with the image receptor with this projection.

12. Which positioning line is placed perpendicular to the image receptor for a parietoacanthial projection?

    _____

13. Where are the petrous ridges located on a well-positioned parietoacanthial projection?

    _____

14. Which paranasal sinuses are demonstrated with an SMV projection of the paranasal sinuses?

_____

15. Where should the CR exit for both the PA parietoacanthial (Waters) and the PA transoral (open-mouth Waters)

projection? _____

16. What is the one major difference in positioning between the parietoacanthial and PA axial transoral projections?

_____

17. Which sinuses are projected through the oral cavity with the PA axial transoral projection?

_____

18. Match each of the following sinus projections with the anatomy best seen (using each choice only once).

_____ 1. Lateral   A. Sphenoid sinus in oral cavity

_____ 2. Parietoacanthial   B. Inferosuperior view of sphenoid and ethmoid sinus

_____ 3. PA Caldwell   C. All four paranasal sinuses demonstrated

_____ 4. PA transoral   D. Best view of maxillary sinuses

_____ 5. SMV for sinuses   E. Best view of frontal and ethmoid sinuses

Review Exercise F: Problem Solving for Technical and Positioning Errors

1. A radiograph of a lateral projection of the facial bones reveals that the mandibular rami are not superimposed. What positioning error led to this radiographic outcome?

_____

2. A radiograph of a parietoacanthial (Waters) projection reveals that the petrous ridges are projected within the maxillary sinuses. Is this an acceptable image? If not, what must be done to improve the image during the repeat exposure?

_____

3. A radiograph of a parietoacanthial (Waters) projection reveals that the distance between the lateral margins of the orbits and the lateral aspect of the skull is not equal. What type of positioning error led to this radiographic outcome?

_____

4. A radiograph of a 30° PA axial projection of the facial bones reveals that the petrous ridges are projected at the level of the inferior orbital margins. Is this an acceptable image for this projection? If not, what must be done to improve the quality of the image during the repeat exposure?

_____

5. A radiograph of a superoinferior projection of the nasal bones reveals that the glabella is superimposed over the nasal bones. What positioning error led to this radiographic outcome, and how can it be corrected during the repeat exposure?

_____

_____

6. A lateral radiograph of the facial bones demonstrates that the bodies of the mandible are not superimposed; one is about 1 cm superior to the other. How would this be corrected on a repeat exposure?

_____

7. A radiograph of a parieto-orbital oblique (Rhese) projection reveals that the optic foramen is located in the upper outer quadrant of the orbit. Is this an acceptable image for this projection? If not, what must be done to correct this problem during the repeat exposure?

_____

_____

8. A radiograph of an axiolateral oblique projection of the mandible reveals that the body of the mandible is severely foreshortened. The body of the mandible is the area of interest. What positioning error led to this radiographic outcome?

_____

_____

9. **Situation:** A patient with a possible fracture of the nasal bones enters the emergency room. The physician is concerned about deviation of the bony nasal septum along with possible nasal bones fracture. What radiographic routine would be best for this situation?

_____

_____

_____

10. **Situation:** A patient with a possible blowout fracture of the right orbit enters the emergency room. In addition to the basic facial bone routine, what single projection would best demonstrate this type of injury?

_____

11. **Situation:** A patient with a possible fracture of the left zygomatic arch enters the emergency room. Neither the AP axial nor the SMV projection demonstrates the left side well. The radiologist is indecisive as to whether this zygomatic arch is fractured. What other projections can the technologist provide to better define this area?

_____

12. **Situation:** As part of a study of the zygomatic arches, the technologist attempts to perform the SMV position. Because of the size of the patient's shoulders, he is unable to flex the neck adequately to place the IOML parallel to the image receptor. What other options does the technologist have to produce an acceptable SMV projection?

_____

13. A radiograph of a PA (Caldwell) projection for sinuses reveals that the petrous ridges are projected into the lower half of the orbits and obscuring the ethmoid sinuses. The technologist used a horizontal x-ray beam for the projection. The skull was positioned to place the OML at a 15° angle from the horizontal plane. What positioning modification is needed to correct this problem during the repeat exposure?

_____

14. A radiograph of a parietoacanthial projection reveals that the distance between the midsagittal plane and the outer orbital margin is not equal. What positioning error is present on this radiograph?

_____

15. A radiograph of an SMV projection for sinuses reveals that the distance between the mandibular condyles and lateral border of the skull is not equal. What specific positioning error is present on this radiograph?

_____

16. A radiograph of a PA transoral projection reveals that the sphenoid sinus is superimposed over the upper teeth and the nasal cavity. How must the position be modified to avoid this problem during the repeat exposure?

_____

17. A radiograph of a parietoacanthial projection reveals that the petrous ridges are projected just below the maxillary sinuses. What positioning error (if any) is present?

_____

18. **Situation:** A patient with a clinical history of sinusitis comes to the radiology department for a sinus study. The patient is quadriplegic and cannot be placed erect. Which single projection will demonstrate any possible air-fluid levels in the sinuses?

_____

19. **Situation:** A patient comes to the radiology department to rule out a possible polyp within the sphenoid sinus. What routine and/or special projection would provide the best overall assessment of the sinuses for this patient?

_____

20. **Situation:** A patient comes to the radiology department with a clinical history of a deviated bony nasal septum. Which facial bone projections will best demonstrate the degree of deviation? (More than one correct answer is possible.)

_____

_____

Review Exercise G: Critique Radiographs of the Facial Bones (see textbook p. 443)

The following questions relate to the radiographs found at the end of Chapter 13 of the textbook. Evaluate these radiographs for the radiographic criteria categories (1 through 5) that follow. Describe the corrections needed to improve the overall image. The major, or "repeatable," error(s) are specific errors that indicate the need for a repeat exposure, regardless of the nature or degree of the other errors.

A. Parietoacanthial (Waters) projection (Fig. C13-132)

Description of possible error:

1. Structures shown: _____

2. Part positioning: _____

3. Collimation and central ray: _____

4. Exposure criteria: _____

5. Anatomic side markers: _____

Repeatable error(s): _____

B. SMV mandible (Fig. C13-133)

Description of possible error:

1. Structures shown: _____

2. Part positioning: _____

3. Collimation and central ray: _____

4. Exposure criteria: _____

5. Anatomic side markers: _____

Repeatable error(s): _____

C. Optic foramina, Rhese method (Fig. C13-134)

Description of possible error:

1. Structures shown: _____

2. Part positioning: _____

3. Collimation and central ray: _____

4. Exposure criteria: _____

5. Anatomic side markers: _____

Repeatable error(s): _____

D. Optic foramina, Rhese method (Fig. C13-135)

Description of possible error:

    1. Structures shown: _____

    2. Part positioning: _____

    3. Collimation and central ray: _____

    4. Exposure criteria: _____

    5. Anatomic side markers: _____

Repeatable error(s): _____

E. Lateral facial bones (Fig. C13-136)

Description of possible error:

    1. Structures shown: _____

    2. Part positioning: _____

    3. Collimation and central ray: _____

    4. Exposure criteria: _____

    5. Anatomic side markers: _____

Repeatable error(s): _____

Review Exercise H: Critique Radiographs of the Paranasal Sinuses (See textbook pp. 444)

The following questions relate to the radiographs found at the end of Chapter 13 of the textbook. Evaluate these radiographs for positioning accuracy as well as exposure factors, collimation, and correct use of anatomical markers. Describe the corrections needed to improve the overall image. The major, or "repeatable," error(s) imply that these specific errors require a repeat exposure be taken regardless of the nature or degree of the other errors. Answers to each critique are given at the end of the laboratory activities.

A. Parietoacanthial transoral (open-mouth Waters) (Fig. C13-137)

Description of possible error:

    1. Structures shown: _____

    2. Part positioning: _____

    3. Collimation and central ray: _____

    4. Exposure criteria: _____

    5. Anatomic side markers: _____

Repeatable error(s): _____

B. Parietoacanthial (Waters) (Fig. C13-138)

Description of possible error:

    1. Structures shown: _____

    2. Part positioning: _____

    3. Collimation and central ray: _____

    4. Exposure criteria: _____

    5. Anatomic side markers: _____

Repeatable error(s): _____

C. Submentovertex (SMV) (Fig. C13-139)

Description of possible error:

    1. Structures shown: _____

    2. Part positioning: _____

    3. Collimation and central ray: _____

    4. Exposure criteria: _____

    5. Anatomic side markers: _____

Repeatable error(s): _____

D. Lateral projection (Fig. C13-140)

Description of possible error:

    1. Structures shown: _____

    2. Part positioning: _____

    3. Collimation and central ray: _____

    4. Exposure criteria: _____

    5. Anatomic side markers: _____

Repeatable error(s): _____

PART III: LABORATORY EXERCISES

You must gain experience in positioning each part of the facial bones before performing the following exams on actual patients. You can get experience in positioning and radiographic evaluation of these projections by performing exercises using radiographic phantoms and practicing on other students (although you will not be taking actual exposures).

The following suggested activities assume that your teaching institution has an energized lab and radiographic phantoms. If not, perform Laboratory Exercises B and C, the radiographic evaluation and the physical positioning activities. (Check off each step and projection as you complete it.)

Laboratory Exercise A: Energized Laboratory

1. Using the skull radiographic phantom, produce radiographs of the following basic routines:

Facial bones	*Temporomandibular joints*	*Zygomatic arches*
_____ Parietoacanthial (Waters)	_____ Submentovertex (SMV)	_____ Modified Law
_____ Modified Waters	_____ Oblique tangential	_____ Schuller method
_____ Lateral	_____ AP axial	_____ AP axial
_____ 15° PA axial (Caldwell)		

Nasal bones	*Mandible*	*Optic foramina*
_____ Lateral	_____ Axiolateral oblique	_____ Parieto-orbital oblique (Rhese)
_____ Superoinferior (tangential)	_____ PA	
_____ SMV	_____ AP axial	

2. Using the skull radiographic phantom, produce radiographs of the following basic routines:

Sinuses

_____ Parietoacanthial (Waters)

_____ Lateral

_____ PA

_____ Submentovertex (SMV)

Laboratory Exercise B: Radiographic Evaluation

1. Evaluate and critique the radiographs produced during the previous experiments, additional radiographs provided by your instructor, or both. Evaluate each radiograph for the following points.

_____ Evaluate the completeness of the study. (Are all pertinent anatomic structures included on the radiograph?)

_____ Evaluate for positioning or centering errors (e.g., rotation, off centering).

_____ Evaluate for correct exposure factors and possible motion. (Are the density and contrast of the images acceptable?)

_____ Determine whether anatomic side markers and an acceptable degree of collimation and/or area shielding are visible on the images.

LABORATORY EXERCISE C: Physical Positioning

On another person, simulate performing all basic and special projections of the facial bones as follows. Include the six steps listed below and described in the textbook. (Check off each step when completed satisfactorily.)

Step 1. Appropriate size and type of image receptor (IR) with correct markers

Step 2. Correct CR placement and centering of part to CR and/or IR

Step 3. Accurate collimation

Step 4. Area shielding of patient where advisable

Step 5. Use of proper immobilizing devices when needed

Step 6. Approximate correct exposure factors, breathing instructions where applicable, and initiating exposure

Projections	Step 1	Step 2	Step 3	Step 4	Step 5	Step 6
Facial bones						
● Parietoacanthial (Waters)	___	___	___	___	___	___
● Modified parietoacanthial	___	___	___	___	___	___
● Lateral facial bones	___	___	___	___	___	___
● 15° PA axial (Caldwell)	___	___	___	___	___	___
Nasal bones						
● Laterals	___	___	___	___	___	___
● Superoinferior nasal bones	___	___	___	___	___	___
Zygomatic arches						
● Submentovertex (SMV)	___	___	___	___	___	___
● Oblique tangential	___	___	___	___	___	___
● AP axial	___	___	___	___	___	___
Optic foramina						
● Parieto-orbital oblique (Rhese)	___	___	___	___	___	___
Mandible						
● PA	___	___	___	___	___	___
● AP axial	___	___	___	___	___	___
● Axiolateral oblique (general survey)	___	___	___	___	___	___
Temporomandibular joints						
● Modified Law	___	___	___	___	___	___
● Schuller method	___	___	___	___	___	___
● AP axial	___	___	___	___	___	___
Paranasal sinus projections						
● Parietoacanthial (Waters)	___	___	___	___	___	___
● Lateral	___	___	___	___	___	___
● PA	___	___	___	___	___	___
● Submentovertex (SMV)	___	___	___	___	___	___
● Parietoacanthial transoral (open-mouth Waters)	___	___	___	___	___	___

Directions: This self-test should be taken only after completing all of the readings, review exercises, and laboratory activities for a particular section. The purpose of this test is not only to provide a good learning exercise but also to serve as a strong indicator of what your final evaluation exam will be. It is strongly suggested that if you do not get at least a 90% to 95% grade on each self-test that you review those areas in which you missed questions before going to your instructor for the final evaluation exam for this chapter.

1. The majority of the hard palate is formed by:
   A. Maxilla
   B. Palatine bones
   C. Zygomatic bone
   D. Mandible

2. Which of the following is *not* an aspect of the maxilla?
   A. Frontal process
   B. Body
   C. Zygomatic process
   D. Ramus

3. Match each of the following definitions or characteristics to the correct facial bone (using each choice only once).

   _____ A. Mandible   1. Contains four processes

   _____ B. Lacrimal bones   2. Forms lower, outer aspect of orbit

   _____ C. Palatine bones   3. Lie just anterior and medial to the frontal process of maxilla

   _____ D. Inferior nasal conchae 4. Unpaired bone in the adult

   _____ E. Nasal bones   5. Located anteriorly in medial aspect of orbit

   _____ F. Maxilla   6. Help to mix air drawn into nasal cavity

   _____ G. Zygomatic bone   7. Possesses a vertical and horizontal portion

4. Identify the seven (cranial and facial) bones that form the bony orbit (Fig.13-11).

   A. _____

   B. _____

   C. _____

   D. _____

   E. _____

   F. _____

   G. _____

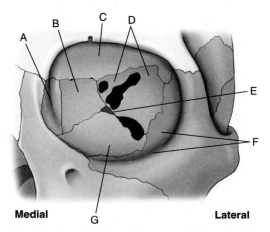

Fig. 13-11. Slightly oblique frontal view of orbit, A-G.

5. On average, how many separate cavities make up the frontal sinus? _____

6. True/False: All of the paranasal sinuses are contained within cranial bones, except the maxillary sinuses.

7. True/False: All of the paranasal sinuses except the sphenoid communicate with the nasal cavity.

8. True/False: In general, all the paranasal sinuses are fully developed by the age of 6 or 7 years.

9. True/False: The frontal sinuses are usually larger in men than in women.

10. Identify the labeled structures on these radiographs of the paranasal sinuses (Figs. 13-12, 13-13, and 13-14)

A. _____   H. _____

B. _____   I. _____

C. _____   J. _____

D. _____   K. _____

E. _____   L. _____

F. _____   M. _____

G. _____

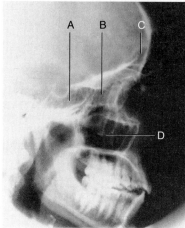

Fig. 13-12. Paranasal sinuses, A-D.

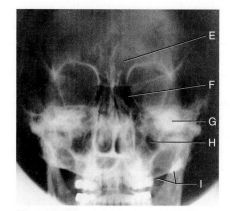

Fig. 13-13. Paranasal sinuses, E-I.

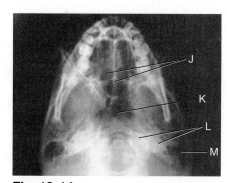

Fig. 13-14. Paranasal sinuses, J-M.

11. Which aspect of the ethmoid bone contains the ethmoid air cells? _____

12. The sphenoid sinus lies directly inferior to the _____

13. True/False: Ultrasound of the sphenoid sinus can be performed to rule out sinusitis.

14. Which one of the following imaging modalities would best demonstrate bony erosion of the maxillary sinus due to acute sinusitis?
    A. CT
    B. MRI
    C. Ultrasound
    D. Conventional radiography

15. True/False: Facial bone studies should be performed erect whenever possible.

16. True/False: A Le Fort fracture produces a "free-floating" zygomatic bone.

17. Which frontal projection of the facial bones best visualizes the region of the maxilla and orbits?

_____

18. For possible cranial trauma, which single projection of the facial bones best demonstrates any possible air-fluid levels in the sinuses if the patient can't stand or sit erect?

_____

19. Which plane is placed parallel to the IR with a true lateral projection of the facial bones?

_____

20. A. What is the angle between the OML and plane of image receptor with a parietoacanthial (Waters) projection?

_____

    B. This will place the _____ positioning line perpendicular to the IR.

21. The CR is centered to exit at the level of the _____ for a well-positioned parietoacanthial projection.
    A. Nasion
    B. Glabella
    C. Inner canthus
    D. Acanthion

22. The CR is centered to exit at the level of the _____ for a well-positioned 15° PA axial projection of the facial bones.
    A. Nasion
    B. Glabella
    C. Midorbits
    D. Acanthion

23. Where are the petrous ridges projected for a properly positioned modified parietoacanthial projection?

_____

24. True/False: The lateral projection of the nasal bones should be performed using a small focal spot, detail screens (IR), and close collimation.

25. True/False: The CR should be angled as needed to be parallel to the glabellomeatal line (GML) for the superoinferior projection of the nasal bones.

300

26. Which positioning line is placed perpendicular to the image receptor for a modified parietoacanthial projection?

_____

27. Where is the CR centered for a lateral projection of the nasal bones?

_____

28. Which positioning line, if placed parallel to the image receptor, will ensure adequate extension of the head for the submentovertex projection for zygomatic arches?

_____

29. How much skull tilt and rotation are required for the oblique inferosuperior (tangential) projection for zygomatic arches? _____

30. How much CR angle is required for the AP axial projection of the zygomatic arches if the IOML is placed perpendicular to the IR? (Hint: This is the same as for an AP axial skull.)

_____

31. The proper method name for the "three-point landing" projection for the optic foramen is the

_____.

32. Where should the optic foramen be located with a well-positioned parieto-orbital projection?

_____

33. What is the maximum amount of CR angulation that should be used for an axiolateral oblique projection of the mandible?

_____

34. Which one of the following factors will prevent superimposition of the ramus on the cervical spine for the axiolateral oblique mandible projection?
   A. Angle CR 10° to 15° cephalad
   B. Have patient open mouth during exposure
   C. Extend chin slightly
   D. Rotate head toward IR

35. How much skull rotation (from lateral position) toward the image receptor is required for the axiolateral oblique projection of the mentum?
   A. 10° to 15°
   B. 30°
   C. 45°
   D. None; keep skull in true lateral position

36. How much CR angulation should be used for a PA axial projection of the mandible?
   A. None
   B. 10° to 15° cephalad
   C. 20° to 25° cephalad
   D. 5° cephalad

37. What structures are better defined when the CR angulation is increased from 35° to 40° caudad for the AP axial projection of the mandible?

_____

38. Where is the CR centered for an SMV projection of the mandible? _____

39. The thyroid dose range for the SMV projection of the mandible is:
    A. 10–50 mrad
    B. 50–100 mrad
    C. 200–300 mrad
    D. 400–500 mrad

40. During a Panorex procedure, it is important to keep the _____ positioning line parallel to the floor.
    A. OML
    B. AML
    C. IOML
    D. GAL

41. What CR angulation is used for the AP axial projection of the TMJ with the OML perpendicular to the image

    receptor? _____

42. True/False: The modified Law method requires a tube angulation of 25°.

43. True/False: The Schuller method requires that the skull be placed in a true lateral position.

44. True/False: A grid is not required for the oblique inferosuperior (tangential) projection for zygomatic arches.

45. Where is the CR centered for a lateral projection of the paranasal sinuses? _____

46. Why should patients remain in an erect position for at least 5 minutes before sinus radiography?

    _____

47. Which projection is best for demonstrating the maxillary sinuses? _____

48. Why should a horizontal CR be used for the erect PA (Caldwell) projection for sinuses rather than the usual

    15° caudad angle? _____

49. A radiograph of a 15° PA projection of the facial bones reveals that the petrous ridges are projected at the level of the midorbital rims. What specific positioning or CR angling error led to this radiographic outcome?

    _____

50. Which positioning line should be perpendicular to the image receptor for the Rhese method projections for optic foramina?
    A. Acanthomeatal line (AML)
    B. Mentomeatal line (MML)
    C. Infraorbitomeatal line (IOML)
    D. Glabellomeatal line (GML)

    _____

51. A radiograph of lateral position for sinuses reveals that the greater wings of the sphenoid bone are not superimposed. What specific positioning error is present?

    _____

52. **Situation:** A patient with severe facial bone injuries comes into the emergency room. The patient is wearing a cervical collar and cannot be moved. What type of positioning routine should be performed for this situation?

_____

53. A superoinferior, tangential projection for the nasal bones was taken with the following factors: 8 × 10-inch (18 × 24-cm) IR crosswise, 85 kV, 13 mAs, 40-inch (102-cm) SID. The resultant radiograph was unsatisfactory because of poor visibility of the facial bones. Which technical factors should be changed for the repeat exposure?

_____

54. **Situation:** A patient with possible facial fractures, including a possible "blow-out" fracture to the right orbit, was brought from the emergency room to the radiology department. What special facial bone projection should be included with the basic facial bone routine of a lateral, parietoacanthial (Waters), and PA axial (Caldwell)?

_____

55. **Situation:** A patient with a clinical history of secondary osteomyelitis comes to the radiology department. Which imaging modalities or procedures can be performed to demonstrate the extent of damage to the sinuses?

_____

_____

Answers to Review Exercises

CHAPTER 1

Review Exercise A: General, Systemic, and Skeletal Anatomy and Arthrology

1. Chemical level
2. A. Epithelial
   B. Connective
   C. Muscular
   D. Nervous
3. A. Skeletal
   B. Circulatory
   C. Digestive
   D. Respiratory
   E. Urinary
   F. Reproductive
   G. Nervous
   H. Muscular
   I. Endocrine
   J. Integumentary
4. 1. C
   2. E
   3. H
   4. G
   5. I
   6. D
   7. J
   8. F
   9. B
   10. A
5. True
6. B. Integumentary
7. C. Integumentary
8. A. Axial skeleton
   B. Appendicular skeleton
9. False (206)
10. False (part of appendicular)
11. True
12. True
13. A. Long bones
    B. Short bones
    C. Flat bones
    D. Irregular bones
14. D. Periosteum
15. C. Medullary aspect
16. C. Periosteum
17. A. Body (diaphysis)
    B. Epiphyses
18. False (25 years)
19. Arthrology

20. A. Synarthrosis
    B. Amphiarthrosis
    C. Diarthrosis
21. A. Fibrous
    B. Cartilaginous
    C. Synovial
22. 1. C
    2. A
    3. C
    4. A
    5. B
    6. C
    7. A
    8. B
    9. B
    10. C
23. A. Plane (gliding)
    B. Ginglymus (hinge)
    C. Trochoidal (pivot)
    D. Ellipsoidal (condyloid)
    E. Sellar (saddle)
    F. Spheroidal (ball and socket)
    G. Bicondylar
24. 1. E
    2. B
    3. F
    4. A
    5. D
    6. G
    7. C
    8. B
    9. C
    10. E
    11. G
    12. D

Review Exercise B: Positioning Terminology

1. Radiograph
2. Central ray
3. Anatomic
4. Median or midsagittal
5. Midcoronal
6. Transverse or axial
7. True
8. False
9. A. Projection
10. C. Position
11. True
12. True

13. Lateral position
14. Left posterior oblique (LPO)
15. Right anterior oblique (RAO)
16. Dorsal decubitus (left lateral)
17. Right lateral
18. Left lateral decubitus (PA)
19. 1. H
    2. G
    3. F
    4. I
    5. B
    6. D
    7. J
    8. C
    9. E
    10. A
20. Anteroposterior (AP)
21. Axial
22. Lordotic position
23. True
24. False (inward, toward midline)
25. 1. B
    2. A
    3. A
    4. A
    5. A
    6. B
    7. B
    8. A
    9. B
    10. A
26. A. Extension
    B. Radial deviation
    C. Plantar flexion
    D. Inversion
    E. Medial (internal) rotation
    F. Adduction
    G. Pronation
    H. Protraction
    I. Elevation
27. 1. F
    2. D
    3. G
    4. E
    5. C
    6. J
    7. I
    8. H
    9. A
    10. B
28. Protraction

29. Radial deviation
30. A. Patient identification and date
    B. Anatomic side markers

Review Exercise C: Positioning Principles

1. False
2. True
3. True
4. False
5. False
6. A. A minimum of two projections 90° from each other
   B. A minimum of three projections when joints are in the prime interest area
7. A. 3
   B. 2
   C. 3
   D. 2
   E. 2
   F. 3
   G. 2
   H. 2
   I. 3
   J. 1 (see text)
8. A. (d) Two
   B. (c) Rather than move the forearm for additional projections, place the cassette and x-ray tube as needed.
9. Palpation
10. A. Ischial tuberosity
    B. Symphysis pubis
11. False (Place as if technologist were facing the patient; patient's right to technologist's left.)
12. True

CHAPTER 2

Review Exercise A: Image Quality in Film-Screen Imaging

1. Silver
2. A. Density
   B. Contrast
   C. Resolution
   D. Distortion
3. Kilovoltage (kV)
4. Milliseconds
5. Density
6. Milliampere seconds (mAs)
7. B. Decrease density to 25%
8. Underexposed
9. Doubling
10. False
11. C. 25% to 30%

12. Anode
13. Cathode
14. Compensating filters
15. A. Wedge filter
    B. Trough filter
    C. Boomerang filter
16. Wedge filter
17. Boomerang filter
18. D. 10 mAs
19. Radiographic contrast
20. Kilovoltage (kV)
21. A. Long-scale contrast (low contrast)
    B. Short-scale contrast (high contrast)
22. Long-scale contrast (low)
23. True
24. True
25. D. 110 kV, 10 mAs
26. B. 8 to 10 kV increase
27. 10 cm
28. A. 2. Off-level grid cut-off
    B. 3. Off-focus grid cut-off
    C. 4. Upside down grid cut-off
29. Resolution or definition
30. Blur or unsharpness
31. A. Focal spot size
    B. Source image receptor distance (SID)
    C. Object image receptor distance (OID)
32. Penumbra
33. False
34. Motion
35. D. Shorten exposure time
36. A. Decrease OID
37. D. 0.3-mm focal spot and 40-inch SID
38. Distortion
39. False (There is always some magnification and distortion caused by OID and divergence of the x-ray beam.)
40. A. Source image receptor distance (SID)
    B. Object image receptor distance (OID)
    C. Object IR alignment
    D. Central ray placement
41. False (increase distortion)
42. False (increase distortion)
43. True
44. C. 44 inches (110 cm)
45. B. 72 inches (180 cm)
46. True
47. False
48. True
49. True
50. False

Review Exercise B: Image Quality in Digital Radiography

1. False
2. True
3. False
4. D. Algorithms
5. C. Digital processing
6. Wide
7. A. Brightness
   B. Contrast
   C. Resolution
   D. Distortion
   E. Exposure index
   F. Noise
8. A. Brightness
9. True
10. False
11. D. Contrast resolution
12. C. Application of processing algorithms
13. B. Contrast resolution
14. A. Acquisition pixel size
    B. Display pixel size
15. Acquisition pixel size
16. False
17. D. 100 to 200 microns
18. B. Display capabilities of the monitor
19. False
20. Exposure index
21. A. mAs
    B. kV
    C. Total detector area irradiated
    D. Objects exposed
22. Sensitivity number
23. Indirectly; directly
24. Underexposure
25. Underexposure
26. Noise
27. Signal-to-noise ratio
28. Low-SNR
29. C. Mottle
30. Post-processing
31. A. Annotation
    B. Edge enhancement
    C. Image reversal
    D. Magnification
    E. Smoothing
    F. Subtraction

Review Exercise C: Applications of Digital Technology

1. A. Image plates (IP)
   B. IP reader
   C. Technologist QC workstation
2. Photostimulable phosphor
3. D. None of the above

4. A. Bar code reader
5. False
6. True
7. True
8. A. Bright light
9. Archiving
10. D. A minimum of 72" (183 cm) required for all CR projections
11. 30
12. False
13. D. Both A and B
14. True
15. True
16. False
17. 1. D
    2. E
    3. A
    4. C
    5. F
    6. B
18. True
19. Picture
    Archiving
    Communication
    System
20. False
21. A. Digital Imaging Communications Medicine
    B. Radiology Information System
    C. Hospital Information System
    D. Healthcare Level 7
22. Teleradiology
23. Integrated Healthcare Enterprise (IHE)
24. A. Display matrix
    B. Exposure latitude
    C. Windowing
    D. Penumbra
    E. Exposure index
    F. Bit depth
    G. Distortion
    H. Kilovoltage
    I. Noise
    J. Telemedicine
    K. Post-processing
25. A. Radiology Information System
    B. Image Receptor
    C. Object Image Distance
    D. Digital Radiography
    E. Automatic Exposure Control
    F. Hospital Information System
26. A. 5
    B. 7
    C. 3
    D. 2
    E. 1
    F. 4
    G. 6

Review Exercise D: Radiation Protection

1. Roentgen
2. Rad
3. Effective dose
4. 5 rem (50 mSv) per year
5. 35 rem (350 mSv)
6. A. Coulombs per kilogram (C/kg) of air
   B. Gray (Gy)
   C. Seivert (Sv)
7. A. 0.03 Gy
   B. 4.48 mGy
   C. 0.38 Sv
   D. 150 mSv
8. A. 0.05 rem (0.5 mSv)
   B. 0.5 rem (5 mSv)
9. 0.1 rem (1 mSv) per year
10. B. 10%
11. A. Thermoluminescent dosimetry
    B. Optically stimulated luminescence
12. As low as reasonably achievable
13. A. Family member (if not pregnant)
14. False (still need to be used)
15. True
16. True
17. False (considers dose levels to all organs)
18. Keep the image intensifier tower as close as possible to the patient.
19. C. Behind the radiologist
20. D. 10 R/min
21. B. 3 to 4 R/min
22. C. Poor communication between technologist and patient
23. A. Carelessness in positioning
    B. Selection of incorrect exposure factors
24. A. AP (more than double because of increased thyroid and breast doses)
    B. Male (from greater dose to gonads because of proximity of testes to primary beam)
    C. Male, shielded: 2 mrad
       Male, unshielded: 6 mrad
       Female, unshielded: 80 mrad
    D. Lungs
    E. Male, unshielded: 322 mrad
       Male, shielded: 42 mrad
       Female, unshielded: 59 mrad
       Female, shielded: 14 mrad
    F. PA chest
    G. Male: AP hip projection without shielding
       Female: AP T spine on 14 × 17

25. B. 0.4 to 0.8 mR/min
26. A. Inherent
    B. Added
27. Aluminum
28. A. Reduces the volume of tissue irradiated
    B. Reduces the accompanying scatter radiation, which adds to patient dose
29. False (2%, not 10%)
30. True
31. True
32. A. Shadow shields
    B. Contact shields
33. C. 1-mm lead equivalent
34. A. 95% to 99%
35. 2 inches; 5 cm
36. Shadow shield
37. True
38. D. Do not use shielding (for initial pelvis projection)
39. Results in some loss of recorded detail
40. A. Skin dose
    B. Midline dose
    C. Gonadal dose
    D. No detectable contribution
41. False (only if it doesn't cover pertinent anatomic parts for that exam)
42. 0.5-mm lead (Pb) equivalent
43. A. Distance
    B. Time
    C. Shielding
44. False
45. False

CHAPTER 3

Review Exercise A: Radiographic Anatomy of the Chest

1. A. Sternum
   B. Clavicles
   C. Scapulae
   D. Ribs
   E. Thoracic vertebrae
2. A. Vertebra prominens
   B. Jugular notch
3. A. Pharynx
   B. Trachea
   C. Bronchi
   D. Lungs
4. A. Thyroid cartilage
   B. Larynx
   C. Sternum
   D. Scapula
   E. Clavicle

5. A. Nasopharynx
   B. Oropharynx
   C. Laryngopharynx
6. Epiglottis
7. Anteriorly
8. Hyoid
9. A. Right
   B. It is larger in diameter and more vertical.
10. A. Carina
    B. T5
11. Alveoli
12. A. Pleura
    B. Parietal pleura
    C. Pulmonary or visceral pleura
    D. Pleural cavity
    E. Pneumothorax
13. A. Base
    B. Hilum (hilus)
    C. Apex (apices)
    D. Costophrenic angle
14. Presence of liver on right
15. A. Thymus gland
    B. Heart and great vessels
    C. Trachea
    D. Esophagus
16. A. Thymus
    B. Arch of aorta
    C. Heart
    D. Inferior vena cava
    E. Superior vena cava
    F. Thyroid
    G. Trachea
    H. Esophagus
17. Pericardial sac or pericardium
18. Ascending, arch, and descending aorta
19. A. Apex of left lung
    B. Trachea
    C. Carina
    D. Heart
    E. Left costophrenic angle
    F. Right hemidiaphragm (or base)
    G. Hilum
    H. Apex of lungs
    I. Hilum
    J. Heart
    K. Right and left hemidiaphragm
    L. Right and left costophrenic angles (superimposed)
20. A. Left main stem bronchus
    B. Descending aorta
    C. T5 (fifth thoracic vertebra)
    D. Esophagus
    E. Region of carina
    F. Right main stem bronchus
    G. Superior vena cava

H. Ascending aorta
I. Sternum

Review Exercise B: Technical Considerations

1. Hypersthenic
2. D. Hyposthenic and asthenic
3. 10 ribs
4. A. Necklace
   B. Bra
   C. Religious medallion around neck
   F. Hair fasteners
   G. Oxygen lines
5. True
6. False
7. 110 to 125 kV
8. E. All of the above
9. Should be able to see faint outlines of at least middle and upper vertebrae and ribs through heart and other mediastinal structures
10. False (Situs inversus may be present.)
11. C. Pigg-O-Stat
12. A. 60 to 70 kV, short exposure time
13. True
14. Second
15. 1. Small pneumothorax
    2. Fixation or lack of normal diaphragm movement
    3. Presence of a foreign body
    4. Distinguishing between opacity in rib or lung
    5. Possible atelectasis (incomplete expansion of the lungs)
16. A. To allow diaphragm to move down farther
    B. To show possible air and fluid levels in the chest
    C. To prevent engorgement and hyperemia of the pulmonary vessels
17. Reduces distortion and magnification of the heart and other chest structures
18. Erect position causes abdominal organs to drop, allowing the diaphragm to move farther down and the lungs to more fully aerate
19. D. Air bronchogram sign
20. C. Symmetric appearance of sternoclavicular joints
21. Extend the chin upward

22. A. Left
    B. Right
    C. Left
23. Prevents upper arm soft tissue from being superimposed over upper chest fields
24. 1½ to 2 inches (5 cm)
25. Vertebra prominens, 8 inches (20 cm) for male, 7 inches (18 cm) for female
26. A. Crosswise
    B. Lengthwise
27. True
28. B. Jugular notch
29. False (should be equal)
30. True
31. False (greater width)
32. True
33. False
34. False
35. 1. F
    2. J
    3. E
    4. I
    5. G
    6. L
    7. K
    8. B
    9. D
    10. C
    11. A
    12. H
36. Atelectasis +
    Lung neoplasm O
    Pulmonary edema + (severe)
    RDS or ARDS (HMD in infants) +
    Secondary tuberculosis (slight increase) +
    Advanced emphysema −
    Large pneumothorax O
    Pulmonary emboli O
    Childhood tuberculosis O
    Asbestosis O
37. B. Myocosis
38. D. AP lordotic

Review Exercise C: Positioning of the Chest

1. Places the heart closer to the image receptor to reduce magnification of the heart
2. T7
3. Scapulae
4. D. Left and right chambers
5. C. Less than 10 mrad
6. True (Both are about 1 mrad.)
7. B. 4

8. Greater than 1 cm (½ to ¾ inch)
9. A. Caudad (±5°)
   B. Sternum
10. Pleural effusion
11. Left lateral decubitus
12. Pneumothorax
13. Right lateral decubitus (affected side up)
14. Rule out calcifications or masses beneath the clavicles
15. AP semiaxial projection, central ray 15° to 20° cephalad
16. A. RAO
    B. LPO
17. Left, 60°
18. Right upper chamber
19. Level of C6-C7, midway between thyroid cartilage and jugular notch
20. A. Thyroid

Review Exercise D: Problem Solving for Technical and Positioning Errors

1. Rotation. The patient is rotated into a slight RAO position.
2. The lungs are underinflated. Explain to the patient the need for a deep inspiration, and take the exposure on the second deep inspiration.
3. A. The 75 kV is too low. The ideal kV range is 110 to 125.
   B. Increase the kV and reduce the mAs for the repeat exposure.
4. Center the central ray higher (to the level of T7, which will be found 7 to 8 inches below the vertebra prominens). Make sure the image receptor is centered to the central ray and the top collimation light border is at the vertebra prominens.
5. B. Decrease the kV moderately (− −).
6. C. Increase the kV slightly (+).
7. Ensure placement of the correct right or left anatomic side marker on the image receptor, because the heart and other thoracic structures may be transposed from right to left.
8. Determine which hemidiaphragm (right or left) is more posterior or more anterior. The left hemidiaphragm can frequently be identified by visualization of the gastric air bubble or the inferior heart shadow, both of which are associated with the left hemidiaphragm.
9. Right lateral decubitus; in a patient with hemothorax (fluid), the side of interest should be down.
10. A. AP and lateral upper airway projections
11. AP lordotic.
12. Inspiration and expiration PA projections and/or a lateral decubitus AP chest with affected side up.
13. C. Erect PA and lateral
14. AP semiaxial projection; CR is angled 15° to 20° cephalad to project the clavicles above the apices and clearly demonstrate the possible tumor.
15. Both the LPO and RAO oblique positions will best demonstrate or elongate the left lung.

CHAPTER 4

Review Exercise A: Abdominopelvic Anatomy

1. Psoas muscles
2. Gastro-
3. A. Duodenum
   B. Jejunum
   C. Ileum
4. Ileum
5. Right Lower, cecum
6. Descending colon, rectum
7. A. Pancreas
   B. Liver
   C. Gallbladder
8. Posteriorly
9. B. Spleen
10. B. Spleen
11. Presence of liver on right
12. Suprarenals (adrenal)
13. False (intravenous urogram [IVU])
14. Peritoneum
15. Retroperitoneal
16. D. Mesentery
17. C. Greater omentum
18. 1. A
    2. C
    3. B
    4. A
    5. C
    6. B
    7. A

8. C
9. B
10. A
11. B
12. B
19. A. RUQ
    B. LUQ
    C. LLQ
    D. LUQ
    E. LUQ
    F. RLQ
    G. LUQ
20. C. Umbilical
21. A. Pubic
22. A. Ischial tuberosity
    B. Greater trochanter
    C. Iliac crest or crest of ilium
    D. Anterior superior iliac spine (ASIS)
    E. Symphysis pubis
23. 1.5 (inches), 3 to 4 (cm), superior; 1.5 (inches), 3 to 4 (cm), inferior
24. Symphysis pubis
25. Inferior costal margin
26. Interspace between L4-5
27. A. Stomach
    B. Jejunum
    C. Ileum
    D. Region of ileocecal
    E. Duodenum
    F. Duodenal bulb
28. A. Stomach
    B. Pancreas
    C. Spleen
    D. Kidney (left)
    E. Liver
    F. Duodenum
    G. Gallbladder

Review Exercise B: Shielding, Patient Dose, Pathology, Exposure Factors, and Positioning

1. A. Patient breathing
   B. Patient movement during exposure
2. Careful breathing instructions
3. Peristaltic action of the bowel
4. Use the shortest exposure time possible.
5. False
6. A. It obscures essential anatomy
7. False
8. B. Female
9. ASISs
   Symphysis pubis
10. C. (70 to 80 kV range)
11. D. All of the above

12. True
13. C. Computed tomography (CT)
14. A. Ultrasound
15. A. Ultrasound
16. 1. E
    2. D
    3. F
    4. C
    5. B
    6. A
    7. G
17. 1. F
    2. E
    3. A
    4. C
    5. D
    6. B
18. Iliac crest
19. Expiration
20. A. Iliac wings
    B. Obturator foramina
       (if visible)
    C. Ischial spines
    D. Outer rib margins
21. Hypersthenic body type
22. True
23. A. (female AP abdomen)
24. C. (35 to 75 mrad)
25. C. Pancreas
26. Increased object image receptor distance (OID) of kidneys on PA
27. Left lateral decubitus (free air best visualized in upper right abdomen in area of liver)
28. To allow intraabdominal air to rise or abnormal fluids to accumulate
29. Dorsal decubitus
30. Lateral position
31. A. AP supine
    B. AP erect or lateral decubitus abdomen
    C. PA erect chest
32. PA chest
33. Two-way abdomen; AP supine abdomen, and left lateral decubitus
34. 2 inches (5 cm) above iliac crest; axilla
35. C. (chest technique)
36. Center and upper left chambers
37. True

Review Exercise C: Problem Solving for Technical and Positioning Errors

1. No. A KUB must include the symphysis pubis on the radiograph to ensure that the bladder is seen. The positioning error involves centering of the central ray to the iliac crest. The technologist should also palpate the symphysis pubis (if permited by institutional policy) or greater trochanter to ensure that it is above the bottom of the cassette.
2. The selected kilovoltage (90 kV) was too high. The technologist needs to lower the kilovoltage to between 70 and 80 kV. The milliamperage and exposure time can be altered to maintain the density.
3. The blurriness may be caused by involuntary motion. To control this motion, the technologist needs to increase the milliamperage and decrease the exposure time (e.g., 400 mA at $\frac{1}{10}$ second).
4. Patient was rotated into a slight right posterior oblique (RPO) position. (The downside ilium will appear wider.)
5. The three-way acute abdominal series, including the anteroposterior (AP) supine and erect abdomen and posteroanterior (PA) erect chest projections.
6. The two-way acute abdomen series: AP supine abdomen and left lateral decubitus
7. A KUB would be performed with the correct exposure factors to visualize the possible stone.
8. A bedside portable left lateral decubitus projection could be performed to demonstrate any fluid levels in the abdomen.
9. A. The erect AP abdomen position best demonstrates air/fluid levels. Ascites produces free fluid in the intraperitoneal cavity.
10. B. Because the patient may have renal calculi in the distal ureters and urinary bladder, gonadal shielding cannot be used.
11. D. Repeat the exposure using two 14- × 17-inch cassettes placed crosswise. The hypersthenic patient often requires this type of IR placement for abdomen studies.
12. B. Decrease the mAs. Because trapped air is easier to penetrate than soft tissue with x-rays, reducing the mAs will prevent overexposing the radiograph.
13. C. KUB and lateral abdomen. With any foreign body study, two projections 90° opposite is recommended to pinpoint the location of the foreign body.

CHAPTER 5

Review Exercise A: Anatomy of Hand and Wrist

1. A. 14
   B. 5
   C. 8
   D. 27
2. A. Proximal phalanx
   B. Distal phalanx
3. A. Proximal phalanx
   B. Middle phalanx
   C. Distal phalanx
4. A. Head
   B. Body (shaft)
   C. Base
5. A. Base
   B. Body (shaft)
   C. Head
6. Interphalangeal joint
7. Metacarpophalangeal (MCP) joints
8. A. Fifth carpometacarpal (CMC) joint
   B. Body of third metacarpal
   C. Head of fifth metacarpal
   D. Fourth metacarpophalangeal (MCP) joint
   E. Head of proximal phalanx of fifth digit
   F. Base of middle phalanx of fourth digit
   G. Distal interphalangeal (DIP) joint of fourth digit
   H. Body of middle phalanx of second digit
   I. Proximal interphalangeal (PIP) joint of second digit
   J. Body of distal phalanx of first digit
   K. Interphalangeal (IP) joint of first digit
   L. Metacarpophalangeal (MCP) joint of first digit
   M. Head of first metacarpal

N. Second carpometacarpal (CMC) joint
O. First carpometacarpal (CMC) joint
9. A. 8
   B. 1
   C. 5
   D. 4
   E. 3
   F. 6
   G. 7
   H. 2
10. Capitate
11. Hamulus or hamular process
12. Scaphoid
13. Either of these two mnemonics is acceptable: (1) Send Letter To Peter To Tell'im (to) Come Home or (2) Steve Left The Party To Take Carol Home
14. A. 3
    B. 9
    C. 2
    D. 5
    E. 1
    F. 8
    G. 6
    H. 7
    I. 4
15. A. Body of first metacarpal (thumb)
    B. Carpometacarpal joint of first digit
    C. Trapezium
    D. Scaphoid
    E. Lunate
    F. Radiocarpal (wrist) joint (between radius and carpals)

Review Exercise B: Anatomy of the Forearm, Elbow, and Distal Humerus

1. A. Radius
   B. Ulna
2. A. U
   B. U
   C. H
   D. H
   E. U
   F. U
   G. U
   H. H
3. Proximal and distal radioulnar joints
4. A. Trochlea
   B. Capitulum
5. Olecranon fossa

6. A. Trochlear sulcus (groove)
   B. (a) Capitulum
      (b) Trochlea
   C. Trochlear notch
7. A. 1
   B. 5
   C. 1
   D. 2
   E. 2
   F. 4
   G. 1
   H. 3
8. Diarthrodial, 4 (four)
9. True
10. Radial collateral ligament
11. A. Ulnar deviation
    B. Radial deviation
12. Ulnar deviation
13. The proximal radius crosses over the ulna.
14. A. Scaphoid fat stripe
    B. Pronator fat stripe
15. A. Elbow flexed 90°
    B. Optimal exposure techniques used
    C. In a true lateral position
16. False (A nonvisible fat pad suggests a negative exam.)
17. True
18. False
19. Posteroanterior (PA) and oblique wrist
20. Lateral wrist
21. A. Radial tuberosity
    B. Radial neck
    C. Capitulum
    D. Lateral epicondyle
    E. Olecranon fossa
    F. Medial epicondyle
    G. Trochlea
    H. Coronoid tubercle
    I. Olecranon process
    J. Superimposed humeral epicondyles
    K. Radial head
    L. Radial neck
    M. Radial tuberosity
    N. Outer ridges of trochlea and capitulum
    O. Trochlear sulcus (groove)
    P. Trochlear notch
22. A. Radial tubercle
    B. Radial neck
    C. Radial head
    D. Capitulum
    E. Lateral epicondyle
    F. Coronoid process
    G. Trochlea
    H. Olecranon process

Review Exercise C: Positioning of the Fingers, Thumb, Hand, and Wrist

1. A. Low to medium (50 to 70 kV for film-screen and 60 kV for CR/DR systems)
   B. Short exposure
   C. Small focal spot
   D. 40 inches (100 cm)
   E. 10 cm
   F. Detail screens (film-screen system)
   G. 5 to 7
   H. 8 to 10; 100%
   I. 3 to 4; 25% to 30%
   J. Soft tissue, trabecular
2. Collimation borders should be visible on all four sides if the image receptor (IR) is large enough to allow this without cutting off essential anatomy.
3. B, D, E, F
4. Child-bearing age or younger
5. True
6. Arthrography
7. PA, PA oblique, and lateral
8. Distal half of metacarpals
9. A. Symmetric appearance of both sides of the shafts of phalanges and distal metacarpals
   B. Equal amounts of tissue on each side of the phalanges
10. A. Perform the medial oblique rather than lateral oblique to decrease OID.
    B. Perform a thumb-down lateral (mediolateral projection) to decrease OID.
11. Proximal interphalangeal (PIP) joint
12. D
13. The AP position produces a decrease in OID and increased resolution.
14. PA oblique
15. 8 × 10 inch (18 × 24 cm)
16. Metacarpophalangeal
17. True
18. C
19. A
20. A. Modified Robert's method
    B. 15° proximal
21. A
22. 1 inch (2.5 cm)
23. True
24. Fan lateral
25. Lateral in extension

26. Norgaard method
27. D
28. 90
29. 45°
30. Anteroposterior (AP) projection (with the hand slightly arched)
31. Excessive lateral rotation from PA
32. B
33. 10 to 15, proximally
34. C
35. 25° to 30°
36. PA projection with radial deviation
37. Carpal canal or Gaynor-Hart projection
38. 45°
39. No difference

Review Exercise D: Pathologic Features of the Fingers, Thumb, Hand, and Wrist

1. A. Barton's fracture
   B. Multiple myeloma
   C. Osteoporosis
   D. Skier's thumb
   E. Achondroplasia
   F. Boxer's fracture
   G. Osteopetrosis
   H. Colles' fracture
2. A. 4
   B. 2
   C. 3
   D. 1
   E. 5
3. Paget's disease (+)
   Joint effusion (0)
   Rheumatoid arthritis (−)
   Osteoporosis (−)
   Osteopetrosis (+)
   Bursitis (0)

Review Exercise E: Positioning of the Forearm, Elbow, and Humerus

1. AP and lateral
2. False
3. Parallel
4. Two AP projections (partially flexed), one with humerus parallel to IR and one with forearm parallel to IR
5. AP oblique with 45° lateral rotation
6. False (because of scatter, divergent rays, or both reaching gonads)

7. AP oblique with 45° medial rotation
8. Lateral, flexed 90°
9. Two projections—central ray perpendicular to humerus and central ray perpendicular to forearm (acute flexion projections)
10. 45° laterally
11. Jones method
12. 45° toward shoulder
13. 45° away from shoulder
14. The rotational position of hand and wrist
15. A. 1
    B. 5
    C. 6
    D. 3
    E. 4
    F. 2

Review Exercise F: Problem Solving for Technical and Positioning Errors

1. Use a small focal spot, minimum 40-inch (102-cm) SID, and detail speed screens to produce a higher-quality study.
2. Rotation
3. Excessive lateral rotation
4. PA forearm projection was performed rather than AP.
5. The central ray needs to be angled 15° proximally, toward the elbow.
6. The elbow is rotated medially.
7. Increase lateral rotation of the elbow to separate the radius from the ulna.
8. The forearm and humerus are not on the same horizontal plane.
9. Coyle method for radial head (lateral elbow, central ray 45° toward shoulder)
10. PA and lateral-in-extension projection
11. AP and lateral forearm projections to include the wrist
12. Two AP projections with acute flexion (Jones method) and a lateral projection
13. Modified Robert's method
14. Carpal canal position (Gaynor-Hart method)
15. Norgaard method—ball catcher's position
16. PA thumb projection—Folio method

17. Tangential projection—carpal bridge projection
18. Trauma axial lateral projection—Coyle method for coronoid process

Review Exercise G: Critique Radiographs of the Upper Limb

A. PA hand (Fig. C5-159) Adult with polydactyl hand (extra digit)
   1. All pertinent anatomic structures included
   2. Fingers flexed preventing clear assessment of joint spaces
   3. No collimation evident on this printed radiograph; centering satisfactory for hand
   4. Under-exposed. If ideal kV range was used, an increase in mAs is required.
   5. No anatomic side marker
   Repeatable error(s): 2 and 4
B. Lateral wrist (Fig. C5-160)
   1. All pertinent anatomic structures included
   2. Upper limb rotated slightly; radius and ulna not directly superimposed; metacarpals not all superimposed
   3. No collimation evident on this printed radiograph; centering slightly off; central ray centered to the distal carpal region; includes too much forearm
   4. Acceptable selected exposure factors
   5. Anatomic side marker evident on this projection
   Repeatable error(s): 2 (rotation) and 3 (centering)
C. AP oblique elbow (Fig. C5-161)
   1. All essential anatomic structures included
   2. Elbow is rotated laterally evident by slight separation of proximal radius and ulna
   3. No collimation borders evident; central ray centering excellent for elbow
   4. Excellent selected exposure factors
   5. No anatomic side marker evident on this projection
   Repeatable error(s): 2 and 5 (unless markers are visible elsewhere on radiograph)

D. PA wrist (Fig. C5-162)
NOTE: This demonstrates a radial deviation for the ulnar side carpals (the opposite of the ulnar deviation for scaphoid).
   1. Part of pisiform cut off laterally
   2. Excellent part positioning with good radial deviation
   3. Central ray centering error—central ray centered over scaphoid and medial carpals; would have excellent collimation if central ray were centered correctly
   4. Excellent exposure factors
   5. Evidence of satisfactory anatomic marker
   Repeatable error(s): 1 and 3
E. PA forearm (Fig. C5-163)
   1. All pertinent anatomic structures not included due to PA projection being performed over AP
   2. Poor part positioning because proximal radius crossing over ulna due to PA projection being performed
   3. No collimation evident on this printed radiograph; acceptable central ray centering, but centered to middle of third metatarsal rather than to third metacarpophalangeal joint
   4. Exposure factors are satisfactory
   5. Anatomic side marker evident
   Repeatable error(s): 1 and 2 (Note: Individual immobilizing infant's hand should wear lead glove or use mechanical restraint)
F. Lateral elbow (Fig. C5-164)
   1. All pertinent anatomic structures demonstrated
   2. Elbow overflexed (beyond 90°) and not true lateral; too much distance between parts of concentric circles 1 and 2; trochlear notch space not open
   3. Satisfactory collimation (i.e., collimation that is evident); central ray centering slightly off center to the elbow joint
   4. Acceptable exposure factors
   5. Anatomic side marker partially off radiograph and unacceptable (unless it is

demonstrated on the actual radiograph)
Repeatable error(s): 2 and 5 (unless marker is more visible on actual radiograph)

CHAPTER 6

Review Exercise A: Anatomy of Proximal Humerus and Shoulder Girdle

1. A. Proximal humerus
    B. Scapula
    C. Clavicle
2. A. Intertubercular groove (bicipital groove)
    B. Greater tubercle (tuberosity)
    C. Head of humerus
    D. Anatomic neck
    E. Lesser tubercle (tuberosity)
    F. Surgical neck
    G. Neutral (Neither the greater nor lesser tubercle is in profile.)
3. A. Sternal extremity
    B. Body (shaft)
    C. Acromial extremity
4. Male
5. A. Lateral angle
    B. Superior angle
    C. Inferior angle
6. Costal
7. Axilla
8. A. Infraspinous fossa
    B. Supraspinous fossa
9. Synovial (diarthrodial)
10. A. Spheroidal
    B. Plane
    C. Plane
11. 1. C
    2. A
    3. A
    4. D
    5. B
    6. C
    7. D
    8. C
12. A. Neck of scapula
    B. Scapulohumeral joint (glenohumeral joint)
    C. Acromion
    D. Coracoid process
    E. Scapular notch
    F. Superior angle
    G. Medial (vertebral)
    H. Lateral (axillary)
    I. Ventral (costal)
    J. Dorsal

K. Spine of scapula
L. Acromion
M. Coracoid process
N. Body (blade, wing, or ala)
O. Inferior angle
13. A. Coracoid process
    B. Scapulohumeral
    C. Acromion
    D. Greater tubercle
    E. Lesser tubercle
    F. Lateral border
    G. Internal (Lesser tubercle is in profile medially.)
    H. Lateral
    I. Perpendicular
    J. Body of scapula
    K. Spine of scapula and acromion
    L. Coracoid process
    M. Body (shaft) of humerus
    N. Scapular Y lateral-anterior oblique projection
14. A. Coracoid process
    B. Glenoid process
    C. Spine of scapula
    D. Acromion
    E. Inferosuperior axial projection
    F. 90°

Review Exercise B: Positioning of Humerus and Shoulder Girdle

1. 1. A
    2. C
    3. B
    4. A
    5. C
    6. A
    7. B
    8. B
    9. A
2. A. Neutral
    B. External
    C. Internal
3. A. True
    B. False
    C. False
    D. False
    E. True
    F. False
    G. True
    H. True
4. A. 70 to 80 kV
5. A. Parent or guardian
6. True
7. False
8. True
9. False
10. True

11. 1. D
    2. B
    3. G
    4. A
    5. C
    6. F
    7. E
12. 1. G
    2. E
    3. F
    4. H
    5. I
    6. B
    7. D
    8. A
    9. C
13. D. Osteoporosis
14. A. AP, external rotation
    B. AP, internal rotation
15. To midscapulohumeral joint, ¾ inch (2 cm) inferior and lateral to coracoid process
16. Transthoracic lateral projection for humerus
17. B. Rotate affected arm externally approximately 45°
18. A. 25° to 30° medially
19. AP oblique; Grashey method
20. A. Tangential (Fisk modification)
21. 10° to 15°
22. D. Scapular Y
23. Supraspinatus outlet tangential projection; Neer method
24. C. Superoinferior axial projection (Hobbs modification)
25. A. 5° to 15°
26. D. 15° cephalad
27. True
28. True
29. True
30. False
31. False
32. True
33. C. Transthoracic lateral
34. D. Scapular Y lateral
35. B. Transthoracic lateral
36. AP apical oblique axial projection
37. Superior
38. More
39. Fracture of clavicle
40. 1. C
    2. B
    3. D
    4. A
    5. C
    6. E

Review Exercise C: Problem Solving for Technical and Positioning Errors

1. Lower kilovoltage peak to 75 kV and double milliamperage seconds (to 40 mAs), which increases radiographic contrast.
2. Increase central ray cephalad angle.
3. Ensure that the affected arm is abducted 90° and use a breathing technique.
4. Supinate the hand and ensure that the epicondyles are parallel to the IR for a true AP.
5. Palpate the scapular borders to ensure true lateral and increase body obliquity if needed to between 50° and 60° from a posteroanterior (PA) position.
6. Increase rotation of affected shoulder toward IR to closer to 45°.
7. Angle the central ray 10° to 15° cephalad to separate the shoulders.
8. The routine includes an anteroposterior (AP) of right shoulder and humerus without rotation (neutral rotation) and a supine, horizontal beam, right transthoracic shoulder. Note: In those cases in which the opposite arm cannot be elevated or extended, a supine posterior oblique scapular Y lateral projection could also be used as a second option for a lateral shoulder position (see Chapter 18).
9. Possible positioning options: Inferosuperior axial projection with exaggerated external rotation and Inferosuperior axial projection (Clements modification)
10. A. AP-internal rotation,
    B. Scapular Y lateral,
    C. Posterior oblique (Grashey method)
11. B. MRI
12. C. Ultrasound
13. The humeral epicondyles were not placed parallel to the plane of the IR.
14. Use breathing exposure technique to create blurring of ribs and lung markings.
15. Transthoracic lateral projection for humerus
16. Anterior dislocation of the proximal humerus

Review Exercise D: Critique Radiographs of the Humerus and Shoulder Girdle

A. AP clavicle (Fig. C6-97)
    1. All of clavicle demonstrated
    2. Rotation of body toward the right, superimposing sternal end over the spine and creating overall distortion of the clavicle and associated joints
    3. Collimation much too loose and not evident at all; central ray centered too low (inferiorly), which also adds to distorted appearance of clavicle
    4. Acceptable but slightly underexposed exposure factors
    5. Missing (or not visible) anatomic side marker
    Repeatable error(s): 2 and 5
B. AP shoulder-external rotation (Fig. C6-98)
    1. All pertinent anatomic structures demonstrated
    2. Greater tubercle is not in profile but note fracture of scapular neck. No rotation of the proximal humerus should be employed. Transthoracic lateral projection should be performed to provide 90° opposite perspective.
    3. No evidence of collimation
    4. Acceptable but slightly over-exposed.
    5. Anatomic side marker is present
    Repeatable error(s): None (considering the degree of trauma). Transthoracic lateral or Scapular Y lateral projection should be performed to provide another perpective.
C. AP scapula (Fig. C6-99)
    1. Lower margin of scapula cut off at bottom edge of radiograph
    2. Acceptable part positioning
    3. Collimation not evident; need to center central ray and cassette to include the entire scapula

4. Underexposed scapula and blurring of ribs, not evident from breathing technique
5. Missing (or not visible) anatomic side marker
   Repeatable error(s): 1, 3, 4, and 5
D. AP humerus (Fig. C6-100)
   1. Distal humerus is not included.
   2. Correct part positioning for AP projection, but centering is off
   3. Evidence of collimation on one side only, indicating incorrect centering; central ray and IR centering too lateral and proximal.
   4. Acceptable
   5. Acceptable; anatomic side marker partially seen on radiograph
      Repeatable error(s): 1 and 3
      Position: AP projection, external rotation

CHAPTER 7

Review Exercise A: Radiographic Anatomy of the Foot and Ankle

1. A. 14
   B. 5
   C. 7
   D. 26
2. A. Phalanges of the foot are smaller.
   B. The joint movements of the foot are more limited than those of the hand.
3. Tuberosity of base of the fifth metatarsal
4. The plantar surface of the foot near the first metatarsophalangeal joint
5. Calcaneus
6. Subtalar or talocalcaneal
7. A. Posterior facet
   B. Anterior facet
   C. Middle facet
8. Sinus tarsi or tarsal sinus
9. 1. B
   2. F
   3. D
   4. G
   5. E
   6. B
   7. G
   8. A
   9. C
   10. B

10. A. Sinus tarsi (tarsal sinus)
    B. Talus
    C. Navicular
    D. Lateral cuneiform
    E. Base of first metatarsal
    F. Body (shaft) of first metatarsal
    G. Sesamoid bone
    H. Metatarsophalangeal (MTP) joint of first digit
    I. Distal phalanx of first digit
    J. Tuberosity at base of fifth metatarsal
    K. Cuboid
    L. Calcaneal tuberosity
    M. Anteroposterior (AP) 45° medial oblique
    N. Tuberosity of calcaneus
    O. Lateral process of calcaneus
    P. Peroneal trochlea (trochlear process)
    Q. Lateral malleolus of fibula
    R. Sustentaculum tali
    S. Talocalcaneal joint
    T. Plantodorsal (axial) projection of calcaneus
11. True
12. B. Cuboid
13. A. Longitudinal arch
    B. Transverse arch
14. A. Talus
    B. Tibia
    C. Fibula
15. Ankle mortise
16. A. Tibial plafond
17. False
18. Sellar
19. A. Tuberosity at base of fifth metatarsal (see fracture on radiograph in Fig. 7-3)
    B. Lateral malleolus of fibula
    C. Distal tibiofibular joint
    D. Medial malleolus
    E. Talus
    F. Calcaneus
    G. Sinus tarsi (tarsal sinus)
    H. Talus
    I. Tibial plafond
    J. Anterior tubercle
    K. Navicular
    L. Cuboid
    M. AP mortise, 15° to 20° medial rotation

Review Exercise B: Radiographic Anatomy of the Lower Leg, Knee, and Distal Femur

1. Tibia
2. Tibial tuberosity

3. Adductor tubercle
4. Fibular notch
5. Tibial plateau
6. D. 10 to 15
7. Apex or styloid process
8. Lateral malleolus
9. Patella
10. A. Intercondylar sulcus
    B. Trochlear groove
11. Intercondylar fossa or notch
12. Because the medial condyle extends lower than the lateral condyle of the femur
13. C. Adductor tubercle
14. A. Medial epicondyle
    B. Lateral epicondyle
15. Popliteal region
16. False
17. True
18. False
19. Quadriceps femoris muscle
20. A. Patellofemoral
    B. Femorotibial
21. A. Fibular (lateral) collateral
    B. Tibial (medial) collateral
    C. Anterior cruciate
    D. Posterior cruciate
22. Medial and lateral menisci
23. A. Suprapatellar bursa
    B. Infrapatellar bursa
24. 1. A
    2. A
    3. C
    4. C
    5. A
    6. A
    7. B
    8. D
    9. A
    10. B
25. 1. C
    2. C
    3. D
    4. D
    5. F
    6. E
26. A. Fibular notch of tibia (also may be identified as distal tibiofibular joint)
    B. Body (shaft) of fibula
    C. Articular facets (or tibial plateau)
    D. Lateral condyle of tibia
    E. Intercondyloid eminence (tibial spine)
    F. Medial condyle of tibia
    G. Tibial tuberosity
    H. Anterior crest of body (shaft of tibia)

I. Medial malleolus
J. Lateral malleolus
K. Body (shaft) of fibula
L. Neck of fibula
M. Head of fibula
N. Apex or styloid process of fibula
O. 10° to 20°
P. Tibial tuberosity
Q. Body (shaft) of tibia
R. Medial malleolus
S. Lateral condyle of femur
T. Patellar surface of femur
U. Medial condyle of femur
V. Patellofemoral joint space
W. Patella
X. Tangential (patellofemoral joint)

27. A. Base of patella
   B. Apex of patella
   C. Tibial tuberosity
   D. Neck of fibula
   E. Head of fibula
   F. Apex or styloid process of fibula
   G. Superimposed medial and lateral condyles
   H. Patellar surface/intercondylar sulcus or trochlear groove
   I. Adductor tubercle
   J. Lateral femoral condyle
   K. Medial femoral condyle

28. A. 1
   B. 4
   C. 2
   D. 3

Review Exercise C: Positioning of the Foot and Ankle

1. True
2. False
3. False
4. True
5. True
6. False
7. A. 9
   B. 8
   C. 10
   D. 7
   E. 1
   F. 5
   G. 6
   H. 3
   I. 2
   J. 4
8. Chondromalacia patellae
9. Rickets

10. A. 7
    B. 3
    C. 8
    D. 1
    E. 5
    F. 4
    G. 2
    H. 6
11. Opens up the interphalangeal and metatarsophalangeal joints
12. Base of third metatarsal
13. Tangential projection
14. 15° to 20°
15. Opens up metatarsophalangeal and certain intertarsal joints
16. D. None; use perpendicular central ray
17. Second to fifth
18. AP oblique with medial rotation
19. AP oblique with lateral rotation
20. Lateromedial
21. AP and lateral weight-bearing projections
22. 40° cephalad
23. Sustentaculum tali
24. 1½ inches (4 cm) inferior to the medial malleolus
25. C. Lateral surface of joint
26. To demonstrate a possible fracture of the fifth metatarsal tuberosity (a common fracture site)
27. 15° to 20° (medially)
28. 45° AP oblique with medial rotation
29. B. Projected over the posterior aspect of the distal tibia
30. AP stress projections

Review Exercise D: Positioning of the Tibia, Fibula, Knee, and Distal Femur

1. AP and lateral projections
2. A fracture may also be present at the proximal fibula in addition to the distal portion.
3. C. Diagonally
4. B. 3° to 5° cephalad
5. A. ½ inch (1.25 cm) distal to apex of patella
6. C. AP oblique, 45° medial rotation
7. Medial (internal)
8. B. 5° cephalad
9. B. 20° to 30°
10. Improper angle of the central ray

11. Overrotation or underrotation of the knee
12. Adductor tubercle on posterolateral aspect of the medial femoral condyle
13. AP or PA weight-bearing knee
14. C. Medial or collateral ligament damage
15. A. Holmblad
16. 40° flexion
17. Distortion caused by central ray angle and increased OID for AP axial projection
18. B. 10° caudad
19. D. 45°
20. C. 60 to 70°
21. D. None. CR is perpendicular to IR
22. True
23. 5° to 10°
24. B. 20 to 30 mrad
25. 30° from horizontal
26. A. 45° to 55°
    B. 90°
27. D. None. CR is perpendicular to IR
28. 1. F
    2. E
    3. D
    4. G
    5. C
    6. A
    7. B
29. A. Rosenberg method
30. C. Béclere method

Review Exercise E: Problem Solving for Technical and Positioning Errors

1. Central ray is not angled correctly; adjust central ray angle to keep it perpendicular to metatarsals.
2. Overrotation of foot (toward the medial direction)
3. Increase cephalad angle of the central ray to correctly elongate the calcaneus.
4. Possibly a spread of the ankle mortise caused by ruptured ligaments
5. Underrotation of the ankle (toward the medial direction). The described appearance is that of a true AP ankle with little or no obliquity.

6. Angling the central ray correctly to keep it parallel to the articular facets (tibial plateau)
7. The wrong oblique position of the knee was obtained. This description is that of a laterally or externally oblique position of the knee.
8. Underrotation of knee (excessive rotation of patella away from the IR)
9. An AP lateral oblique projection with 30° of external rotation will separate the bases of the first and second metatarsals.
10. Repeat the AP projection to ensure the ankle joint is demonstrated.
11. Rotation of the affected limb or incorrect CR angle to match the degree of flexion of the lower limb
12. Decrease the amount of flexion of the knee to only 5° to 10°.
13. An AP or PA weight-bearing bilateral knee projection will best evaluate the joint spaces.
14. AP and lateral weight-bearing foot projections
15. AP and lateral weight-bearing projections
16. Intercondylar fossa projections, including the PA axial projections (Holmblad, Rosenberg, and/ or Camp-Coventry methods) demonstrate the entire knee joint and intercondylar fossa region, which may be hiding "joint mice."
17. The lateral knee projection will best demonstrate any separation of the tibial tuberosity from the shaft of the tibia.
18. By angling the central ray 5° to 7° cephalad, the medial femoral condyle will be superimposed with the lateral condyle. If CR angulation was used on the initial projection, increase the amount of angle with the repeat exposure.
19. The superoinferior sitting tangential method is best suited for this patient. While remaining in the wheelchair, the patient's knees can be flexed, the IR can be positioned on a foot stool, and the CR is placed vertically above the knees.

20. The most common error with the tangential (inferosuperior) projection is overflexion of the knee which will draw the patella into the intercondylar sulcus. Flexion of the lower limb should not exceed 45°. Another possible error is that the CR is not parallel to the joint space.

Review Exercise F: Critique Radiographs of the Distal Lower Limb

A. Bilateral tangential patella (Fig. C7-142)
1. Portion of each patella superimposed over intercondylar sulcus of femur
2. Excessive flexion of knee most likely cause of superimposition of patella over femur
3. Evidence of collimation; correct central ray centering and IR placement; may be an error in central ray angle, which would have contributed to the superimposition
4. Underexposed
5. Anatomic side marker present Repeatable error(s): 1, 2, and 3 (possibly 4)

B. Lateral calcaneus (Fig. C7-143)
1. Obvious compound fracture of calcaneus. All pertinent anatomy seen.
2. Positioning is acceptable but foot is plantar flexed
3. Off centering of part to IR-too anterior. Better centering would lead to more concise collimation
4. Acceptable exposure factors
5. Anatomic side marker visible Repeatable error(s): None

C. AP mortise ankle (Fig. C7-144)
1. Note: Tri-malleolar fracture. All pertinent anatomy demonstrated.
2. Because of the severity of the fracture, lower limb should have not been rotated medially.
3. No collimation evident. Centering is correct.
4. Acceptable exposure factors
5. No anatomic side marker visible Repeatable error(s): None. If repeated, the ankle must not be

rotated and a side markers must be used.

D. AP lower limb (pediatric) (Fig. C7-145)
1. Note fracture of distal femur. All anatomy demonstrated
2. Positioning is correct for AP projection
3. No collimation nor gonadal shielding used. Centering is correct for entire lower limb. Unprotected hand used to immobilize the lower limb: Unacceptable practice
4. Acceptable exposure factors
5. Anatomic side marker visible Repeatable error(s): 3 (not a repeatable error in this situation)

E. Lateral knee (Fig. C7-146)
1. All pertinent anatomic structures included but patellofemoral joint not open* (presence of superimposition of patella over lateral condyle because of rotation)
2. Rotation of anterior knee away from cassette (underrotation); almost total superimposition of proximal fibula; visibility of adductor tubercle identifies medial condyle as being posterior; overflexed knee (should be flexed only 15° to 20° rather than the almost 45° used in this radiograph)
3. No evidence of collimation; correct central ray centering and IR placement
4. Acceptable exposure factors
5. Anatomic side marker present Repeatable error(s): 1 and 2

F. Lateral knee (Fig. C7-147)
1. Closure of patellofemoral joint space caused by positioning error
2. Excessive rotation of anterior knee toward cassette (overrotation); separation of proximal fibula from tibia; outline of adductor tubercle on medial condyle also anterior to lateral condyle; knee slightly underflexed
3. No evidence of collimation; correct central ray centering and IR placement
4. Acceptable exposure factors
5. Anatomic side marker present Repeatable error(s): 1 and 2

CHAPTER 8

Review Exercise A: Anatomy of Femur, Hips, and Pelvic Girdle

1. Femur
2. Fovea capitis
3. Medial; posteriorly
4. 15 to 20
5. True
   A. Right and left hip bones, sacrum, and coccyx
   B. Right and left hip bones
   C. Ossa coxae and/or innominate bones
6. A. Ilium
   B. Ischium
   C. Pubis
7. Acetabulum, mid teens
8. A. Crest of ilium (iliac crest)
   B. Anterior superior iliac spine (ASIS)
9. Ischial tuberosity
10. Symphysis pubis
11. Obturator foramen
12. A. 1 inch (2½ cm)
    B. 1½ to 2 inches (4 to 5 cm)
13. Pelvic brim
14. A. False pelvis
    B. True pelvis
15. A. Supports the lower abdominal organs and fetus
    B. Forms the actual birth canal
16. A. Inlet
    B. Cavity
    C. Outlet
17. 1. B
    2. B
    3. A
    4. A
    5. C
    6. A
    7. C
    8. A
18. Cephalopelvimetry
19. Sonography (ultrasound)
20. 1. F
    2. F
    3. M
    4. M
    5. M
    6. F
21. A. Synovial, diarthrodial, spheroidal
    B. Synovial, amphiarthrodial, N/A
    C. Cartilaginous, amphiarthrodial, N/A
    D. Cartilaginous, amphiarthrodial, N/A

22. A. Crest, IL
    B. ASIS, IL
    C. Greater trochanter
    D. Body, IS
    E. Superior ramus, P
    F. Ischial tuberosity, IS
    G. Inferior ramus, P
    H. Obturator foramen
    I. Body, P
    J. Body, IL
    K. Wing (ala), IL
    L. Right sacroiliac (SI) joint
    M. Ischial spine, IS
    N. Sacrum
    O. Body, IL
    P. Posterior superior iliac spine (PSIS), IL
    Q. Posterior inferior iliac spine, IL
    R. Greater sciatic notch, IL
    S. Ischial spine, IS
    T. Lesser sciatic notch, IS
    U. Ischial tuberosity, IS
    V. Ramus, IS
    W. Inferior ramus, P
    X. Acetabulum, IS, IL, P
    Y. Anterior inferior iliac spine, IL
    Z. ASIS, IL

Review Exercise B: Positioning of Femur, Hips, Pelvis, and Sacroiliac Joints

1. A. ASIS
   B. Symphysis pubis (or greater trochanter if palpation of this landmark is not permitted by institution)
2. Approximately 2½ inches (6 to 7 cm) below the midpoint of the line
3. ASIS; 1 to 2 inches (3 to 5 cm); symphysis pubis and/or greater trochanter; 3 to 4 inches (8 to 10 cm)
4. 15 to 20
5. Lesser trochanter should not be visible, or should only be slightly visible, on the radiograph.
6. The patient's foot is rotated externally.
7. AP pelvis
8. It covers anatomic structures of primary interest.
9. Yes. Use a shaped ovarian shield with top of shield at level of ASIS and bottom at symphysis pubis.

10. Yes. The top of the shield should be placed at the inferior margin of the symphysis pubis.
11. It reduces patient dose approximately 30%.
12. It reduces radiographic contrast.
13. B. DDH (development dysplasia of hip)
14. True
15. A. Sonography
16. D. Nuclear medicine
17. A. 7
    B. 5
    C. 4
    D. 2
    E. 6
    F. 1
    G. 3
18. C. Compensating filter
19. A. CT
20. True. If an AP and lateral femur study is ordered, both joints must be demonstrated
21. Midway between ASIS and symphysis pubis
22. B. Upper right and left chambers
23. Rotation toward left side
24. Right rotation
25. A. T
    B. NT
    C. NT
    D. T
    E. T
26. B. PA axial oblique
27. Females (nearly 3 times more)
28. 40° to 45°
29. Midfemoral neck
30. 35 × 43 cm (14 × 17 inches) crosswise
31. 1 inches (2½ cm) superior to the symphysis pubis
32. B. 30° to 45° cephalad
33. A. Acetabular fractures
34. D. 45°
35. D. 12° cephalad
36. C. PA 35° to 40° toward affected side
37. True
38. Traumatic
39. It is flexed and elevated to prevent it from being superimposed over the affected hip.
40. C. Use of gonadal shielding
41. True
42. True
43. 15 to 20
44. A. Posterior oblique projections of acetabulum (Judet method)
    B. 0° (perpendicular)

45. AP axial outlet projection (Taylor method)
46. 1. D
    2. C
    3. F
    4. E
    5. B
    6. A
47. D. 20° to 30° from vertical
48. True
49. 15° from the vertical
50. False

Review Exercise C: Problem Solving for Technical and Positioning Errors

1. Rotate the lower limbs 15° to 20° internally to place the proximal femurs in a true AP position. (With general chronic pain, the lower limbs can usually be rotated safely.)
2. The patient is rotated toward the left—left posterior oblique (LPO).
3. Repeat the exposure using a 20° to 25° cephalad central ray angle. (It will separate the greater trochanter from the femoral neck.)
4. If possible, elevate the patient at least 2 inches (or 5 cm) by placing sheets or blankets beneath the pelvis.
5. A greater central ray angle is required. Female patients require a central ray angle of 30° to 45°.
6. The PA axial oblique (Teufel method) or posterior oblique (Judet method) can be taken to demonstrate aspects of the acetabulum more completely
7. When using automatic exposure control (AEC) for an AP pelvis projection, the left or right ionization chambers must be activated. The center chamber is over the less dense pelvic cavity, which may lead to an underexposed image.
8. Ensure that the central ray is centered to near the midline of the grid cassette and that the face of the cassette is perpendicular to the central ray.
9. Yes. Any orthopedic appliance or prosthesis must be seen in its entirety in both projections.

10. AP pelvis and axiolateral left hip. The AP pelvis radiograph should be taken initially without leg rotation; the radiograph must be reviewed by the physician and checked for fractures or dislocations before attempting an internal rotation of the left leg for the axiolateral (inferosuperior) projection.
11. AP pelvis and modified axiolateral—Clements-Nakayama method
12. Posterior oblique—Judet method
13. AP pelvis projection and possibly posterior oblique (Judet method) projections to provide another perspective of the ASIS region (Note: Perform projections on 14 × 17-inch (35 × 43-cm) IR to demonstrate entire pelvis). Decrease kV to 65 to 70 (from standard 80 to 90 kV).
14. Palpate both ASIS and ensure they are equal distance from tabletop.
15. AP pelvis and bilateral "frog-leg" (modified Cleaves) projections

Review Exercise D: Critique Radiographs of the Femur and Pelvis

A. AP Pelvis (Fig. C8-76)
   1. All anatomy of the pelvis is demonstrated
   2. The lesser trochanters are visible, which indicates the lower limbs were not rotated 15° to 20° medially
   3. No collimation evident (acceptable) and CR centering was slightly off laterally (to the patient's right)
   4. Exposure factors are acceptable
   5. Anatomic side marker evident
   Repeatable error(s): 2
B. AP Pelvis (Fig. C8-77)
   1. All anatomy of pelvis is demonstrated.
   2. No rotation of lower limbs evident by presence of lesser trochanters. But due to pelvic ring fracture involving pubis,

inadvisable to rotate lower limbs. Fracture may have extended into acetabulum. Slight tilt of pelvis.
   3. No collimation evident (acceptable) and CR centering is acceptable.
   4. Exposure factors are aceptable.
   5. No anatomic side marker visible.
   Repeatable error(s): 5 (Unsure side of fracture)
C. Unilateral "frog-leg" projection (performed cystography (Fig. C8-78)
   1. All pertinent anatomy is demonstrated.
   2. Lower limb should not have been rotated into frog-leg position due to severity of fracture.
   3. No collimation evident and is needed to reduce exposure to abdomen. Note: Patient's right upper limb is in field. Centering is too low.
   4. Exposure factors are acceptable.
   5. Anatomic side marker is evident.
   Repeatable error(s): 2 and 3 (if exposure is to be repeated for other reasons).
D. Bilateral frog-leg (2-year-old) (Fig. C8-79)
   1. Left hip (assuming that this is the left side because the side marker is not visible) obscured by artifact (superimposition of patient's hand)
   2. Tilted pelvis (and note that the gonadal shield placement is useless for either males or females—a serious error for a small child)
   3. No visible collimation, which should be visible for this pediatric patient; central ray centering/film placement too high for pelvis centering but acceptable for bilateral hip projection
   4. Very low contrast (may have been caused by not using a grid)
   5. No visible anatomic side marker
   Repeatable error(s): 1

CHAPTER 9

Review Exercise A: Radiographic Anatomy of the Cervical and Thoracic Spine

1. A. 7
   B. 12
   C. 5
   D. 1
   E. 1
   F. 26
2. A. Thoracic
   B. Sacral
3. A. Cervical
   B. Lumbar
4. 1. B and D
   2. A and C
   3. A and C
   4. B and D
   5. A
5. Lordosis
6. Scoliosis
7. Body; vertebral arch
8. Lamina
9. Intervertebral
10. Vertebral (spinal) canal
11. A. Medulla oblongata
    B. Lower border of L1
    C. Conus medullaris
12. Spinal nerves and blood vessels
13. A. Spinous process
    B. Lamina
    C. Transverse process
    D. Facet of superior articular process
    E. Pedicle
    F. Vertebral foramen
    G. Spinous process
    H. Facet of superior articular process
    I. Pedicle
    J. Body
    K. Inferior articular process
    L. Superior articular process
    M. Zygapophyseal joint
    N. Facet for head of rib articulation
    O. Intervertebral foramen
    P. Facet for rib articulation
    Q. Costovertebral joints
    R. Costotransverse joints
14. C. Zygapophyseal joints
15. True
16. False (between C1 and C2 visualized on a frontal or AP projection)
17. A. Annulus fibrosus
    B. Nucleus pulposus
18. Herniated nucleus pulposus (HNP)
19. A. C1: Atlas
    B. C2: Axis
    C. C7: Vertebra prominens
20. A. Transverse foramina
    B. Bifid spinous process
    C. Overlapping vertebral bodies
21. Articular pillar
22. Lateral mass
23. 90; 70 to 75
24. Atlanto-occipital articulation
25. Dens or odontoid process
26. Rotation of the skull
27. Presence of facets for articulation with ribs
28. T5 to T8
29. A. Body, C4
    B. Dens (odontoid), C2
    C. Posterior arch and tubercle, C1
    D. Zygapophyseal joint, C5-6
    E. Spinous process (vertebra prominens), C7
    F. Posterior arch and tubercle, C1
    G. Pedicle, C4
    H. Intervertebral foramen, C4-5
30. 15° cephalad

Review Exercise B: Positioning of the Cervical and Thoracic Spine

1. A. Manubrium
   B. Jugular (suprasternal) notch
   C. Body
   D. Sternal angle
   E. Xiphoid process
2. 1. H
   2. E
   3. F
   4. B
   5. D
   6. C
   7. A
   8. G
3. Thyroid gland, parathyroid glands, and female breasts
4. A. Increase in exposure latitude
   B. Decrease in patient dose
5. True
6. False (Lead masking should be used even if close collimation is used.)
7. True
8. True
9. A. Keep vertebral column parallel to image receptor (IR)
10. B. Using a small focal spot
    C. Increasing SID
11. A. 9
    B. 10
    C. 4
    D. 8
    E. 2
    F. 6
    G. 1
    H. 7
    I. 5
    J. 3
12. A. Erect (AP/PA) and lateral spine including bending laterals
    B. Lateral cervical
    C. AP open mouth C1-2, tomography—following lateral projection
    D. Scoliosis series
    E. Lateral cervical spine
    F. Lateral of affected spine
13. Spondylitis is an inflammatory process of the vertebrae. Spondylosis is a condition of the spine characterized by rigidity of a vertebral joint.
14. True
15. Myelography
16. Nuclear medicine
17. Lower margin of upper incisors and base of skull
18. To open up the intervertebral disk spaces
19. C. Base of skull
20. A. Compensates for increased object image receptor distance (OID); reduces magnification
    B. Less divergence of x-ray beam to reduce shoulder superimposition of C7
21. 15° cephalad
22. Right intervertebral foramina (upside)
23. Left intervertebral foramina (downside)
24. Rotate the skull into a near lateral position
25. 60 to 72 inches (150 to 180 cm)
26. Expiration; for maximum shoulder depression
27. Lateral, horizontal beam projection
28. Twining method
29. To T1; 1 inch (2.5 cm) above the jugular notch, or at vertebra prominens
30. C4 to T3
31. D. Hyperextension and flexion lateral positions

32. If unable to demonstrate the upper portion of the dens with the AP "open mouth" projection
33. AP "wagging jaw" projection (Ottonello method)
34. Correct use of anode-heel effect; use of compensating (wedge) filter
35. To blur out rib and lung markings that obscure detail of thoracic vertebrae
36. Right (downside)
37. C. Swimmer's lateral projection
38. A. 90 kV, 7 mAs
39. True (anterior oblique <5 mrad; posterior oblique <69 mrad)
40. B. Articular pillar (lateral masses of C-spine)
41. C. 20° to 30° caudad
42. Lead mat or masking
43. Mentomeatal line (MML)
44. Right
45. 20° from lateral position

Review Exercise C: Problem Solving for Technical and Positioning Errors

1. Excessive extension of the skull
2. Increase central ray angulation to 15° cephalad.
3. When the lower intervertebral foramina are narrowed while the upper foramina are well demonstrated, the positioning error most often is under rotation of the upper body. The upper body must be rotated 45°.
4. Initiate exposure during suspended expiration and increase SID to 72 inches (183 cm).
5. Reduce mAs and increase exposure time to produce more blurring of the mandible.
6. Use of a breathing technique to blur lung markings and ribs more effectively
7. Utilize a compensating (wedge) filter with thicker part of filter placed over the upper thoracic spine to equalize the density along the thoracic spine.
8. Angle CR 3° to 5° caudad.
9. Horizontal beam lateral projection
10. Hyperextension and flexion lateral positions
11. Perform either the (AP) Fuchs or (PA) Judd method.
12. Cervicothoracic (swimmer's) lateral projection
13. AP axial—vertebral arch (pillar) projection
14. AP open mouth projection. The patient's mouth must be carefully opened without any movement of the cervical spine.
15. Scoliosis series

Review Exercise D: Critique Radiographs of the Cervical and Thoracic Spine

A. AP open mouth (Fig. C9-91)
   1. Upper aspect of dens obscured by base of skull
   2. Overextension of skull, causing superimposition of base of skull over dens
   3. Collimation is poor, resulting in excessive exposure to face, eyes, and neck region; central ray and IR placement is too high
   4. Acceptable exposure factors
   5. Anatomic side marker
      Repeatable error(s): 1, 2 and 3
B. AP open mouth (Fig. C9-92)
   1. Upper aspect of dens and joint space obscured by front incisors
   2. Overflexion of skull causing superimposition of front incisors over top of dens
   3. Collimation too loose, resulting in excessive exposure to face, eyes, and neck region; slightly low central ray and IR
   4. Acceptable exposure factors
   5. No evidence of anatomic side marker
      Repeatable error(s): 1 and 2
C. AP axial projection (Fig. C9-93)
   1. Distorted vertebral bodies and intervertebral joint spaces; base of skull superimposed over upper cervical spine
   2. Overextension of skull and/or excessive central ray cephalic angle, which probably led to poor definition of vertebral bodies and joint spaces
   3. Evidence of collimation; slightly low central ray centering but correct IR placement
   4. Acceptable exposure factors
   5. Evidence of anatomic side marker
      Repeatable error(s): 1 and 2
      Note: Unsure of the origin of the artifact seen on lower, left cervical spine region
D. Right Posterior Oblique (Fig. C9-94)
   1. Lower intervertebral joint spaces and foramina not clearly demonstrated.
   2. Appears that body is underrotated from AP position (with appearance of upper rib cage suggesting underrotation rather than overrotation), an error that led to narrowing and obscuring of the lower intervertebral foramina.
   3. Collimation is evident. CR is centered too low.
   4. Acceptable exposure factors
   5. Anatomic side marker is evident
      Repeatable error(s): 1, 2, and 3
E. Lateral (trauma) (Fig. C9-95)
   1. Aspect of C1 and dens cut off; C7-T1 not demonstrated
   2. Need to depress shoulders (because chin cannot be adjusted as a result of the trauma)
   3. No evidence of collimation except along anterior, upper margin; central ray centered too posterior, causing upper cervical spine to be cut off; IR placement centered too low
   4. Acceptable exposure factors (poor contrast resulting from using a nongrid technique)
   5. No evidence of anatomic side marker
      Repeatable error(s): 1, 2, and 3
F. AP for odontoid process-Fuch's method (Fig. C9-96)
   1. Upper part of odontoid process is not demonstrated.
   2. The skull and neck is under extended, which produces a poor image of the dens within the foramen magnum. There is slight rotation of the skull.
   3. The CR is centered too high and collimation is absent.
   4. Slightly under-exposed
   5. No evidence of anatomic side marker
      Repeatable errors: 1, 2, 3, and 5

321

CHAPTER 10

Review Exercise A: Anatomy of the Lumbar Spine, Sacrum, and Coccyx

1. Pars interarticularis
2. B. Intervertebral foramina
3. Lateral position
4. A. Pedicle
   B. Transverse process
   C. Superior articular process and facet
   D. Lamina
   E. Spinous process
   F. Zygapophyseal joints
   G. Intervertebral foramina
5. Lesser (50° for upper and 30° for lower)
6. Pelvic sacral foramina
7. Promontory
8. Cornu
9. 30°
10. Coccyx
11. Base
12. A. Synovial, diarthrodial, plane, or gliding
    B. Cartilaginous, amphiarthrodial (slightly movable), none
13. A. Intervertebral disk space, L1-2
    B. Spinous process, L2
    C. Transverse process, L3
    D. Region of lamina (body), L4
    E. Left ala of sacrum
    F. Left sacroiliac joint
    G. Body of L1
    H. Pedicles of L2
    I. Intervertebral foramina, L3-4
    J. Intervertebral disk space, L5-S1
    K. Sacrum
    L. Inferior articular process, L3 (leg)
    M. Zygapophyseal joint, L4-5
    N. Pars interarticularis, L3 (neck)
    O. Pedicle, L3 (eye)
    P. Transverse process, L3 (nose)
    Q. Superior articular process, L3 (ear)
14. A. Left zygapophyseal joints
    B. Left zygapophyseal joints
    C. Intervertebral foramina
    D. Right zygapophyseal joints
    E. Right zygapophyseal joints
15. 50°, 30°, 45°

Review Exercise B: Topographic Landmarks and Positioning of the Lumbar Spine, Sacrum, and Coccyx

1. 1. C
   2. E
   3. A
   4. B
   5. D
2. False
3. True
4. False (not used for females if the shield would obscure essential anatomy)
5. False (PA would open spaces better.)
6. False (should be slightly flexed)
7. True
8. False
9. A. 4
   B. 1
   C. 1
   D. 5
   E. 2
10. A. 8
    B. 3
    C. 1
    D. 2
    E. 4
    F. 7
    G. 6
    H. 5
11. Iliac crest
12. A. Sacroiliac (SI) joints are equidistant from the spine.
    B. Spinous process should be midline to the vertebral column.
13. 30°
14. Right (upside)
15. Pedicle
16. Excessive rotation
17. Lateral
18. 5° to 8°, caudad
19. With the sag or convexity of the spine closest to the IR
20. Reduces lumbar curvature, which opens the intervertebral disk space
21. True
22. 1½ inches (4 cm) inferior to iliac crest and 2 inches (5 cm) posterior to ASIS
23. 30° cephalad
24. True
25. False (lower margin 1 to 2 inches [3 to 5 cm] below iliac crest)
26. True
27. A. 1000 to 1200 mrad
28. The convex side of the spine
29. Pelvis
30. Hyperextension and hyperflexion projections
31. 15° cephalad
32. A PA (prone) with 15° caudad central ray angle
33. 2 inches (5 cm) superior to the symphysis pubis
34. False (need different central ray angles for AP projections; can combine lateral but not AP projections)
35. AP of sacrum and coccyx
36. Place lead blocker on table top behind patient.
37. Left
38. 25° to 30°
39. D. 35° cephalad
40. 1 inch (2.5 cm) medial from upside ASIS

Review Exercise C: Problem Solving for Technical and Positioning Errors

1. Rotation of the spine
2. Insufficient rotation of the spine (should be to midvertebral bodies).
3. If the patient has a wide pelvis, the central ray can be angled 5° to 8° caudad.
4. Place additional support beneath the spine, or use a 5° to 8° caudad angle.
5. An increase in central ray angle is required to separate the coccyx from the symphysis pubis.
6. Decrease rotation of the body and spine.
7. AP or PA and collimated lateral projections would provide the best view of the L3 region. The central ray should be about 2 inches (5 cm) above the iliac crest.
8. A. Use high kV technique.
   B. Perform a PA rather than an AP projection.
   C. Use breast shields.
9. Perform a PA rather than an AP projection and reverse the direction of the central ray from caudad to cephalad.
10. A lateral L5-S1 position would demonstrate the degree of

forward displacement of L5 onto S1.
11. The CR should be angled 15° to 20° cephalad.
12. Although AP and lateral projections of the lumbar spine are helpful, posterior or anterior oblique positions will best demonstrate advanced signs of spondylolysis.
13. B. MRI
14. Hyperflexion and hyperextension lateral positions
15. Basic lumbar spine projections should be performed erect

Review Exercise D: Critique Radiographs of the Lumbar Spine, Sacrum, and Coccyx

A. Lateral lumbar spine (Fig. C10-83)
1. Posterior elements of upper lumbar spine cut off
2. Patient too far posterior
3. Evident and acceptable collimation (could be collimated a little more tightly if centering were correct); central ray centering too anterior, causing posterior elements to become cut off
4. Acceptable but slightly underexposed exposure factors
5. Anatomic side marker cut off
   Repeatable errors: 1, 2, and 3
B. Lateral lumbar spine (Fig. C10-84)
1. All structures demonstrated. Note: This patient has a transitional vertebrae, which produces six lumbar vertebrae. Also, there is calcification of the abdominal aorta.
2. Poor visibility of upper intervertebral joint spaces due to poor positioning of upper thoracic. Often if the shoulders are not superimposed there is closure of the upper joint spaces.
3. Collimation not evident; acceptable central ray centering and IR placement
4. Overexposed exposure factors
5. No evidence of anatomic side marker (it may have been placed too low on IR)
   Repeatable errors: 2 and 5

C. Lateral L5-S1 (Fig. C10-85)
1. All pertinent anatomic structures included
2. Excellent part and central ray centering
3. Additional collimation needed; S1 joint space not open; may need waist support or central ray caudal angle
4. Underexposed L5-S1 joint space region
5. Evidence of anatomic side marker (better to place up and posterior to spine)
   Repeatable errors: 3 and 4
D. Oblique lumbar spine (Fig. C10-86)
1. Posterior elements of upper lumbar spine cut off
2. Overrotated upper aspect of lumbar spine (eye of "Scottie dog" [pedicles] posterior and not centered to body)
3. Evidence of collimation; central ray centered too anterior; posterior elements of lumbar spine to become cut off
4. Acceptable exposure factors
5. Evidence of anatomic side marker
   Repeatable errors: 1, 2, and 3
E. Oblique lumbar spine (Fig. C10-87)
1. Entire lumbar spine demonstrated
2. Underrotated lumbar spine (eye of "Scottie dog" [pedicles] too anterior)
3. Collimation too loose and not evident (should be visible on sides); central ray centering and IR placement correct
4. Acceptable but slightly overexposed exposure factors
5. No evidence of anatomic side marker
   Repeatable error: 2

CHAPTER 11

Review Exercise A: Anatomy of the Bony Thorax, Sternum, and Ribs

1. A. Sternum
   B. Thoracic vertebra
   C. 12 pairs of ribs

2. A. Jugular (suprasternal) notch
   B. Facet for sternoclavicular joint
   C. Facet for first rib
   D. Manubrium
   E. Sternal angle
   F. Xiphoid process
   G. Costocartilage of seventh rib (last of "true" ribs)
   H. Tenth rib
   I. Costocartilage of second rib
   J. Clavicle
3. Body
4. 40
5. 6 inches (15 cm)
6. A. T9 or 10
   B. T4-5
7. Sternoclavicular joint
8. Costocartilage
9. True ribs connect to the sternum by their own costocartilage. False ribs are connected to the sternum via the costocartilage of the seventh rib.
10. True
11. False (called the sternal end)
12. D. Tubercle
13. A. Artery
    B. Vein
    C. Nerve
14. A. Posterior vertebral ends
    B. 3 to 5 inches (7.5 to 12.5 cm)
    C. First (anterior sternal end)
    D. Eighth or ninth
    E. 11
15. 1. B
    2. A
    3. B
    4. A
    5. A
    6. A
16. Synovial
17. A. True ribs, 1 through 7
    B. False ribs, 8 through 12
    C. Floating ribs, 11 through 12
18. Each rib attaches to the sternum by its own costocartilage.
19. They do not connect to anything anteriorly (thus the term "floating" ribs).
20. A. Vertebral end (posterior)
    B. Tubercles (for articulation with vertebrae)
    C. Axillary or angle portion of rib
    D. Costal groove
    E. Sternal end (anterior)
    F. Neck
    G. Head

Review Exercise B: Positioning of the Ribs and Sternum

1. True
2. False (less obliquity)
3. Approximately 15°
4. A. Low (65 to 70)
   B. Low
   C. High (3 to 4 seconds) with breathing technique
5. It blurs lung markings and ribs, which improves the visibility of the sternum.
6. Increase in patient dose, especially skin dose
7. CT or nuclear medicine
8. A. Recumbent
   B. Expiration
   C. Medium (70 to 80)
9. Above
10. Away from
11. PA and anterior obliques (Placing the area of interest closest to the IR is one recommended routine.)
12. AP and RPO (to shift spine away from area of interest)
13. By taping a small, metallic "BB" over the site of the injury
14. Erect PA and lateral chest
15. B
16. A
17. C
18. A
19. False
20. True
21. RAO; it places the sternum over the heart to provide a uniform background for added visibility of the sternum.
22. Midsternum (midway between jugular notch and xiphoid process)
23. LPO (oblique supine position)
24. 60 to 72 inches (152 to 183 cm); reduces magnification created by the long object image receptor distance (OID)
25. B. The entire sternum should lie over the heart shadow adjacent to the spine.
26. B. Level of T2-3
27. A. Suspend respiration on inspiration.
28. 10° to 15° from PA position
29. LAO
30. A. The nature of the trauma or patient complaint
   B. The location of the rib pain or injury
   C. Whether or not the patient has been coughing up blood
31. 3 to 4 inches (8 to 10 cm) below the jugular notch, level of T7
32. RAO or LPO elongates the left axillary ribs (and shifts the spine away from the injury site)
33. PA and LAO (to elongate the right axillary rib region)
34. 45°
35. A. 1 to 5 mrad
36. False (only about one third, or 33%)
37. True (Note: A greater difference in breast dose exists for posterior versus anterior rib projections than for thyroid doses because of the more anterior surface placement of the breasts compared with the thyroid.)
38. True. The gonadal dose is so low that it is not listed on the dose charts for rib projections.
39. C. 38 inches (15 cm)
40. B. Hemothorax

Review Exercise C: Problem Solving for Technical and Positioning Errors

1. Underrotation of the patient
2. Lower the kV to 65 for higher contrast and to prevent overpenetration of the sternum.
3. Increase the exposure time (and lower the mA) to allow for greater blurring of the lung markings.
4. Have the patient bring the breasts to the side; hold them in this position with a wide bandage.
5. CT
6. 15° to 20° RAO sternum with breathing technique; lateral sternum on inspiration; and 10° to 15° LAO of sternoclavicular joint with suspended inspiration
7. Suspend respiration during inspiration to move the diaphragm below the eighth ribs.
8. LPO and horizontal beam lateral projections (may use 15° to 20° mediolateral central angle if patient cannot be in oblique position)
9. Erect PA and LAO (or RPO) position with suspended inspiration
10. Recumbent PA (or AP if the patient cannot assume prone position) and RAO (or LPO) positions with suspended expiration
11. Because of patient condition, it is best to perform all positions erect and initiate exposure on full inspiration for upper ribs and full expiration for lower ribs. AP projections and both oblique positions (RPO and LPO) must be performed. It is recommended that kV (manual technique employed) for all projections be lowered because of the advanced osteoporosis.
12. A limited rib series will indicate which ribs are fractured (and whether this has led to flail chest). Since the patient is restricted to a backboard, the oblique positions may not be possible.

Review Exercise D: Critique Radiographs of the Bony Thorax

A. Bilateral ribs above diaphragm (Fig. C11-46)
   1. Ninth through eleventh ribs are cut off at left lateral margin.
   2. Tilt of body toward projected ribs Nos. 9 and 10 below collimation field
   3. CR centering is acceptable
   4. Acceptable exposure factors
   5. Anatomic side marker is evident
      Repeatable errors: 1 and 2
B. Oblique sternum (Fig. C11-47)
   1. All pertinent anatomic structures included
   2. Sternum is overrotated; sternum away from the spine and rotated beyond heart shadow and distorted (Note: Because of additional patient dose, some departments may choose not to repeat this projection since the outline of the sternum is visible.)
   3. Collimation not completely evident; central ray centering and IR placement correct
   4. Acceptable exposure factors and processing
   5. No evidence of anatomic side marker
      Repeatable errors: 2

C. Ribs below diaphragm
(Fig. C11-48)
1. Right lower ribs cut off; only lower three pair of ribs demonstrated, indicating diaphragm is too low from poor expiration
2. No elevation of diaphragm; need to take exposure during expiration with the patient in a recumbent position to raise the diaphragm to the highest level
3. No evidence of collimation; acceptable central ray centering, but IR should have been placed crosswise to prevent lateral margins of ribs from being cut off
4. Acceptable exposure factors and processing
5. Anatomic side marker evident but placed a little low and almost off the radiograph
Repeatable errors: 1 and 3
D. Lateral sternum (Fig. C11-49)
1. Lower aspect of sternum cut off
2. Acceptable part positioning
3. No evidence of collimation; central ray centering and IR placement too high, causing lower sternum to be cut off
4. Acceptable exposure factors
5. No evidence of markers
Repeatable errors: 1 and 3

CHAPTER 12

Review Exercise A: Anatomy of the Cranium

1. A. 8
   B. 14
2. A. Frontal
   B. Right parietal
   C. Left parietal
   D. Occipital
3. A. Right temporal
   B. Left temporal
   C. Sphenoid
   D. Ethmoid
4. A. Frontal
   B. Right parietal
   C. Right temporal
   D. Sphenoid
   E. Ethmoid
   F. Left temporal
   G. Left parietal
   H. Occipital

5. A. Frontal
   B. Ethmoid
   C. Sphenoid
   D. Left temporal
   E. Left parietal
   F. Occipital
   G. Right parietal
   H. Right temporal
6. A. Crista galli
   B. Cribriform plate
   C. Perpendicular plate
   D. Lateral labyrinth (mass)
   E. Middle nasal conchae (turbinate)
7. Cribriform plate
8. Perpendicular plate
9. A. Anterior clinoid processes
   B. Lesser wing
   C. Greater wing
   D. Sella turcica
   E. Dorsum sellae
   F. Posterior clinoid process
   G. Clivis
   H. Foramen rotundum
   I. Foramen ovale
   J. Foramen spinosum
   K. Foramen magnum
   L. Optic foramen
   M. Lateral pterygoid process (plate)
   N. Pterygoid hamulus
   O. Medial pterygoid process (plate)
   P. Superior orbital fissure
   Q. Body of sphenoid (sinus)
10. Sella turcica
11. Dorsum sellae
12. Optic foramen
13. Medial and lateral pterygoid processes
14. Lateral
15. Orbital or horizontal portion
16. A. Coronal
    B. Squamosal
    C. Lambdoidal
    D. Sagittal
    E. Bregma
    F. Lambda
    G. Pterion
    H. Asterion
    I. Anterior (bregma)
    J. Posterior (lambda)
    K. Sphenoid (pterion)
    L. Mastoid (asterion)
17. Fibrous or synarthrodial
18. Sutural or wormian; lambdoidal
19. Supraorbital margin (SOM)
20. Ethmoidal notch

21. Right and left parietals
22. Occipital
23. External occipital protuberance, or inion
24. Occipital condyles, or lateral condylar portions
25. A. Squamous
    B. Mastoid
    C. Petrous
26. False (petrous portion)
27. Top of the ear attachment (TEA)
28. Internal acoustic meatus
29. Fig. 12-15
    A. Supraorbital margins of right orbit
    B. Crista galli of ethmoid
    C. Sagittal suture—posterior skull
    D. Lambdoidal suture—posterior skull
    E. Petrous ridge
    Fig. 12-16
    A. External acoustic meatus (EAM)
    B. Mastoid portion of temporal bone
    C. Occipital bone
    D. Lambdoidal suture
    E. Clivus
    F. Dorsum sellae
    G. Posterior clinoid processes
    H. Anterior clinoid processes
    I. Vertex of skull
    J. Coronal suture
    K. Frontal bone
    L. Orbital plates of frontal bone
    M. Cribriform plate
    N. Sella turcica
    O. Body of sphenoid bone: sphenoid sinus

Review Exercise B: Specific Anatomy and Pathology of the Temporal Bone

1. A. Squamous
   B. Mastoid
   C. Petrous
2. Petrous portion
3. Auricle or pinna
4. 1 inch (or 2.5 cm)
5. Tympanic membrane (eardrum)
6. Auditory ossicles
7. Eustachian or auditory tube
8. To equalize the atmospheric pressure within the middle ear
9. Aditus
10. Tegmen tympani

11. Malleus
12. Stapes
13. Incus
14. Oval or vestibular window
15. A. Hearing
    B. Equilibrium
16. Round or cochlear window
17. True
18. A. Malleus
    B. Incus
    C. Stapes
    D. Oval window
    E. Cochlea
    F. Round window
    G. Eustachian tube
    H. Tympanic cavity
    I. Tympanic membrane
    J. EAM or canal
19. A. 5
    B. 3
    C. 1
    D. 6
    E. 2
    F. 4
20. A. Expansion of the internal
    acoustic canal
21. B. CT

Review Exercise C: Skull Morphology, Topography, and Positioning of the Cranium

1. A. Mesocephalic (c)
   B. Brachycephalic (b)
   C. Dolichocephalic (a)
2. Mesocephalic, 47
3. ±40
4. False (These are other terms for the infraorbitomeatal line.)
5. 7° to 8°; 7° to 8° (same degrees of difference)
6. 1. G
   2. E
   3. J
   4. N
   5. H
   6. K
   7. D
   8. F
   9. B
   10. I
   11. O
   12. L
   13. C
   14. A
   15. M
7. 70 to 85 kV
8. True
9. True

10. C. 200 to 300 mrad
11. A. Rotation
    B. Tilt
    C. Excessive flexion
    D. Excessive extension
    E. Incorrect central ray angulation
12. A. Rotation
    B. Tilt
13. True
14. A. Computed tomography (CT)
15. B. Ultrasound
16. D. Nuclear medicine
17. A. 3
    B. 5
    C. 6
    D. 1
    E. 2
    F. 4
    G. 7
18. A. Paget's disease
19. Occipital
20. A. OML
21. C. Foramen magnum
22. D. Rotation
23. IOML; 37
24. Dorsum sellae and posterior clinoids should be projected into the foramen magnum.
25. 25° cephalad
26. 2 inches (5 cm) above the EAM
27. B. Rotation
28. In the lower one third of the orbits
29. Excessive flexion or insufficient central ray angle
30. 0° posteroanterior (PA)
31. Rule out any possible cervical fractures or subluxation.
32. ¾ inch (2 cm) anterior and ¾ inch (2 cm) superior to the EAM
33. B. IOML
34. A. 30° caudal to IOML
35. D. Lateral
36. C. 25° to 30° PA axial
37. C. Lateral
38. A. 1½ inches (4 cm) superior to the nasion
39. C. 37° caudad
40. A. CT

Review Exercise D: Problem Solving for Technical and Positioning Errors

1. Rotation of skull present; rotation of skull toward left
2. Excessive extension or excessive caudad central ray angle—

projects the petrous ridges lower than expected (should be in the lower third of the orbit)
3. Rotation of the skull
4. Insufficient extension of the skull, or central ray was not perpendicular to IOML
5. Skull tilt
6. Skull rotation
7. Central ray angled less than 37° to the IOML, or less than 30° to the OML (would be caused by 30° angle to IOML)
8. Collimated, lateral projection of the sella turcica
9. Right lateral projection of the skull
10. Should perform the PA axial projection (Haas method)
11. Horizontal beam (dorsal decubitus) lateral position—will demonstrate a possible air-fluid level in the sphenoid sinus
12. Ultrasound (sonography)—a noninvasive means of evaluating the newborn's cranium
13. Either MRI or CT can be performed.
14. Overangulation of the CR
15. No repeat exposure is required. Due to elongation of the facial mass with the AP axial projection for skull, cutting off aspects of the mandible is acceptable.

Review Exercise E: Critique Radiographs of the Cranium

A. Lateral skull: 4-year-old (Fig. C12-74)
1. Foreign bodies (earrings) obscuring essential anatomic structures
2. Correct part positioning, but patient's hand seen supporting mandible; can use positioning sponge if needed to support skull
3. No evidence of collimation; correct central ray and IR placement
4. Appears underexposed on this printed copy (may be a repeatable error if actual radiograph also appears this light)
5. No evidence of anatomic side marker
   Repeatable errors: 1 and possibly 4

B. Lateral skull: 54-year-old, posttraumatic injury (Fig. C12-75)
  1. Vertex of the skull just slightly cut off (may be repeatable error because of proximity to the site of trauma)
  2. Tilted and rotated skull (separation of the orbital plates from the tilt; separation of the greater wings of the sphenoid, the rami of the mandible, and the EAMs—all indicating rotation)
  3. No evidence of collimation; slightly high central ray centering if the photo borders are also the collimation borders, which would add to the tilt appearance
  4. Acceptable exposure factors
  5. No evidence of anatomic side marker
     Repeatable errors: 1 and 2
C. AP axial (Towne) skull: (C12-76)
  1. Entire occipital bone and foramen magnum demonstrated
  2. Correct part positioning
  3. No evidence of collimation; overangled central ray; anterior arch of C1 projected into the foramen magnum rather than the dorsum sellae
  4. Acceptable but slightly underexposed exposure factors
  5. No evidence of anatomic side marker
     Repeatable errors: 3
D. AP or PA skull (Fig. C12-77) AP 15° cephalad projection, as indicated by the large size of the orbits, which was caused by magnification from increased OID (can compare with radiograph that follows)
  1. All pertinent anatomic structures demonstrated but with some foreshortening of frontal bone
  2. Petrous ridges not in the lower third of orbits; position requires more flexion or less central ray angle as an AP; skull slightly rotated (note distance between orbits and lateral margins of skull)
  3. No evidence of collimation; less central ray angle needed (see previous answer; can also compare with correctly angled

central ray on PA radiograph in Fig. C12-87)
  4. Acceptable exposure factors
  5. No evidence of anatomic side marker
     Repeatable errors: 2 and 3
E. AP or PA skull (Fig. C12-78) PA 15° Caldwell projection
  1. All pertinent anatomic structures not demonstrated; patient ID marker and side marker obscuring skull
  2. Correct part positioning
  3. Evidence of collimation (circular cone); size of cassette too small for the skull; correct central ray placement and angle (petrous ridges in lower third of orbit)
  4. Acceptable exposure factors
  5. Evidence of anatomic side marker, but placed over skull; patient ID marker over upper right cranium—both repeatable errors
     Repeatable errors: 1 and 5

CHAPTER 13

Review Exercise A: Radiographic Anatomy of the Facial Bones

1. A. Middle nasal conchae
2. Maxilla
3. A. Frontal process
   B. Zygomatic process
   C. Alveolar process
   D. Palatine process
4. Frontal process
5. Acanthion
6. Horizontal portion of the palatine bones
7. Frontal and ethmoid
8. Zygomatic or malar bones
9. D. Sphenoid
10. Lacrimal bones
11. Conchae, turbinates
12. False (Most of the nose is made up of cartilage.)
13. Septal cartilage, vomer (pushed laterally to one side)
14. A. 3
    B. 8
    C. 6
    D. 7
    E. 5
    F. 1
    G. 2
    H. 4

15. A. Nasal bones
    B. Lacrimal bones
    C. Zygomatic bones
    D. Maxillary bones
    E. Inferior nasal conchae
    F. Mandible
16. Vomer and palatine bones
17. A. Pterygoid hamulus, sphenoid
    B. Right palatine process, right maxilla
    C. Left palatine process, left maxilla
    D. Horizontal portions, right and left palatine bones
18. A. Perpendicular plate of ethmoid
    B. Vomer
    C. Septal cartilage
19. A. Condyle
    B. Neck
    C. Ramus
    D. Gonion or mandibular angle
    E. Body
    F. Mental foramen
    G. Mentum or mental protuberance
    H. Alveolar process
    I. Coronoid process
    J. Mandibular notch
    K. Temporal bone
    L. Temporomandibular joint (TMJ)
    M. External auditory meatus (EAM)
    N. Mastoid process
20. A. Lacrimal (facial)
    B. Ethmoid (cranial)
    C. Frontal (cranial)
    D. Sphenoid (cranial)
    E. Palatine (facial)
    F. Zygomatic (facial)
    G. Maxilla (facial)
21. H. Optic foramen
    I. Superior orbital fissure
    J. Inferior orbital fissure
    K. Sphenoid strut
22. 30, 37
23. Inferior orbital fissure
24. A. Superior orbital fissure
25. B. Optic nerve

Review Exercise B: Radiographic Anatomy of the Paranasal Sinuses

1. Antrum of Highmore
2. Maxillary
3. Between the inner and outer tables of the skull, posterior to the glabella

4. 6 years
5. Lateral masses or labyrinths
6. B. Osteomeatal complex
7. Sphenoid sinus
8. A. Nasal cavity (fossae)
   B. Maxillary sinuses
   C. Right temporal bone
      (squamous portion)
   D. Frontal sinuses
   E. Ethmoid sinuses
   F. Sphenoid sinuses
   G. Maxillary sinuses
   H. Ethmoid sinuses
   I. Frontal sinuses
   J. Squamous portion of left
      temporal bone
   K. Mastoid portion of left
      temporal bone
   L. Sphenoid sinus
   M. Roots of upper teeth
      (alveolar process)
      Fig. 13-9
9. A. Sphenoid sinus
   B. Maxillary sinuses
   C. Ethmoid sinuses
   D. Frontal sinus
      Fig. 13-10
   E. Frontal sinuses
   F. Sphenoid sinus
   G. Ethmoid sinuses
   H. Maxillary sinuses
10. Infundibulum
11. True
12. B. Prone

Review Exercise C: Positioning of the Facial Bones

1. False (may also be performed
   erect)
2. True
3. False (decrease of 25% to 30%)
4. True
5. False (It is used for this.)
6. False (Strong magnets in MRI
   prohibit this.)
7. Blow-out fracture
8. Tripod
9. Dense petrous pyramids
   superimpose the orbits, obscuring
   facial bone structures.
10. C. Zygoma
11. Waters method
12. Orbits including infraorbital
    rims, bony nasal septum,
    maxillae, zygomatic bones, and
    arches
13. B. 30°
14. Orbital rims and orbital floors

15. A. Reduces OID of facial bones
    B. Reduces exposure to anterior
       facial bones and neck structures
       such as thyroid glands
16. A. IR is placed lengthwise for
       facial bones but crosswise for
       the cranium.
    B. CR is centered to the zygoma
       for facial bones and 2 inches
       (5 cm) above the EAM for the
       cranium.
17. Mentomeatal; 37
18. Acanthion
19. Nasion
20. Lips–meatal; 55
21. True
22. False (toward the affected side)
23. True
24. False (Thyroid gland dose is
    significant.)
25. Maxillary sinuses; inferior orbital
    rims
26. Glabelloalveolar (GAL)
27. Zygomatic arches
28. 1 inch (2.5 cm) superior to glabella
    to pass through midarches
29. A. Rhese method
    B. Three-point landing
30. A. Cheek, nose, chin
    B. 53°
    C. Acanthiomeatal
    D. Lower outer
31. 1. E
    2. C
    3. F
    4. A
    5. D
    6. B

Review Exercise D: Positioning of the Mandible and Temporomandibular Joints (TMJ)

1. Submentovertex (SMV)
2. Axiolateral oblique
3. Extend the chin
4. A. 30°
   B. 45°
   C. 0°, true lateral
   D. 10° to 15°
   E. 25° cephalad
5. Insufficient cephalic CR angle or
   head tilt
6. Acanthion (at lips for PA
   projection)
7. Orbitomeatal line (OML)
8. True
9. False (cephalad)
10. Condyloid process

11. A. 35° caudad
    B. 42° caudad
12. Glabella
13. SMV projection
14. Panoramic tomography (Panorex)
15. Narrow, vertical slit diaphragm
16. Infraorbitomeatal line (IOML)
17. Curved, nongrid cassette
18. True
19. True
20. B. Schuller
21. 25 to 30; caudad
22. A. Modified Law
    B. 15
    C. 15
23. 40° caudad
24. Midsagittal

Review Exercise E: Positioning of the Paranasal Sinuses

1. 65-80 kV
2. A. Perform positions erect when
      possible
   B. Use horizontal x-ray beam
3. True
4. True
5. False
6. A. Lateral
   B. PA Caldwell
   C. Parietoacanthial (Waters)
   D. SMV
7. Lateral
8. Horizontal x-ray beam
9. Frontal and anterior ethmoid
10. 15°
11. A. Maxillary
    B. 37
12. Mentomeatal line (MML)
13. Just below the maxillary sinuses
14. Sphenoid, ethmoid, and maxillary
    sinuses
15. Level of the acanthion
16. The mouth (oral cavity) is open
    with the PA transoral projection.
17. Sphenoid sinuses
18. 1. C
    2. D
    3. E
    4. A
    5. B

Review Exercise F: Problem Solving for Technical and Positioning Errors

1. Rotation of the head
2. No. The petrous ridges should be
   projected just below the maxillary

sinuses. The patient's head needs to be extended more.

3. Rotation of the head

4. Yes, this image meets the evaluation criteria for a 30° PA axial projection.

5. Excessive flexion of the head and neck or incorrect CR angle will project the glabella into the nasal bones. The CR must be parallel to the glabelloalveolar line.

6. The head was tilted. Ensure that the MSP is parallel to the image receptor.

7. No. Increase extension of the head and neck. The AML should be placed perpendicular to the IR to ensure that the optic foramen is open and is projected into the lower outer quadrant of the orbit (head rotation is correct).

8. Insufficient rotation of the head toward the IR. The head should be rotated 30° (from lateral position) toward the IR to prevent foreshortening of the body.

9. PA Waters and R and L laterals. The parietoacanthial (Waters) or the optional PA axial projections would demonstrate any possible septal deviation. The lateral projections would demonstrate any possible fracture of the nasal bones or anterior nasal spine. (The superoinferior projection would provide an axial perspective but is considered an optional projection in most departments and not part of the routine unless specifically requested.)

10. Modified parietoacanthial (modified Waters) projection

11. Perform the oblique inferosuperior (tangential) projections. These projections are most ideal to demonstrate a depressed fracture of the zygomatic arch. (Bilateral projections are generally taken for comparison.)

12. Angle CR to place it perpendicular to the IOML. Angle image receptor to maintain a perpendicular relationship between the CR and image receptor. This will prevent distortion of the anatomy.

13. The head and neck need to be extended more to project the petrous ridges below the ethmoid sinuses.

14. Rotation of the head

15. Tilt of the head

16. Increase extension of the head and neck to project the entire sphenoid sinus through the oral cavity.

17. None. The petrous ridges should be below the floors of the maxillary sinuses on a well-positioned parietoacanthial projection.

18. The most diagnostic projection is the horizontal beam lateral projection to demonstrate any air-fluid levels.

19. The PA transoral special projection in addition to the routine four sinuses projection series (the lateral, PA Caldwell, parietoacanthial, and SMV)

20. PA, PA axial, and parietoacanthial projections will demonstrate a possible bony nasal septal deviation.

Review Exercise G: Critique Radiographs of the Facial Bones

A. Parietoacanthial (Waters) projection(C13-132)
1. Pertinent anatomy is all included but not well demonstrated due to positioning and exposure errors.
2. Skull is underextended. This led to the petrous ridges being projected into the lower maxillary sinuses. Also, skull appears to be rotated.
3. Collimation is not evident. CR and image receptor appears correct.
4. Facial bone region appears to be overexposed with very poor contrast.
5. Anatomic side marker is not evident.
Repeatable error(s): 2 and 4

B. SMV mandible (C13-133)
1. Pertinent anatomy is included but not well demonstrated due to positioning error.
2. Skull is underextended and/or CR angle is incorrect. (IOML was not parallel to IR and not perpendicular to CR.) Mandible is foreshortened and rami projected into temporal bone.
3. Collimation is not evident. CR centering and IR placement is correct.
4. Image appears to be slightly underexposed.
5. Anatomic side marker is not evident.
Repeatable error(s): 2 (possibly 4)

C. Optic foramina, Rhese method (C13-134)
1. Optic foramen is included but is slightly distorted.
2. Skull is rotated excessively toward a PA. (The skull is rotated more than 53° from the lateral position. This led to the optic foramen being projected into the middle lower aspect of the orbit.)
3. Collimation is not evident. CR and IR placement are correct.
4. Exposure factors are acceptable.
5. Anatomic side marker is not evident.
Repeatable error(s): 2 (The foramen is well demonstrated, and this may not be a repeatable error by itself.)

D. Optic foramina, Rhese method (C13-135)
1. Optic foramen is distorted and totally obscured.
2. Skull appears to be overextended. (The AML was not perpendicular.) This projects the optic foramina into the infraorbital rim structure. Skull also appears to be underrotated, toward a lateral position. (If the skull is rotated less than 53° from the lateral position, the optic foramen will be projected into the lateral margin of the orbit.)
3. Collimation is evident and appears satisfactory. CR and IR placement are correct.
4. Exposure factors are acceptable.
5. Anatomic side marker is not evident.
Repeatable error(s): 1 and 2

E. Lateral facial bones (C13-136)
  1. Very distal end of mandible is cut off. Probably would not justify repeat exposure unless this was a specific area of interest.
  2. Skull is rotated. (Note the separation of rami of mandible, greater wings of sphenoid, and orbits).
  3. Collimation is evident and acceptable (except for cutoff of lower tip of mandible). CR and IR placement are acceptable.
  4. Exposure factors appear to be satisfactory.
  5. Anatomic side marker is not evident.
     Repeatable error(s): 2 (possibly 1)

Review Exercise H: Critique Radiographs of the Paranasal Sinuses

A. Parietoacanthial transoral (openmouth Waters) (C13-137)
  1. Sphenoid and maxillary sinuses not well demonstrated. Petrous ridges are projected into lower aspect of maxillary sinuses. The base of skull is superimposed over sphenoid sinus.
  2. Skull is underextended, leading to errors previously described. (Chin not elevated sufficiently.)

  3. Collimation is not centered to film. CR is centered too low (inferior) according to circular collimation on top, but this is not a repeatable error by itself. Film appears centered high, not aligned with CR.
  4. Exposure factors are acceptable.
  5. Anatomical side marker is not evident.
     Repeatable errors: 1 and 2
B. Parietoacanthial (Waters) (C13-138)
  1. Maxillary sinuses not well demonstrated. Petrous ridges are projected into lower aspect of maxillary sinuses. Artifacts appear to be either surgical clips and devices or external hair pins or clips.
  2. Skull is underextended and severely rotated.
  3. Collimation is not evident. CR centering and film placement are slightly now.
  4. Exposure factors are acceptable.
  5. Anatomical side marker is not evident.
     Repeatable errors: 1 and 2
C. Submentovertex (SMV) (C13-139)
  1. Maxillary and ethmoid sinuses not well demonstrated and partially cut off. Mandible is superimposed over sinuses.

  2. Skull is grossly underextended and tilted. (Also some rotation.)
  3. Collimation would have been OK if centering would have been correct. CR centering is off laterally. This led to cutoff of the anatomy.
  4. Exposure factors are acceptable.
  5. Anatomical side marker is not evident.
     Repeatable errors: 1, 2, and 3 (CR centering)
D. Lateral projection (C13-140)
  1. Part of ethmoid and maxillary sinuses not well demonstrated due to superimposed mandible. Earrings were not removed.
  2. Skull is underextended and slightly rotated to the right.
  3. Collimation is acceptable. CR centering and film placement are acceptable but slightly anterior.
  4. Exposure factors are acceptable for the sphenoid/ethmoid sinuses.
  5. Anatomical side marker is not evident.
     Repeatable errors: 1 and 2

Self-Test Answers

CHAPTER 1

General Anatomy, Terminology, and Positioning Principles

Self-Test A: General, Systemic, and Skeletal Anatomy and Arthrology

1.
   A. Integumentary
   D. Osseous
2. C. 206
3. B. Circulatory
4. B. Urinary
5. D. Integumentary
6. B. Axial and appendicular
7. A. Spongy or cancellous
8. C. Hyaline or articular cartilage
9. D. Diploe
10. A. Diaphysis
11. C. Epiphyses
12. A. Fibrous
13. B. Cartilaginous
14. C. Distal tibiofibular joint
15.
   1. C
   2. A
   3. B
   4. D
   5. C
   6. A
   7. D
   8. C
16. D. Fibrous
17.
   1. E
   2. A
   3. F
   4. C
   5. B
   6. D
   7. G
   8. D
   9. C
   10. E

Self-Test B: Positioning Terminology

1. C. Midcoronal
2. False
3. C. Sagittal plane
4.
   1. E
   2. I
   3. G
   4. J
   5. A
   6. K
   7. C
   8. H
   9. B
   10. F
   11. L
   12. D
5.
   1. L
   2. G
   3. F
   4. J
   5. A
   6. H
   7. D
   8. C
   9. B
   10. K
   11. I
   12. E
6. D. Projection
7. A. LAO
8. C. Ventral decubitus
9. D. Anteroposterior
10. C. RPO
11. D. AP oblique with lateral rotation
12. A. Dorsoplantar
13. D. Fowler's
14. B. PA oblique with medial rotation
15. A. Tangential
16. C. Transthoracic
17. D. Parietoacanthial
18. C. AP Chest with 20° cephalic angle
19. A. Radiographic view
20.
   1. D
   2. H
   3. I
   4. F
   5. J
   6. C

7. A
8. G
9. B
10. E

Self-Test C: Positioning Principles

1. False
2. False
3. False
4. True
5.
   1. B
   2. B
   3. A
   4. A
   5. B
   6. A
   7. A
   8. B
   9. A
   10. A
6. B. KUB
7. C. Two
8. C. Two
9. C. Two
10. B. Three
11. C. Two
12. C. Two
13. B. Three
14. C. PA, oblique and lateral projections
15. A. PA and lateral projections
16. D. Palpation

CHAPTER 2

Image Quality, Digital Technology, and Radiation Protection

Self-Test A: Image Quality in Film-Screen Imaging

1. C. Kilovoltage
2. A. Density
3. B. Milliamperage seconds (mAs)
4. False
5. B. Decrease to 5 mAs
6. B. Kilovoltage (kV)
7. C. 110 kV 2 mAs

8. A. 60 kV, 30 mAs
9. True
10. False
11. C. 60 kV and 5 mAs
12. D. All of the above
13. False
14. D. Shortening the exposure time
15. D. 0.3 mm focal spot and 40-inch SID
16. B. Compensating filter
17. B. Boomerang
18. A. Wedge
19. A. Off-level grid cutoff
20. C. AP abdomen
21. D. Distortion
22. C. 72-inch SID and 3-inch OID
23. False
24. B. Parallel
25. C. Focal spot size

Self-Test B: Image Quality in Digital Radiography

1. A. Pixels
2. D. Algorithms
3. False
4. True
5. True
6. B. Brightness
7. C. Processing algorithms
8. A. Contrast resolution
9. B. Display pixel size
10. False
11. True
12. D. Exposure index
13. A. Noise
14. True
15. False
16. B. Scatter radiation
17. C. Post-processing
18. A. Smoothing
19. B. Contrast
20. False

Self-Test C: Applications of Digital Technology

1. A. CR provides a wide exposure latitude
2. C. Bright light
3. D. Bar code reader
4. D. Photostimulable phosphor
5. A. Laser
6. False
7. C. 30
8. False
9. True
10. True

11. False
12. True
13. True, film-screen images can be scanned in
14. C. Radiology information system
15. A. A set of standards to ensure communication among digital imaging systems
16. D. Teleradiology
17. B. Penumbra
18. C. Display matrices
19. B. 11 × 14 inches IR
20. D. Smoothing

Self-Test D: Radiation Protection

1. B. Gray
2. D. Roentgen
3. D. 5 rem or 50 mSv
4. A. 250 mSv
5. B. 0.1 rem or 1 mSv
6. D. 10 R/minute
7. C. 3 to 4 R/minute
8. A. Absorb lower energy x-rays
9. B. AP thoracic spine (14 × 17 collimation)
10. C. 50% to 90%
11. C. Shadow shield
12. False
13. True
14. True
15. False (2%)
16. D. Collimation
17. C. Increase kV and lower mAs
18. D. Behind radiologist
19. A. Bucky slot shield
20. B. .05 rem (0.5 mSv)
21. False
22. False
23. True
24. D. ALARA does not apply to digital imaging (False)
25. False

CHAPTER 3

Chest

1.
   1. E
   2. C
   3. D
   4. B
   5. A
2. D. Vertebra prominens
3. C. Jugular notch
4. A. Right and left bronchi
5. B. Carina

6. D. Hilum
7. B. Alveoli
8. B. Hilar pleura
9. B. Hemothorax
10. A. Costophrenic angle
11. C. Epiglottis
12. D. Asthenic
13. D. 125 kV, 600 mA, $\frac{1}{60}$ sec, 72 inch SID
14.
   A. 8
   B. 10
   C. 1
   D. 5
   E. 4
   F. 11
   G. 9
   H. 13
   I. 7
   J. 3
   K. 6
   L. 12
   M. 2
15.
   A. Superior portion (apex) of left lung
   B. Jugular notch (superior margin of manubrium)
   C. Trachea
   D. Esophagus
16.
   A. Esophagus
   B. Descending aorta
   C. T4-T5 vertebra
   D. Trachea
   E. Superior vena cava
   F. Ascending aorta
   G. Sternum
   H. Left lung region
17. A. Pigg-O-Stat
18. C. 65 kVp, short exposure time
19. A. To reduce patient dose
20. D. To reduce chest rotation
21. A. Remove scapulae from lung fields
22. C. 3 to 4 inches (8 to 10 cm) below jugular notch
23. A. Dyspnea.
24. A. Atelectasis
25. C. Pulmonary edema
26. B. Pulmonary emboli
27. D. Tuberculosis
28. A. Be reduced
29. C. Rotation into an LAO position
30. Yes, 10 ribs showing is acceptable. (Some healthy patients can inhale deeper and show 11 ribs.)

31. Yes. The costophrenic angles must be visualized on both the PA and lateral projections.
32. D. Raise upper limbs higher
33. No. This separation is acceptable and is caused by the divergent x-ray beam.
34. B. Perform AP semiaxial projection
35. C. Yes. Decrease exposure factors
36. A. Left lateral decubitus
37. C. 60° LAO
38. D. Left lateral decubitus
39. Radiograph C3-90
    A. (a), (c), (f) (slight rotation is evident)
    B. Criterion (a)
    C. (a), (f), (g)
40. Radiograph C3-92
    A. (b), (c), (f)
    B. Criteria (b) and (f)
    C. (a), (d), (e)

CHAPTER 4

Abdomen

1. D. Peritoneum
2. C. Psoas muscles
3. A. Duodenum
4. C. Ileocecal valve
5.
    1. D
    2. H
    3. G
    4. F
    5. C
    6. A
    7. I
    8. B
    9. E
6. D. Kidney
7. C. Ureter
8. D. Gallbladder
9. D. Mesentery
10.
    A. RLQ
    B. RUQ
    C. LUQ
    D. LUQ
    E. RUQ
    F. LLQ
    G. RLQ
    H. RUQ and LUQ
    I. RUQ
11. C

12.
    1. A
    2. A
    3. B
    4. A
    5. B
    6. A
    7. C
    8. B
    9. C
    10. B
13. A. T9-10
14.
    1. 3
    2. 7
    3. 1
    4. 6
    5. 5
    6. 2
    7. 4
15. B. Greater trochanter
16. A. Iliac crest
17. A. Short exposure time
18. D. Ascites
19. B. Paralytic ileus
20. A. Intussusception
21. D. Ulcerative colitis
22. C. Pneumoperitoneum
23. B. Diaphragm
24. B. Ascites
25. D. Ileus
26.
    A. Iliac crest
    B. L4 lumbar spine
    C. Psoas muscles
    D. Coccyx
    E. Pubic symphysis
    F. Obturator foramen
27.
    A. Liver
    B. Gallbladder
    C. Duodenum
    D. Stomach
    E. Left colic flexure of large intestine
    F. Pancreas
    G. Spleen
    H. Left kidney
    I. Abdominal aorta
    J. Inferior vena cava
28. B. 78 kV, 600 mA, 1/30 sec, grid, 40 inches SID
29. C. Rotation toward the right
30. A. Upon expiration
31. B. Use two cassettes placed crosswise
32. D. 5 minutes
33. B. Diaphragm
34. A. Left lateral decubitus

35. D. AP erect abdomen
36. B. Left lateral decubitus
37. C. Dorsal decubitus
38. B. AP erect abdomen
39. B. Left lateral decubitus
40. A. Sonography
41. D. Nuclear medicine
42. D. Collimation
43.
    A. True
    B. False (250 to 300 range)
    C. False (AP is about 35% greater than PA)
    D. True (testes are out of primary field)
44. Radiograph C4-49
    A. (a), (b), (c)
    B. Criteria (a) and (c)
    C. (b), (c),
45. Radiograph C4-51
    A. (a), (b), (d) ,(e)
    B. Criterion (a), (b), (d-decrease exposure time)
    C. (b), (c), (e)

CHAPTER 5

Upper Limb

1.
    A. A. 14
    B. B. 8
    C. B. 27
2.
    A. 7
    B. 4
    C. 2
    D. 5
    E. 1
    F. 6
3.
    A. 11
    B. 13
    C. 4
    D. 15
    E. 7
    F. 17
    G. 5
    H. 18
    I. 12
    J. 1
    K. 16
    L. 8
    M. 2
    N. 3
    O. 9
    P. 14
    Q. 6
    R. 10

4. C. Hamate
5. D. Trapezium
6. A. Scaphoid
7. D. Scaphoid and trapezium
8.
   A. 6
   B. 3
   C. 8
   D. 2
   E. 5
   F. 11
   G. 9
   H. 1
   I. 4
   J. 7
   K. 10
9. C. PA-Radial deviation
10. C. Scaphoid
11. A. PA–Ulnar deviation
12. B. Scaphoid
13. D. Ulna
14. A. Anterior aspect of distal humerus
15. C. Lateral and medial epicondyle
16. A. Medial aspect of coronoid process
17. A. Head of ulna
18.
   A. 4
   B. 3
   C. 2
   D. 1
   E. 4
19.
   A. 2
   B. 1
   C. 4
   D. 3
   E. 2
   F. 9
   G. 7
   H. 5
   I. 4
   J. 1
   K. 10
   L. 1
   M. 3
   N. 6
   O. 8
20.
   A. 5
   B. 3
   C. 8
   D. 7
   E. 11
   F. 1
   G. 2
   H. 4

I. 10
J. 9
K. 6
21. True
22. False (lateral)
23. B. Causes the proximal radius to cross over the ulna
24. A. Supinated
25. B. Pronated
26.
   A. 3
   B. 4
   C. 1
   D. 2
   E. 1
   F. 4
   G. 2
27. False
28. B. Parallel to long axis of the IR
29. D. Soft-tissue structures within certain synovial joints
30.
   1. F
   2. H
   3. G
   4. E
   5. B
   6. D
   7. A
   8. C
31. C. Advanced osteoporosis
32. A. Affected PIP joint
33. D. All of the above
34. B. Third MCP joint
35. A. Increased OID
36. C. Bennett's fracture
37. True
38. False
39. D
40. True
41. C. Decrease obliquity of hand
42. A. Rotate upper limb medially
43. C. Rotate wrist laterally 5° to 10°
44. A. Insufficient medial rotation
45. B. Place humerus/forearm in same horizontal plane
46. B. Wrist
47. C. Wrist/forearm
48. D. 68 to 70 kV or 10 mAs
49. A. Coyle method
50. AP elbow projection
   A. (c), (e), (f)
   B. Criteria (e) and (f)
   C. (a), (e), (f)
51. PA wrist projection
   A. (b) Radial deviation

B. (a), (b)
C. Criteria (a) and (b)
D. (b)

CHAPTER 6

Humerus and Shoulder Girdle

1. D. (While both terms are correct [B and C], scapulohumeral joint is the preferred term)
2. C. Acromioclavicular
3. B. Medial angle
4. D. Coracoid process
5. False
6. A. Scapular spine
7. C. Acromion
8. B. Spheroidal
9.
   A. 3
   B. 6
   C. 5
   D. 8
   E. 12
   F. 10
   G. 7
   H. 2
   I. 9
   J. 4
   K. B. External rotation
   L. 2
   M. 12
   N. 3
   O. 6 or 11
   P. 13 or 5
   Q. 1
   R. 8
   S. A. Inferosuperior axial projection
10. A. Center and right AEC chambers activated
11. True
12. True
13. D. Nuclear medicine
14. A. Ultrasound
15.
   1. D
   2. E
   3. C
   4. F
   5. G
   6. A
   7. B
16. D. Scapular Y (Neer method)
17. A. Osteoarthritis
18. B. Rheumatoid arthritis
19. A. External rotation

20. C. 1 in (2.5 cm) inferior to coracoid process
21. C. Internal rotation
22. B. 25° to 30° medially
23. B. Use exaggerated, external rotation
24. B. Perpendicular to IR
25. D. Grashey method
26. C. 10° to 15°
27. B. Reduced OID
28. A. Scapular Y lateral (Neer method)
29. B. Transthoracic lateral for humerus
30. A. 10° to 15° caudad
31. C. Scapulohumeral dislocations
32. A. Scapulohumeral joint space
33. A. 5° to 15° toward axilla
34. C. Posterior oblique (Grashey method)
35. D. AC joints
36. B. Fractured clavicle
37. B. 8 to 10 lb
38. False
39. True
40.
    1. B. (66 mrad)
    2. C. (3 to 8 mrad)
    3. C. (1 to 3 mrad)
    4. B. (45 mrad)
    5. A. (1005 mrad)
    6. C. (10 mrad)
    7. C. (1 mrad)
    8. C. (0 mrad)
41. D. Rotate body more toward affected side
42. C. Garth method
43. A. Increase CR angulation
44. A. AC joint series—non-weight and weight-bearing projections
45. D. Tangential projection-Fisk method
46. A. Wrong direction of CR angle
47. B. Perform the projection with the patient's upper chest prone on the table (arm is extended upward)
48. C. AP and transthoracic lateral of humerus
49. AP clavicle (C6-97)
    A. (b), (c), (e), (f)
    B. Criteria (b), (e), (f)
    C. (a), (b), (f)
50. AP scapula (C6-99)
    A. (a), (b), (d), (e)
    B. Criteria (a), (b), (d), (e)
    C. (a), (b), (d), (e)

CHAPTER 7

Lower Limb

1. B. Tail
2. False (proximal aspect or tuberosity is commonly fractured)
3. A. Plantar surface near head of first metatarsal
4. D. Navicular
5. C. Intermediate cuneiform
6. B. Subtalar joint
7. B. Tibial plafond
8. False (the lateral aspect of the ankle joint would not be open)
9.
    1. D
    2. G
    3. B
    4. F
    5. A
    6. E
    7. C
10.
    A. 3
    B. 4
    C. 5
    D. 1
    E. 2
    F. C. AP ankle
11.
    A. 6
    B. 8
    C. 5
    D. 2
    E. 3
    F. 1
    G. 7
    H. 4
    I. 9
    J. 2
    K. 5
12. A. Fig. 7-11
13. A. Affected MTP joint
14. B. 10° to 15° posterior (toward calcaneus)
15. C. Tangential
16. D. 30° to 40°
17. D. Dorsoplantar projection
18. A. 10° posterior (more or less angle may be applied based on the height of the arch)
19. C. AP oblique-medial rotation
20. D. Intercondylar tubercles
21. A. Intercondylar fossa
22. A. (5° to 7°)

23. True
24. B. Base
25. C. Cruciates
26. C. Menisci
27.
    A. 3
    B. 9
    C. 6
    D. 8
    E. 1
    F. 4
    G. 2
    H. 10
    I. 5
    J. 7
28. B. AP oblique-medial rotation
29.
    A. 3
    B. 5
    C. 1
    D. 6
    E. 2
    F. 3
    G. 5
    H. 1
    I. 4
    J. 7
30. B. Under rotation toward IR
31. True
32. C. Over rotation of knee toward IR
33. D. Osgood-Schlatter disease
34. D. Lisfranc injury
35. A. Osteogenic sarcoma
36. B. Runner's knee
37. C. Base of third metatarsal
38. B. AP oblique (15° to 20° medial rotation)
39. D. Interepicondylar
40. B. Proximal tibiofibular
41. True
42. D. All of the above
43. D. Bilateral Merchant
44. C. Requires overflexion of knee
45. B. Lateral rotation of lower limb
46. C. Increase CR angle to 45° caudad
47. A. Increase CR angulation to 40°
48. A. Superoinferior (sitting) tangential projection
49. B. Excessive medial rotation
50. Weight-bearing foot study

CHAPTER 8

Femur and Pelvis

1.
   - A. Left hip bone
   - B. Right hip bone
   - C. Sacrum
   - D. Coccyx
2.
   - A. Ilium
   - B. Ischium
   - C. Pubis
3. D. All of the above
4. Obturator foramen
5. B. Lesser trochanter
6.
   - A. Body
   - B. Ramus
7. Brim of the pelvis (pelvic brim)
8.
   1. B
   2. A
   3. A
   4. B
   5. A
   6. B
   7. B
9. Acute; less than 90°
10.
   - A. Greater trochanter
   - B. Neck of femur
   - C. Acetabulum
   - D. Anterior superior iliac spine (ASIS)
   - E. Crest of ilium
   - F. Ischial spine
   - G. Superior ramus of pubis
   - H. Symphysis pubis
   - I. Ischial tuberosity
   - J. Female
   - K. Neck of femur
   - L. Lesser trochanter
   - M. Greater trochanter
   - N. Ischial tuberosity
   - O. Axiolateral (inferosuperior) projection or Danelius-Miller method
   - P. Ala (wing) of left ilium
   - Q. Body of left ilium
   - R. Body of left pubis
   - S. Inferior ramus of left ischium
   - T. Greater trochanter
   - U. Lesser trochanter
   - V. Neck of right femur
   - W. AP bilateral frog-leg projection (modified Cleaves method)

11.
   1. M
   2. M
   3. F
   4. F
   5. F
   6. M
12. A. Ischial spines
13. Fovea capitis
14. C. Sacroiliac joints
15. D. Compensating filter
16. A. Sonography
17. C. Fractured proximal femur
18. D. Ankylosing spondylitis
19.
   1. F
   2. B
   3. A
   4. E
   5. D
   6. C
20. C. Limited view of the lesser trochanter in profile
21. B. 200 to 500
22. True
23. A. Bilateral modified Cleaves
24. D. 30° to 45° cephalad
25. D. 35° to 40° toward affected side
26. A. 12° cephalad
27. True
28. False. (Midway between ASIS and symphysis pubis)
29. False. (Trauma projection)
30. D. None. CR is perpendicular.
31. B. AP axial projection
32. The AP axial outlet projection (Taylor method) will elongate the pubis and ischium and define this region more completely.
33. It is soft tissue from the unaffected thigh. This leg must be flexed and elevated high enough to keep it from superimposing the affected hip.
34. Only abduct the femurs 20° to 30° from the vertical rather than 45° to minimize distortion of the femoral neck.
35. No. It is an acceptable image because the lesser trochanters should not be visible at all or only minimally on a well-positioned AP hip projection.
36. AP pelvis and bilateral "frog-leg"
37. B. Reverse central ray angle
38. Rotation of pelvis toward the patient's left. The elevated or

upside obturator foramen will become more narrowed as compared to the opposite side.
39. Multiple answers are correct: Posterior oblique projections (Judet method) will demonstrate possible pelvic ring and acetabular fractures and AP axial "outlet" and AP axial "Inlet" projections will demonstrate possible fractures involving the ischium and pubis.
40. Reduce CR angle to 12° cephalad

CHAPTER 9

Cervical and Thoracic Spine

1. Lower border of first lumbar (L1) vertebrae
2. Five
3. A. Thoracic; D. Sacral
4. True
5. Kyphosis
6. Scoliosis
7. Herniated nucleus pulposus (HNP)
8. Intervertebral foramina
9. Zygapophyseal joints
10. B. Nucleus pulposus
11. False (vertebral artery and vein)
12. False (C-spine possesses bifid spinous processes)
13. 45°
14. Transverse atlantal ligament
15. Zygapophyseal joint
16. Demifacets
17. C. T11; D. T12
18. A. Each has three foramina (one in each transverse process in addition to the vertebral foramina).
    B. Bifid spinous processes
19. Presence of facets for articulation with ribs
20. Lateral position
21.
   - A. Anterior arch (with anterior tubercle), C1 (atlas)
   - B. Dens (odontoid process), C2
   - C. Transverse atlantal ligament, C2
   - D. Transverse foramen, C1
   - E. Superior facets (atlanto-occipital articulation), C1
   - F. Posterior arch, C1
   - G. Dens (odontoid process), C2

H. Transverse process, C1
I. Articular pillar (lateral mass), C2
J. Right zygapophyseal joint, C2 to C3
K. Bifid, spinous process, C4
L. Vertebra prominens (spinous process), C7
M. Superior articular process, T10
N. Intervertebral disk space, T10 to T11
O. Facet for costovertebral joint, T11
P. Right zygapophyseal joint, T11 to T12
Q. Right intervertebral foramen, T12 to L1
R. Facet of inferior articular process, L2
S. Lower thoracic (T10, 11, and 12) and upper lumbar (L1 and 2).
T. Evident by facets for articulation with ribs on upper three but not on lower two. (Note also that the last two thoracic vertebrae do not have facets on transverse processes for costotransverse joints, characteristic of T11 and T12.)

22.
A. Lateral mass (articular pillar), C1
B. Zygapophyseal joint, C1 to C2
C. Body, C2
D. Spinous process (superimposed by body), C2
E. Inferior articular process, C2
F. Dens (odontoid process), C2
G. Upper incisors (teeth)
23. Lateral position
24. Left zygapophyseal joints (downside joints)
25. 1. B
   2. A
   3. C
   4. D
   5. F
   6. E
26. D. Nuclear medicine
27. B. Clay shoveler's fracture
28. A. Scoliosis and/or kyphosis
29. False. Most common at the L4 to L5 level

30.
A. Close side collimation
B. Place a lead mat on tabletop behind patient
31. AP open-mouth projection
32.
A. 15° to 20° cephalad
B. 15° caudad
C. 15° cephalad
33. B. Left anterior oblique (LAO)
34.
A. Suspend respiration on full expiration
B. Have patient hold 5 to 10 lb in each hand.
35. Cervicothoracic lateral or "swimmer's" projection
36.
A. AP projection-Fuchs method
B. PA projection-Judd method
37. Tilt and/or rotation of the spine
38. Not keeping spine parallel to the film and/or not aligning the CR perpendicular to spine
39. Yes. (The technologist needs to assume there may be a fracture present. A horizontal beam lateral projection should be taken for all suspected trauma to the cervical spine. A physician must examine the radiograph and clear the patient for the remaining projections.)
40. AP open-mouth projection. Note that a horizontal beam lateral projection must be taken and cleared first.
41. C. 100 to 200 mrad
42. D. 4 times greater
43. D. 900 to 1000 mrad
44. C. 10 to 15 times greater
45. Excessive flexion of skull
46. AP and lateral cervical spine projections
47. Hyperflexion and hyperextension lateral positions
48. D. Collimate as close as possible
49. A. CT
50. D. C7

CHAPTER 10

Lumbar Spine, Sacrum, and Coccyx

1. C. Larger and more blunt
2. C. Promontory
3. B. 25 to 30
4. 45°

5. C. Between superior and inferior articular processes
6.
A. Left superior articular process
B. Left ala or wing of sacrum
C. Pelvic (anterior) sacral foramina
D. Apex of sacrum
E. Right and left superior articular processes
F. Sacral promontory (also seen on frontal view)
G. Auricular surface (for sacro-iliac joint)
H. Coccyx
I. Apex of coccyx
J. Horn (cornu) of coccyx
K. Horn (cornu) of sacrum
L. Median sacral crest
7.
A. Spinous process
B. Lamina
C. Transverse process
D. Pedicle (also shown on lateral view)
E. Vertebral foramen
F. Body (also shown on lateral view)
G. Superior articular process
H. Inferior articular process
I. Region of articular facets (R and L sides superimposed as seen on a lateral view)
J. Intervertebral notch or foramen
8. Large vertebral body and large, blunt spinous process
9. Synovial, plane (gliding)
10.
A. Superior articular process (ear)
B. Transverse process (nose)
C. Pedicle (eye)
D. Inferior articular process (leg)
E. Pars interarticularis (neck)
F. Zygapophyseal joint (between L-4/5)
11. Zygapophyseal
12. B. Lower costal margin
13. False (would obscure essential anatomy since the ovaries are located near the lower lumbar spine).
14. False (ovaries are slightly anterior, thus AP results in about 30% greater gonadal dose than PA).

15. Opens the intervertebral disk space by reducing the normal lumbar curvature of the spine.
16. False. The lead blocker should be used with digital imaging to prevent secondary scatter from reaching the sensitive image receptor. Scatter radiation produces greater "noise" in the processed image.
17. True
18. C. Compression fracture
19. B. Spina bifida
20. A. Ankylosing spondylitis
21. 1 to 1.5 inches (3 to 4 cm) above the iliac crest
22. Right, or the upside joints
23. 50° from plane of table
24. A patient with a wide pelvis and narrow thorax
25. B. 5° to 8°, caudad
26. A. 35°, cephalad
27. Level of ASIS at the midline of the body
28. True
29. PA (AP) projection, Ferguson method (with and without block under convex side of curve)
30. Hyperextension and hyperflexion lateral projections
31. 2 inches (5 cm) superior to symphysis pubis
32.
    A. Close collimation
    B. Place a lead mat on tabletop behind patient
33. To reduce gonadal dose
34. C. 1000 to 1500 mrad
35. Rotation to the patient's right.
36. Decrease rotation of the spine
37. Insufficient cephalad CR angulation or the CR was angled in the wrong direction
38. A lateral projection (may include a coned down spot AP/PA and lateral of the L3 region)
39. AP, lateral, L5-S1 spot lateral and right and left 30° oblique positions
40. Decrease rotation of body for oblique positions to no more than 25° to 30° with the CR centered to the upside SI joint.

CHAPTER 11

Bony Thorax—Sternum and Ribs

1.
    A. Manubrium
    B. Body
    C. Xiphoid process
2. Xiphoid process
3. Sternal angle
4. D. Manubrium
5. A. True rib attaches directly to the sternum with its own costocartilage.
6. D. Does not possess costocartilage
7. True rib
8. D. Sternal angle
9. D. All of the above
10.
    1. A
    2. A
    3. B
    4. A
    5. B
11.
    A. Left clavicle
    B. Left sternoclavicular (SC) joint
    C. First rib (sternal end)
    D. Manubrium
    E. Sternal angle
    F. Body
    G. Xiphoid process
    H. Jugular notch
    I. Manubrium
    J. Sternal angle
    K. Body
    L. Xiphoid process
12.
    A. Suspended inspiration
    B. Low to medium kV (65 to 70)
    C. Erect (if patient is able)
13. 40 inches (100 cm). There must be a minimum of 15 inches (38 cm) between the patient's skin and the collimator.
14. B. Breathing technique (if patient is cooperative)
15.
    A. Place the area of interest closest to IR.
    B. Rotate the spine away from the area of interest for axillary ribs
16.
    A. Pneumothorax
    B. Hemothorax

17.
    A. 15° to 20°
    B. More
18. C. Patients with history of multiple myeloma
19. D. Blunt trauma
20.
    A. 66 mrad (50 to 100 range)
    B. 3 mrad (2 to 5 range)
21. C. (LPO)
22. B. Drawn back
23. The SC joints are equal distance from the midline of spine
24. 10° to 15°
25. Midway between the xiphoid process and lower rib cage
26. B. 65 to 70 kV
27. A. LAO
28. Overrotation of the sternum. A large-chested patient only requires approximately 15° of rotation. Overrotation will lead to foreshortening along the width of the sternum and will shift the sternum away excessively from the spine.
29. Rotation of the upper body from a true lateral will cause the ribs to be superimposed over the sternum.
30.
    A. AP and RPO performed recumbent
    B. Suspend upon expiration
31.
    A. PA and RAO performed recumbent
    B. Expose upon inspiration
32. 10° to 15° RAO will project the right SC joint adjacent to the spine.
33. LPO and horizontal beam lateral positions. (See Chapter 18 for details.)
34. PA and lateral chest study
35. False. (AEC is generally not recommended for rib routines due to the need for high-contrast, optimum detail exposures, which can generally be better achieved manually.)
36. False. Exposure is made with suspended respiration upon expiration.
37. PA and LAO positions taken erect if possible.
38. Recumbent AP and LPO positions

39. RAO and lateral sternum (possibly a chest examination as well)
40. Nuclear medicine bone scan

CHAPTER 12

Skull and Cranial Bones

1. C. Occipital
2. C. Squamous
3.
   A. Right parietal
   B. Left parietal
   C. Sphenoid
   D. Ethmoid
4. Parietal tubercles or eminences
5. External occipital protuberance or inion
6.
   A. 5
   B. 6
   C. 3
   D. 7
   E. 2
7. Petrous portion or petrous pyramids
8. True
9. True
10. Clivus
11. Lateral labyrinth or masses
12. Crista galli
13. Left pterion
14. Squamosal suture
15. Sutural or wormian bones
16.
    1. C
    2. C
    3. B
    4. C
    5. D
    6. D
    7. A
    8. D
    9. E
    10. A
    11. B
    12. E
    13. A
    14. C
    15. E
17.
   A. Orbital or horizontal portion, frontal
   B. Supraorbital margin (SOM), frontal
   C. Crista galli, ethmoid
   D. Sagittal suture
   E. Midlateral orbital margin (zygomatic-facial)
   F. Petrous ridge, temporal
   G. Petrous portion, temporal
   H. Petrous ridge, temporal
   I. Dorsum sellae, sphenoid
   J. Posterior clinoid processes, sphenoid
   K. Orbital or horizontal portion, frontal
   L. Sella turcica (body), sphenoid
   M. Sphenoid sinus, sphenoid
18. C. Brachycephalic
19. A. Mesocephalic
20.
   A. External acoustic meatus (EAM)
   B. Angle (gonion) of mandible
   C. Mental point (mentum)
   D. Acanthion
   E. Nasion
   F. Glabella
   G. Glabellomeatal line (GML)
   H. Orbitomeatal line (OML)
   I. Infraorbitomeatal line (IOML)
   J. Acanthomeatal line (AML)
   K. Lips-meatal line (LML)
   L. Mentomeatal line (MML)
21. B. TEA
22. A. Pinna
23. B. IOML
24. B. 7° to 8°
25. A. Rotation
26.
   A. 5
   B. 6
   C. 2
   D. 4
   E. 1
   F. 3
27. D. Multiple myeloma
28. A. Computed tomography (CT)
29. B. MRI
30. Squamous portion
31. Petrous portion
32. Tympanic membrane
33. A. Malleus
34. Eustachian or auditory tube
35. Auditory nerve and blood vessels
36. Epitympanic recess; mastoid
37. Encephalitis
38. C. Stapes
39. Membranous
40. Cochlea, vestibule, semicircular canals
41. A. Malleus
   B. Incus
   C. Stapes
   D. Internal acoustic meatus—for auditory nerve and blood vessels
   E. Cochlea
   F. Eustachian or auditory tube
   G. Tympanic cavity
   H. Tympanic membrane or ear drum
   I. External acoustic meatus (EAM)
42. C. Cholesteatoma
43. True
44.
   A. AP axial projection (Towne method)
   B. PA axial projection (Haas method)
45.
   A. 37° caudad
   B. 30° caudad
46. 2 inches (5 cm) superior to the EAM
47. Interpupillary
48. Superior to the mastoid processes and symmetrical
49. 1½ inch (4 cm) inferior to the mandibular symphysis, midway between the gonions
50.
   A. 37° caudad
   B. 30° caudad
51. Increase CR angle approximately 7° caudad
52. Rotation
53. Increase extension of the skull to place the OML perpendicular to the IR (this will project the petrous ridges into the lower one third of the orbits).
54. Horizontal beam (dorsal decubitus) lateral skull projection will demonstrate any possible air-fluid levels in the sphenoid sinus.
55. Perform the AP projection with a 15° cephalad CR angle to the OML.
56. Use the IOML instead of OML and increase CR angle an additional 7° caudad for a total of 37°.
57. Decrease CR angle based on the skull line used (OML-30°; IOML-37°)
58. Tilt of the skull

59. Rotation of the skull to the patient's right
60. Extend the skull further to place the IOML parallel to the IR

CHAPTER 13

Facial Bones and Paranasal Sinuses

1. A. Maxilla
2. D. Ramus
3.
   A. 4
   B. 5
   C. 7
   D. 6
   E. 3
   F. 1
   G. 2
4.
   A. Lacrimal
   B. Ethmoid
   C. Frontal
   D. Sphenoid
   E. Palatine
   F. Zygomatic
   G. Maxilla
5. 1 to 2 sinuses
6. True
7. False
8. False
9. True
10. A. Sphenoid sinuses
    B. Ethmoid sinuses
    C. Frontal sinuses
    D. Maxillary sinuses
    E. Frontal sinuses
    F. Ethmoid and sphenoid sinuses superimposed
    G. Petrous portion of temporal bone
    H. Maxillary sinuses
    I. Base of skull
    J. Ethmoid sinuses
    K. Sphenoid sinus
    L. Petrous portion of temporal bone
    M. Mastoid portion of temporal bone
11. Lateral masses or labyrinth
12. Sella turcica
13. True
14. A. CT
15. True
16. False (The tripod fracture does this.)
17. Parietoacanthial (Waters) projection (dense petrous pyramids are projected below the maxillary sinuses)
18. Horizontal beam (cross-table) lateral projection
19. Midsagittal plane
20.
    A. 37°
    B. Mentomeatal line (MML)
21. D. Acanthion
22. A. Nasion
23. Lower half of the maxillary sinuses
24. True
25. False (glabelloalveolar, GAL)
26. Lips-meatal line (LML)
27. ½ inch (1.25 cm) inferior to nasion
28. Infraorbitomeatal line (IOML)
29. 15° rotation and 15° tilt toward the affected side
30. 37° caudad
31. Parieto-orbital oblique projection or Rhese method
32. Lower outer quadrant of the orbit
33. 25° cephalad
34. C. Extend chin slightly
35. C. 45°
36. C. 20° to 25° cephalad
37. Temporomandibular fossae
38. 1½ inches (4 cm) inferior to mandibular symphysis (or midway between angles of mandible)
39. C. 200 to 300 mrad
40. C. IOML
41. 35° caudad
42. False (15° caudad)
43. True
44. True
45. Midway between outer canthus and EAM
46. To allow any fluid in the sinuses to settle
47. Parietoacanthial (Waters) projection
48. To demonstrate any air-fluid levels without distortion
49. Excessive flexion of the head, or insufficient caudal CR angle
50. A. Acanthomeatal (AML)
51. Rotation of the skull
52. Reverse parietoacanthial (Waters) projection with the use of cephalic CR angle to keep CR parallel to MML. In addition, horizontal beam lateral projection must be included as part of the positioning routine.
53. Reduce kVp to 50 to 60 range and increase mAs accordingly.
54. Modified parietoacanthial (modified Waters) or a PA axial projection with a 30° caudad angle will best demonstrate the floor of the orbit. Note that the modified Waters is more commonly performed for possible blow-out fractures over the standard parietoacanthial (Waters) projection.
55. Routine radiographic sinus series can be performed, but CT of the sinuses may best demonstrate bony erosion.